T0227024

Stroke in Atrial Fibrillation

Editors

SAMUEL J. ASIRVATHAM
RANJAN K. THAKUR
ANDREA NATALE

CARDIAC ELECTROPHYSIOLOGY CLINICS

www.cardiacEP.theclinics.com

Consulting Editors
RANJAN K. THAKUR
ANDREA NATALE

March 2014 • Volume 6 • Number 1

ELSEVIER

1600 John F. Kennedy Boulevard • Suite 1800 • Philadelphia, Pennsylvania, 19103-2899

http://www.theclinics.com

CARDIAC ELECTROPHYSIOLOGY CLINICS Volume 6, Number 1
March 2014 ISSN 1877-9182, ISBN-13: 978-0-323-28699-2

Editor: Adrianne Brigido
Developmental Editor: Barbara Cohen-Kligerman

Cardiac Electrophysiology Clinics (ISSN 1877-9182) is published quarterly by Elsevier Inc., 360 Park Avenue South, New York, NY 10010-1710. Months of issue are March, June, September, and December. Subscription prices are $200.00 per year for US individuals, $293.00 per year for US institutions, $105.00 per year for US students and residents, $225.00 per year for Canadian individuals, $331.00 per year for Canadian institutions, $285.00 per year for international individuals, $354.00 per year for international institutions and $150.00 per year for Canadian and foreign students/residents. To receive student/resident rate, orders must be accompanied by name of affilliated institution, date of term, and the signature of program/residency coordinator on institution letterhead. Orders will be billed at individual rate until proof of status is received. Foreign air speed delivery is included in all Clinics subscription prices. All prices are subject to change without notice. **POSTMASTER:** Send address changes to Cardiac Electrophysiology Clinics, Elsevier Health Sciences Division, Subscription Customer Service, 3251 Riverport Lane, Maryland Heights, MO 63043. **Customer Service: 1-800-654-2452 (US and Canada). From outside of the US and Canada, call 314-477-8871. Fax: 314-447-8029. E-mail: JournalsCustomerService-usa@elsevier.com (for print support); JournalsOnlineSupport-usa@elsevier.com (for online support).**

Reprints. For copies of 100 or more of articles in this publication, please contact the Commercial Reprints Department, Elsevier Inc., 360 Park Avenue South, New York, NY 10010-1710. Tel.: 212-633-3874; Fax: 212-633-3820; E-mail: reprints@elsevier.com.

Printed and bound by CPI Group (UK) Ltd, Croydon, CR0 4YY

Contributors

CONSULTING EDITORS

RANJAN K. THAKUR, MD, MPH, MBA, FHRS
Professor of Medicine and Director, Arrhythmia Service, Thoracic and Cardiovascular Institute, Sparrow Health System, Michigan State University, Lansing, Michigan

ANDREA NATALE, MD, FACC, FHRS
Executive Medical Director, Texas Cardiac Arrhythmia Institute, St. David's Medical Center, Austin, Texas; Consulting Professor, Division of Cardiology, Stanford University, Palo Alto, California; Adjunct Professor of Medicine, Heart and Vascular Center, Case Western Reserve University, Cleveland, Ohio; Director, Interventional Electrophysiology, Scripps Clinic, San Diego, California; Senior Clinical Director, EP Services, California Pacific Medical Center, San Francisco, California

EDITORS

SAMUEL J. ASIRVATHAM, MD, FACC, FHRS
Professor of Medicine, Division of Cardiovascular Diseases, Department of Internal Medicine; Division of Pediatric Cardiology, Department of Pediatrics and Adolescent Medicine, St. Mary's Hospital, Mayo Clinic College of Medicine, Rochester, Minnesota

RANJAN K. THAKUR, MD, MPH, MBA, FHRS
Professor of Medicine and Director, Arrhythmia Service, Thoracic and Cardiovascular Institute, Sparrow Health System, Michigan State University, Lansing, Michigan

ANDREA NATALE, MD, FACC, FHRS
Executive Medical Director, Texas Cardiac Arrhythmia Institute, St. David's Medical Center, Austin, Texas; Consulting Professor, Division of Cardiology, Stanford University, Palo Alto, California; Adjunct Professor of Medicine, Heart and Vascular Center, Case Western Reserve University, Cleveland, Ohio; Director, Interventional Electrophysiology, Scripps Clinic, San Diego, California; Senior Clinical Director, EP Services, California Pacific Medical Center, San Francisco, California

AUTHORS

SAMUEL J. ASIRVATHAM, MD, FACC, FHRS
Professor of Medicine, Division of Cardiovascular Diseases, Department of Internal Medicine; Division of Pediatric Cardiology, Department of Pediatrics and Adolescent Medicine, St. Mary's Hospital, Mayo Clinic College of Medicine, Rochester, Minnesota

CONOR BARRETT, MD
Al-Sabah Arrhythmia Institute, St. Luke's Hospital, New York

LUKE J. BURCHILL, MBBS, PhD
Cleveland Clinic, Cleveland, Ohio

J. DAVID BURKHARDT, MD
Texas Cardiac Arrhythmia Institute, St. David's Medical Center, Austin, Texas

DAVIDE CASTAGNO, MD
Division of Cardiology, Department of Medical Sciences, Città della Salute e della Scienza, University of Turin, Turin, Italy

JOSE MARIA CASTELLANO, MD, PhD
The Mount Sinai Medical Center, Cardiovascular Institute, New York, New York; National Center for Cardiovascular Research (CNIC), Madrid, Spain

JOHN CATANZARO, MD, FACC
Cardiac Electrophysiology, Columbia St Mary's Cardiovascular Physicians, Columbia St Mary's Healthcare, Milwaukee, Wisconsin

FEDERICO CESARANI, MD
Division of Radiology, Cardinal Guglielmo Massaia Hospital, Asti, Italy

JASON CHINITZ, MD
The Mount Sinai Medical Center, Cardiovascular Institute, New York, New York

LAURA CORSINOVI, MD, PhD
Division of Cardiology, Department of Medical Sciences, Città della Salute e della Scienza, University of Turin, Turin, Italy

ZOLTAN CSANADI, MD, PhD
Department of Cardiology, University of Debrecen, Debrecen, Hungary

STEPHAN DANIK, MD
Al-Sabah Arrhythmia Institute, St. Luke's Hospital, New York

EMILE G. DAOUD, MD, FHRS
Professor, Internal Medicine, Electrophysiology Section, Division of Cardiovascular Medicine, Ross Heart Hospital, The Wexner Medical Center at the Ohio State University Medical Center, Columbus, Ohio

PEERAWUT DEEPRASERTKUL, MD
Sparrow Thoracic and Cardiovascular Institute, Michigan State University, Lansing, Michigan

SANJAY DESHPANDE, MD, FACC
Chief, CV Electrophysiology, Columbia St Mary's Cardiovascular Physicians, Columbia St Mary's Healthcare, Milwaukee, Wisconsin

CHRISTOPHER V. DESIMONE, MD, PhD
Division of Cardiovascular Diseases, Mayo Clinic, Rochester, Minnesota

LUIGI DI BIASE, MD, PhD
Department of Cardiology, University of Foggia, Foggia, Italy; Texas Cardiac Arrhythmia Institute, St. David's Medical Center, Austin, Texas; Albert Einstein College of Medicine, Montefiore Hospital, Bronx, New York; Department of Biomedical Engineering, University of Texas, Austin, Texas

ELISA EBRILLE, MD
Department of Cardiology, University of Turin, Turin, Italy

PAUL A. FRIEDMAN, MD, FACC, FHRS
Consultant Electrophysiologist, Division of Cardiovascular Diseases and Professor of Medicine, College of Medicine, Mayo Clinic, Rochester, Minnesota

VALENTIN FUSTER, MD, PhD
The Mount Sinai Medical Center, Cardiovascular Institute, New York, New York; National Center for Cardiovascular Research (CNIC), Madrid, Spain

FIORENZO GAITA, MD
Professor, Division of Cardiology, Department of Medical Sciences, Città della Salute e della Scienza, University of Turin, Turin, Italy

PILAR GALLEGO, MD, PhD
University of Birmingham Centre for Cardiovascular Sciences, City Hospital, Birmingham, United Kingdom; Department of Hematology and Clinical Oncology, Hospital Universitario Morales Meseguer, Murcia, Spain

PHILIP GREENLAND, MD
Professor of Medicine and Preventive Medicine, Department of Preventive Medicine, Bluhm Cardiovascular Institute, Northwestern University Feinberg School of Medicine, Chicago, Illinois

MAHMOUD HOUMSSE, MD, FHRS
Assistant Professor, Internal Medicine, Electrophysiology Section, Division of Cardiovascular Medicine, Ross Heart Hospital, The Wexner Medical Center at the Ohio State University Medical Center, Columbus, Ohio

SYED I. HUSSAIN, MD
Assistant Professor of Neurology, Department of Neurology and Ophthalmology, Michigan State University, Lansing, Michigan

RICCARDO IEVA, MD
Department of Cardiology, University of
Foggia, Foggia, Italy

SAURABH JHA, MD, MS
Cleveland Clinic, Cleveland, Ohio

ALLAN L. KLEIN, MD, FASE
Cleveland Clinic, Cleveland, Ohio

GEORGE KLEIN, MD
University Hospital, London Health Sciences
Centre, London, Ontario, Canada

ZACHARY LAKSMAN, MD
University Hospital, London Health Sciences
Centre, London, Ontario, Canada

GREGORY Y.H. LIP, MD
University of Birmingham Centre for
Cardiovascular Sciences, City Hospital,
Birmingham, United Kingdom

ENOCH B. LULE, MD
Fellow, Cardiac Electrophysiology, Sparrow
Thoracic and Cardiovascular Institute,
Michigan State University, Lansing, Michigan

MALINI MADHAVAN, MBBS
Division of Cardiovascular Diseases, Mayo
Clinic, Rochester, Minnesota

SIVA K. MULPURU, MD
Division of Cardiovascular Diseases,
Department of Internal Medicine, Mayo Clinic,
Rochester, Minnesota

EDINA NAGY-BALÓ, MD
Department of Cardiology, University of
Debrecen, Debrecen, Hungary

ANDREA NATALE, MD, FACC, FHRS
Executive Medical Director, Texas Cardiac
Arrhythmia Institute, St. David's Medical
Center, Austin, Texas; Consulting Professor,
Division of Cardiology, Stanford University,
Palo Alto, California; Adjunct Professor of
Medicine, Heart and Vascular Center, Case
Western Reserve University, Cleveland, Ohio;
Director, Interventional Electrophysiology,
Scripps Clinic, San Diego, California; Senior
Clinical Director, EP Services, California Pacific
Medical Center, San Francisco, California

ROD PASSMAN, MD, MSCE
Professor of Medicine and Preventive
Medicine, Department of Preventive Medicine,
Bluhm Cardiovascular Institute, Northwestern
University Feinberg School of Medicine,
Chicago, Illinois

MARTINA PIANELLI, MD
Division of Cardiology, Department of Medical
Sciences, Città della Salute e della Scienza,
University of Turin, Turin, Italy

ALEJANDRO A. RABINSTEIN, MD
Department of Neurology, Mayo Clinic,
Rochester, Minnesota

ANMAR RAZAK, MD
Assistant Professor of Neurology, Department
of Neurology and Ophthalmology, Michigan
State University, Lansing, Michigan

MICHAEL P. RILEY, MD, PhD
Assistant Professor of Medicine, Hospital of
the University of Pennsylvania, Philadelphia,
Pennsylvania

VANESSA ROLDÁN, MD, PhD
Department of Hematology and Clinical
Oncology, Hospital Universitario Morales
Meseguer, Murcia, Spain

JAVIER SANCHEZ, MD
Texas Cardiac Arrhythmia Institute, St. David's
Medical Center, Austin, Texas

PASQUALE SANTANGELI, MD
Clinical Cardiac Electrophysiology, University
of Pennsylvania, Philadelphia, Pennsylvania;
Department of Cardiology, University of
Foggia, Foggia, Italy; Texas Cardiac
Arrhythmia Institute, St. David's Medical
Center, Austin, Texas

FRANCESCO SANTORO, MD
Department of Cardiology, University of
Foggia, Foggia, Italy

MARCO SCAGLIONE, MD
Division of Cardiology, Cardinal Guglielmo
Massaia Hospital, Asti, Italy

AMIT B. SHARMA, MD
Fellow, Cardiac Electrophysiology, Sparrow
Thoracic and Cardiovascular Institute,
Michigan State University, Lansing, Michigan

SHALINI SHARMA, MD
Fellow, Department of Radiology, Michigan
State University, Lansing, Michigan

**FAISAL F. SYED, BSc(Hons), MBChB,
MRCP**
Fellow in Cardiovascular Diseases, Division of
Cardiovascular Diseases and Assistant
Professor of Medicine, College of Medicine,
Mayo Clinic, Rochester, Minnesota

**RANJAN K. THAKUR, MD, MPH, MBA,
FHRS**
Professor of Medicine and Director, Arrhythmia
Service, Thoracic and Cardiovascular Institute,
Sparrow Health System, Michigan State
University, Lansing, Michigan

TODD T. TOMSON, MD
Department of Preventive Medicine, Bluhm
Cardiovascular Institute, Northwestern
University Feinberg School of Medicine,
Chicago, Illinois

MARIA CONSUELO VALENTINI, MD
Division of Neuroradiology, Città della Salute e
della Scienza, Turin, Italy

ALBERT L. WALDO, MD
The Walter H. Pritchard Professor of
Cardiology, Professor of Medicine and
Professor of Biomedical Engineering, Division
of Cardiovascular Medicine, University
Hospitals Case Medical Center, Case
Western Reserve University, Cleveland,
Ohio

SAMUEL WANN, MD, MACC
Cardiologist, Columbia St Mary's
Cardiovascular Physicians, Columbia St
Mary's Healthcare, Milwaukee, Wisconsin

JONATHAN WILLNER, MD
The Mount Sinai Medical Center,
Cardiovascular Institute, New York,
New York

TEERAPAT YINGCHONCHAROEN, MD
Cleveland Clinic, Cleveland, Ohio

Contents

Atrial fibrillation is the single most common sustained cardiac dysrhythmia in the United States, and a major cause of hospitalization, stroke, disability, and death. The rapidly increasing prevalence of atrial fibrillation is largely attributable to the aging of the population. Because atrial fibrillation may be intermittent and asymptomatic or minimally symptomatic at onset, its prevalence is difficult to establish. Implanted loop recorders, pacemakers, and defibrillators have enabled precise assessment of the heart rhythm over long periods of time. The incidence of asymptomatic atrial fibrillation is higher than is perceived by patients, and carries with it an increased risk of stoke.

Atrial fibrillation is the most common sustained cardiac arrhythmia and is associated with a high risk of stroke and thromboembolism. Increasing evidence suggests that the thrombogenic tendency inherent to atrial fibrillation is related to several underlying pathophysiological mechanisms, including reduced flow in the left atrium, changes in vessel walls, and changes in blood constituents. This article reviews the mechanisms of stroke, available risk stratification tools and therapies available for prevention of stroke in patients with atrial fibrillation.

This article reviews the role of cardiac imaging in stroke prevention, defining how imaging tools can be useful in this field. Cardioembolic sources during atrial fibrillation are discussed. New closure devices can be implanted in the left atrial appendage and routinely monitored with imaging modalities. Acute and chronic left ventricular dysfunction is reviewed, identifying the possible mechanism of thrombus formation and its early detection. Valvular evaluation of native heart disease and possible implications for stroke risk are defined.

Atrial fibrillation (AF) is the most common supraventricular arrhythmia in the United States. The incidence and prevalence of AF are increasing as the population ages and associated risk factors become more prevalent. Stroke is the most severe complication of AF. Various risk stratification schemes to guide therapy and the associated risk of bleeding are described. AF is also associated with cognitive decline, which may be secondary to recurrent microemboli; microbleeds secondary to

understanding of how risk can be minimized, are explained. This article provides a platform for newer study, changes in the way procedures are done, and possibly vascular-based stroke-reduction strategies.

Patients undergoing atrial fibrillation ablation are anticoagulated before, during, and following their procedure to reduce the serious risk of a thromboembolic complication. Despite this well established recommendation, there remains debate about the optimal nature of anticoagulation and a continuing evolution in practice patterns. This article addresses issues related to anticoagulation in atrial fibrillation ablation focusing on the preprocedural, intraprocedural, and postprocedural periods.

Atrial fibrillation (AF) is one of the most common cardiac arrhythmias and relates to high morbidity and mortality due to thromboembolic events, especially ischemic stroke. During the last 15 years, transcatheter ablation has emerged as an effective therapeutic option to treat AF but carries a risk of possible complications. The occurrence of cerebrovascular accidents, both symptomatic and silent, is one of the most frequent and severe. Transcatheter AF ablation entails a relevant risk of silent cerebral ischemia detected by means of magnetic resonance imaging, and many efforts have been directed to improve the safety of this procedure.

Transcatheter treatment of atrial fibrillation (AF) is a complex intervention performed in patients who are at inherently increased risk of a thromboembolic complication, including stroke. It is therefore not surprising that cerebrovascular accidents have been among the most feared complications since the inception of AF ablation. While improvements have been made to limit the incidence of thromboembolic events during catheter ablation of AF, the optimal strategy to minimize such complications has yet to be determined. It is hoped that larger trials using periprocedural anticoagulation strategies can be undertaken to definitively address these important concerns.

Early detection of atrial fibrillation (AF) before an AF-related stroke potentially allows for prevention, but the best methods are uncertain. Population screening trials have demonstrated the ability to increase detection in older individuals by systematic screening. The subset of patients with implantable cardiac rhythm management devices are at particular risk. Remote monitoring has substantially reduced the time to detection. Although primary prevention of stroke is a priority, detection in patients with cryptogenic stroke represents another opportunity for therapeutic intervention. Evidence that early detection actually leads to improved stroke outcomes is still being gathered.

Atrial fibrillation (AF) is associated with embolic stroke. AF can be asymptomatic and the first detection of AF may be from the stored electrograms of cardiac implantable electronic devices. These devices can digitally record and store intracardiac electrograms that satisfy criteria for AF. Current guidelines do not address management of device-detected AF and, in particular, whether these episodes should prompt the initiation of anticoagulation/antiplatelet therapy. This article reviews the data regarding management of device-detected AF.

Current anticoagulant therapies aimed at stroke prevention in atrial fibrillation (AF) are increasingly challenged by a complex patient population at significant risk of bleeding. Mounting evidence shows that left atrial appendage (LAA) closure is an effective strategy for reducing stroke risk in patients with nonvalvular AF, without the need for anticoagulation. Several approaches and devices have been developed in recent years, each with their own set of advantages and disadvantages. This article reviews these approaches, identifies pertinent aspects, and outlines necessary or ongoing research in establishing LAA closure as a safe and effective approach to stroke risk reduction.

This article outlines current evidence and indications for electrocardiographic monitoring in documenting subclinical atrial fibrillation (AF) in patients with cryptogenic stroke. Longer monitoring improves detection rates of subclinical AF. Incorporation of risk factors predicting patients at higher risk of stroke can be used to target populations suitable for longer-term monitoring. Although longer duration of AF is expected to increase the risk of stroke, the exact cutoff for duration of clinical significance is not yet established. It seems probable that a combination of clinical risk factors and duration of AF will provide the best prediction of future clinical stroke.

Approximately 800,000 strokes occur in the United States every year, resulting in 200,000 deaths. Strokes may be ischemic (80%) or hemorrhagic (20%). Strokes caused by atrial fibrillation (AF) are thromboembolic, and AF is the leading cause of ischemic stroke. Rapid distinction between these forms of strokes is critical because approaches to treatment are different. The goal for acute ischemic stroke is reperfusion of ischemic brain tissue, whereas the treatment of hemorrhagic stroke is supportive therapy and correction of the underlying conditions. The treatment of acute ischemic strokes is similar to treatment of acute myocardial infarction, which requires timely reperfusion for optimal results.

CARDIAC ELECTROPHYSIOLOGY CLINICS

FORTHCOMING ISSUES

June 2014
Electrocardiography of Complex Arrhythmias: Electrocardiographic and Intracardiac Electrogram Correlation
Mohammad Shenasa and Edward Gerstenfeld, *Editors*

September 2014
Implantable Devices: Design, Manufacturing and Malfunction
Kenneth A. Ellenbogen and Charles J. Love, *Editors*

December 2014
Cardiac Sodium Channel Disorders
Hugues Abriel, *Editor*

RECENT ISSUES

December 2013
Clinical and Electrophysiologic Management of Syncope
Antonio Raviele and Andrea Natale, *Editors*

September 2013
Remote Monitoring and Physiologic Sensing Technologies
Samuel J. Asirvatham, K.L. Venkatachalam, and Suraj Kapa, *Editors*

June 2013
Mapping of Atrial Tachycardias Post-Atrial Fibrillation Ablation
Ashok J. Shah, Michel Haissaguerre, and Shinsuke Miyazaki, *Editors*

ISSUES OF RELATED INTEREST

Interventional Cardiology Clinics October 2013 (Vol. 2, No. 4)
Interventional Pharmacology
George D. Dangas, *Editor*
Available at: http://www.interventional.theclinics.com/home

Heart Failure Clinics January 2014 (Vol. 10, No. 1)
Heart Failure in Adult Congenital Heart Disease
Alexander R. Opotowsky and Michael J. Landzberg, *Editors*
Available at: http://www.heartfailure.theclinics.com

DOWNLOAD Free App!

Review Articles
THE CLINICS

NOW AVAILABLE FOR YOUR iPhone and iPad

Preface
Stroke in Atrial Fibrillation

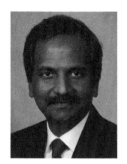 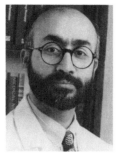 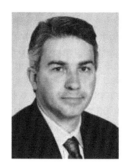

| Samuel J. Asirvatham, MD, FACC, FHRS | Ranjan K. Thakur, MD, MPH, MBA, FHRS | Andrea Natale, MD, FACC, FHRS |

Editors

Atrial fibrillation (AF) is the most common sustained arrhythmia in humans, and its prevalence appears to be increasing. AF is important because it may cause symptoms and limit physical functioning, thereby reducing quality of life; it is associated with higher mortality in subsets of patients with preexisting heart disease and is also associated with a significantly higher risk of strokes. The association between AF and stroke has been known for quite some time, but we have developed a nuanced understanding of this association and medical science has progressed far enough that we can have a significant impact on preventing strokes due to AF and reducing morbidity and mortality due to AF strokes. At the same time, much remains yet to be learned and new research is unfolding many more questions.

Approximately 800,000 strokes occur in the United States annually, resulting in approximately 200,000 deaths. It is the leading cause of disability in adults. Strokes are broadly classified as ischemic (>80%) or hemorrhagic; AF strokes are primarily ischemic events due to cardiogenic thromboemboli. Of all ischemic strokes, 30% to 40% remain unexplained as to an underlying cause; these are considered cryptogenic strokes, and AF may account for more than 25% of these.

So, AF and stroke are inextricably linked. On the national level, AF already requires considerable health care resources, but the increasing prevalence of this arrhythmia urgently demands more effective therapeutic strategies for treatment and prevention of complications such as stroke. This issue of *Cardiac Electrophysiology Clinics* summarizes what we already know about AF strokes, explores emerging knowledge, and points out gaps that await further research.

We are grateful to our colleagues around the world, who are leaders in their respective areas, for their contributions. We begin by exploring the magnitude of the problem and mechanisms of stroke in AF. The issue of cryptogenic stroke is discussed in detail along with tools to help look for AF to define the underpinning cause. Recent research has shed some light on the temporal relationship between AF and stroke—much more work is needed to understand the time lag between AF episodes and stroke. New oral anticoagulants for stroke prevention will undoubtedly reduce the burden of AF stroke morbidity and mortality. Several articles deal with various anticoagulation issues in AF patients. AF strokes are caused by thrombi originating in the left atrial appendage—a novel way to prevent these strokes may be to occlude the os of the left atrial

Card Electrophysiol Clin 6 (2014) xiii–xiv
http://dx.doi.org/10.1016/j.ccep.2013.12.001
1877-9182/14/$ – see front matter © 2014 Elsevier Inc. All rights reserved.

appendage to prevent embolization; this approach is discussed in detail. A surprising finding has been that AF ablation, while effective, may cause silent or minimally symptomatic cerebral lesions—their etiology, implications, and prevention are of great interest and discussed in detail from both the electrophysiologist's perspective as well as the neurologist's perspective. Neurological implications of AF, such as stroke and cognitive decline, are discussed in detail. Finally, if a stroke occurs, neurointerventionists may be able to cannulate cerebral arteries and remove the thrombi, thereby restoring blood flow and neurologic function; several cases are illustrated to show what is possible and the potential consequences.

We hope the reader will find this issue of *Cardiac Electrophysiology Clinics* imminently readable and a comprehensive summary of current thinking about stroke due to AF. Electrophysiologists and cardiologists—as well as internists, family physicians, and neurologists—will find this issue helpful because all of us comanage patients with this pervasive arrhythmia and its consequences.

Samuel J. Asirvatham, MD, FACC, FHRS
Department of Internal Medicine and
Pediatric Cardiology
St. Mary's Hospital
Mayo Clinic College of Medicine
200 First Street SW
Rochester, MN 55905, USA

Ranjan K. Thakur, MD, MPH, MBA, FHRS
Thoracic and Cardiovascular Institute
Sparrow Health System
Michigan State University
1200 East Michigan Avenue, Suite 580
Lansing, MI 48912, USA

Andrea Natale, MD, FACC, FHRS
Texas Cardiac Arrhythmia Institute
Center for Atrial Fibrillation
St. David's Medical Center
1015 East 32nd Street, Suite 516
Austin, TX 78705, USA

E-mail addresses:
asirvatham.samuel@mayo.edu (S.J. Asirvatham)
thakur@msu.edu (R.K. Thakur)
andrea.natale@stdavids.com (A. Natale)

Atrial Fibrillation
Prevalence and Scope of the Problem

Sanjay Deshpande, MD[a], John Catanzaro, MD[a],
Samuel Wann, MD, MACC[b],*

KEYWORDS

- Heart • Atrial fibrillation • Prevalence • Dysrhythmia

KEY POINTS

- Stroke is 5 times more common in individuals with atrial fibrillation, and 3 times more common in patients with heart failure, resulting in marked increases in morbidity and mortality.
- The rapidly increasing prevalence of atrial fibrillation is largely attributable to the aging of the population.
- Because atrial fibrillation may be intermittent and asymptomatic or minimally symptomatic at onset, its prevalence is difficult to establish.
- In the past, atrial fibrillation has been classified as intermittent or paroxysmal, persistent or sustained, and long-standing or permanent.
- More recently, implanted loop recorders, pacemakers, and defibrillators have enabled more precise assessment of the heart rhythm over long periods of time.
- The incidence of asymptomatic atrial fibrillation is higher than is perceived by the patients and carries with it an increased risk of stoke even if the atrial fibrillation is asymptomatic and intermittent.

The banal use of atrial fibrillation as a diagnosis in clinical medicine belies the magnitude of its footprint. Atrial fibrillation is a major public health problem in the United States. It is the single most common sustained cardiac dysrhythmia, and a major cause of hospitalization, stroke, disability, and death. The human and economic costs of atrial fibrillation are enormous. The US Centers for Disease Control and Prevention estimates that more than 2.66 million Americans had atrial fibrillation in 2010, and expects that as many as 12 million people will have atrial fibrillation in 2050. This projection is based on the aging population; the increase in chronic cardiovascular and other diseases, including obesity and diabetes;

as well as more frequent diagnosis from increased/improved monitoring. Most of the data are derived from longitudinal follow-up of a predominantly white population both from the United States and Europe. This article focuses on the epidemiologic context of the clinical aspects of patients with atrial fibrillation to facilitate a better understanding and care of these patients.

GENDER AND RACE

Men have a 1.5-fold higher risk for developing atrial fibrillation than women after adjustment for age and predisposing conditions. Atrial fibrillation seems to be less common in African Americans,

The authors have no relevant conflicts of interest to disclose.

[a] Cardiac Electrophysiology, Columbia St. Mary's Cardiovascular Physicians, Watertower Medical Commons, Suite 206, 2350 North Lake Drive, Milwaukee, WI 53211, USA; [b] Columbia St. Mary's Cardiovascular Physicians, Watertower Medical Commons, Suite 400, 2350 North Lake Drive, Milwaukee, WI 53211, USA

* Corresponding author.

E-mail address: samuelwann@gmail.com

Card Electrophysiol Clin 6 (2014) 1–4

http://dx.doi.org/10.1016/j.ccep.2013.10.006

even in the setting of heart failure[1] and despite[2] a preponderance of risk factors such as hypertension. The lifetime risk of developing atrial fibrillation is slightly higher in men of European descent (26%) than in women of European descent (23%).[3]

AGE AT DIAGNOSIS

Atrial fibrillation is uncommon before the age of 60 years. The rapidly increasing prevalence of atrial fibrillation is largely attributable to the aging of the population. More than 12% of patients with atrial fibrillation are between 75 and 84 years old, whereas only 1% of patients with atrial fibrillation are less than 60 years old.[4] Age combined with other risk factors is more proarrhythmic.[5,6] More than one-third of patients with atrial fibrillation are older than 80 years (Go), presenting additional management challenges caused by common age-associated comorbidities and frailty.

Body Habitus

A tall stature and obesity are independently associated with an increased incidence of atrial fibrillation. It is thought that this is a direct reflection of left atrial size but, in obesity, diabetes and ventricular diastolic dysfunction are likely contributory.[1] Because the obesity epidemic will contribute to the increased future incidence of atrial fibrillation, targeting obesity may have the opposite effect.

Family History

Although uncommon, genetic susceptibility to atrial fibrillation is supported by parental atrial fibrillation predisposing the offspring by a factor of 2 to 3. These patients with atrial fibrillation are typically young, and the influence of genetic predisposition in the elderly remains unclear at this time.

Habits

An athletic lifestyle, particularly one involving endurance activities, is a risk for atrial fibrillation, especially in young patients (primarily from high vagal tone). Cigarette smoking seems to be significant factor in women and alcohol abuse is also related to the occurrence of atrial fibrillation.[1] All of these are potentially modifiable factors with a likely positive impact.

DIAGNOSIS AND PROGNOSIS

In the past, the diagnosis and classification of atrial fibrillation as paroxysmal, persistent, or permanent has generally relied on symptoms, assessment of the peripheral pulse, 12-lead electrocardiograms, or short external electrocardiographic monitoring.

Because atrial fibrillation may be intermittent and asymptomatic or minimally symptomatic, its prevalence is difficult to establish. Implanted loop recorders, pacemakers, and defibrillators have recently enabled detection of subclinical atrial fibrillation by review of longitudinal data.

The incidence of asymptomatic atrial fibrillation is higher than is perceived by patients, and carries with it an increased risk of stoke despite its apparent silence.[7,8] There is an irrational proclivity, despite clear data, to avoid prescribing appropriate anticoagulants in asymptomatic or minimally symptomatic atrial fibrillation.[9] Adherence to prescribed guidelines regarding anticoagulation contributes significantly to stroke reduction.

Stroke is the most severe consequence of atrial fibrillation, and is 5 times more common in individuals with atrial fibrillation.[1] Although most strokes are caused by documented cerebrovascular disease, about 1 in 7 strokes are caused by atrial fibrillation, and subclinical atrial fibrillation is suspected as the cause of 1 in 4 ischemic strokes.[7–10]

An important unanswered question is how long anticoagulation should be maintained after successful ablation of atrial fibrillation. It is generally recommended that anticoagulation be maintained indefinitely in patients with CHADS[2] (congestive heart failure [CHF], hypertension, age ≥75 years, diabetes mellitus, prior stroke or TIA, or thromboembolism) scores of 2 or greater, regardless of the success of the ablation procedure, and some cardiologists stop anticoagulants after 3 months after successful ablation of atrial fibrillation in patients with CHADS[2] scores of 0 to 1.[11]

Atrial fibrillation is also associated with an increased risk of death independent of embolic stroke,[12] in part because of the presence of multiple comorbidities such as heart failure, hypertension, and coronary artery disease, all of which can be life limiting. However, atrial fibrillation independently increases the risk of sudden death from ventricular tachyarrhythmias.[13]

Associated Cardiovascular Disease

Systemic hypertension is the most notable risk factor in the development of atrial fibrillation. CHF, valvular heart disease, and myocardial infarction all increase the likelihood of future atrial fibrillation. The relationship of atrial fibrillation and heart failure (causes or consequence) remains to be determined on a case-by-case basis. CHF is associated with an approximate 5-fold risk of atrial fibrillation. Young patients with more recent onset of atrial fibrillation and uncontrolled rates are typically more likely to have CHF as the consequence.

Restoration of sinus rhythm or optimal rate control has been shown to reverse left ventricular systolic dysfunction. Atrial fibrillation in the setting of acute myocardial infarction implies a worse short-term prognosis. Left atrial enlargement, left ventricular hypertrophy (LVH), and diastolic dysfunction echocardiographic correlates with atrial fibrillation. Appropriate therapy directed toward systemic hypertension associated with LVH has been shown to reduce atrial fibrillation when concomitant regression of LVH was documented.[1]

Atrial fibrillation is common after cardiac surgery, is typically multifactorial, and is more likely with valvular heart disease. Both β-blocker and amiodarone use has been effective in prophylaxis.

Associated Noncardiovascular Diseases

Diabetes, coupled with obesity and the metabolic syndrome, is strongly associated with atrial fibrillation in the absence of structural cardiovascular disease.[14]

Sleep apnea can predispose to atrial fibrillation by metabolic and autonomic abnormalities, as well as structural cardiovascular changes. Treatment of sleep apnea should be considered before cardioversion is attempted, to minimize the possibility of recurrence.

Hyperthyroidism, both clinically overt and subclinical, is associated with a higher risk of developing atrial fibrillation, and the latter is particularly relevant in the elderly.

ECONOMIC IMPACT

The estimated cost of treating Americans with atrial fibrillation is US$26 billion per year.[15–18] The direct medical costs incurred in treating patients with atrial fibrillation are 73% higher than costs in control subjects, and do not fully account for total medical costs of related conditions resulting from atrial fibrillation, particularly the costs associated with long-term care of patients with debilitating strokes. Also not accounted for in this estimate is the cost to society and individuals of lost wages caused by disability related to atrial fibrillation and stroke. As the population ages, it is inevitable that the prevalence of atrial fibrillation and its costs will increase.

SUMMARY

Atrial fibrillation is a major public health problem in the United States.[18–20] It is the single most common sustained cardiac dysrhythmia, and a major cause of hospitalization, stroke, disability, and death. The human and economic costs of atrial fibrillation are enormous. The US Centers for Disease Control and Prevention estimates that more than 2.66 million Americans had atrial fibrillation in 2010, and expects that as many as 12 million people will have atrial fibrillation in 2050.[16] Stroke is 5 times more common in individuals with atrial fibrillation, and 3 times more common in patients with heart failure, resulting in marked increases in morbidity and mortality.[1] The estimated cost of treating Americans with atrial fibrillation is US$26 billion per year.[18] **Fig. 1** summarizes various clinical factors associated with atrial fibrillation.

The rapidly increasing prevalence of atrial fibrillation is largely attributable to the aging of the population. More than 12% of patients with atrial fibrillation are between 75 and 84 years old, whereas only 1% of patients with atrial fibrillation are less than 60 years old.[4] More than one-third of patients with atrial fibrillation are older than 80 years,[17] presenting additional management challenges caused by common age-associated comorbidities and frailty. The lifetime risk of

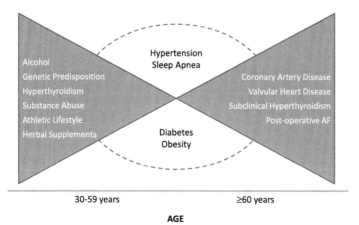

Fig. 1. The epidemiologic basis of atrial fibrillation.

developing atrial fibrillation is slightly higher in men of European descent (26%) than in women of European descent (23%).[3] Atrial fibrillation is less common in African Americans[2] despite a preponderance of risk factors such as hypertension.

Because atrial fibrillation may be intermittent and asymptomatic or minimally symptomatic at onset, its prevalence is difficult to establish. In the past, atrial fibrillation was classified as intermittent or paroxysmal, persistent or sustained, and long-standing or permanent. This classification has generally relied on symptoms, assessment of the peripheral pulse, occasional electrocardiograms, or short periods of external electrocardiographic monitoring. More recently, implanted loop recorders, pacemakers, and defibrillators have enabled more precise assessment of the heart rhythm over long periods of time. The incidence of asymptomatic atrial fibrillation is higher than is perceived by patients, and carries with it an increased risk of stoke even if the atrial fibrillation is asymptomatic and intermittent.[7,8]

REFERENCES

1. Kannel WB, Wolf PA, Benjamin EJ, et al. Prevalence, incidence, prognosis and predisposing conditions for atrial fibrillation: population-based estimates. Am J Cardiol 1998;82:2N–9N.

2. Alonso A, Agarwal SK, Soliman EZ, et al. Incidence of atrial fibrillation in whites and African-Americans: the Atherosclerosis Risk in Communities (ARIC) study. Am Heart J 2009;158:111–7.

3. Lloyd-Jones DM, Wang TJ, Larson MG, et al. Lifetime risk for development of atrial fibrillation: the Framingham Heart Study. Circulation 2004;31:1042–6.

4. Wolf PA, Benjamin EJ, Belanger AJ, et al. Lifetime risk for development of atrial fibrillation: the Framingham Study. Am Heart J 1996;131:790–5.

5. Fuster V, Ryden L, Asinger R, et al. ACC/AHA/ESC guidelines for the management of patients with atrial fibrillation. J Am Coll Cardiol 2001;38:1231–66 Circulation 2001;104(17):2118–50 and Eur Heart J 2001;22(20):1852–923.

6. Wann LS, Curtis AB, January CT, et al. 2011 ACCF/AHA/HRS focused update on the management of patients with atrial fibrillation (updating the 2006 guideline): a report of the American College of Cardiology Foundation/American Heart Association Task Force on Practice Guidelines. J Am Coll Cardiol 2011;57:223–42 Circulation 2011;123:104–23.

7. Healey JS, Connolly SJ, Gold MR, et al. Subclinical atrial fibrillation and the risk of stroke. N Engl J Med 2012;366:120–9.

8. Ott A, Breteler MM, de Bruyne MC, et al. Atrial fibrillation and dementia in a population-based study. The Rotterdam Study. Stroke 1997;28:316–21.

9. Santini M, Gasparini M, Landolina M, et al. Device-detected atrial tachyarrhythmias predict adverse outcome in real-world patients with implantable biventricular defibrillators. J Am Coll Cardiol 2011;57:167–72.

10. Roger VL, Go AS, Lloyd-Jones DM, et al. Heart disease and stroke statistics – 2012 update: a report from the American Heart Association. Circulation 2012;125:e2–220.

11. Mardigyan V, Verma A, Dirnie D, et al. Anticoagulation management pre- and post atrial fibrillation ablation: a survey of Canadian centres. Can J Cardiol 2013;29:219–23.

12. Benjamin EJ, Wolf PA, D'Agostino RB, et al. Impact of atrial fibrillation on the risk of death: the Framingham Heart Study. Circulation 1998;98:946–52.

13. Chen LY, Sotoodehnia N, Buzkova P, et al. Atrial fibrillation and the risk of sudden cardiac death – the Atherosclerosis Risk in Communities Study and Cardiovascular Health Study. JAMA Intern Med 2013;173:29–31.

14. Mohanty S, Mohanty P, Biase LD. Impact of metabolic syndrome on procedural outcomes in patients with atrial fibrillation undergoing catheter ablation. J Am Coll Cardiol 2012;59:1295–301.

15. Stewart S, Hart CL, Hole DJ, et al. A population-based study of the long-term risks associated with atrial fibrillation: 20-year follow-up of the Renfrew-Paisley study. Am J Med 2002;313:359–64.

16. Kakkar AK, Mueller I, Bassard JP, et al. International longitudinal registry of patients with atrial fibrillation at risk of stroke: Global Anticoagulant Registry in the FIELD (GARFIELD). Am Heart J 2012;163:13–9.

17. Kim MH, Johnston SS, Chu BC, et al. Estimation of total incremental health care costs in patients with atrial fibrillation in the United States. Circ Cardiovasc Qual Outcomes 2011;4:313–20.

18. Office of information products and data analytics OIPDA, CMS Administrative Claims Data, January 2011-December 2011, from the Chronic Condition Warehouse, 2012.

19. Centers for Disease Control and Prevention. Atrial fibrillation fact sheet. Available at: http://www.cdc.gov/dhdsp/data_statistics/fact_sheets/fs_atrial_fibrillation.htm. Accessed November 18, 2013.

20. Go AS, Hylek EM, Phillips KA, et al. Prevalence of diagnosed atrial fibrillation in adults. National implications for rhythm management and stroke prevention: the Anticoagulation and Risk Factors in Atrial Fibrillation (ATREA) Study. JAMA 2001;285:2370–5.

Mechanisms of Stroke in Atrial Fibrillation

Jose Maria Castellano, MD, PhD[a,b,*], Jason Chinitz, MD[a],
Jonathan Willner, MD[a], Valentin Fuster, MD, PhD[a,b]

KEYWORDS

• Atrial fibrillation • Stroke • Thromboembolism • Cardiac arrhythmia

KEY POINTS

• Atrial fibrillation (AF) is the most common form of arrhythmia and its prevalence is projected to increase. The risk of stroke in patients with AF is increased by 5-fold, and strokes in association with AF are more often fatal, disabling, and associated with greater morbidity and recurrence than other causes of stroke.
• The causes of thrombus formation in the context of AF are multifactorial and include changes in flow, atrial anatomy, prothrombotic alterations in blood constituents, and inflammation.
• Improved risk stratification is critical to distinguish which patients may be safely treated without anticoagulation.

INTRODUCTION

Atrial fibrillation (AF) is the most common sustained cardiac rhythm disorder, affecting 1% to 2% of the general population.[1] Its incidence increases dramatically with age, from less than 0.5% at 40 to 50 years, to 10% in octogenarians.[2] The prevalence of AF is likely to increase even further over the next 50 years, mainly due to the increasing mean age of the general population, the obesity epidemic, and improvements in the management of cardiovascular disease, such that by 2050, sixteen million Americans are predicted to have AF.[1]

The yearly incidence of stroke in patients with nonvalvular AF is about 5%, which is 5 times higher than that in matched populations without any form of arrhythmia.[3] Strokes associated with AF are often fatal, and patients who survive are left more disabled, suffer greater morbidity, have longer hospital stays, are less likely to be discharged to their own homes, and are more likely to suffer a recurrence than patients with other causes of stroke. As a result, the risk of death from AF-related stroke is 2-fold that of stroke in patients without AF, and the cost of care is increased 1.5-fold.[4] Moreover, the risk of AF-related stroke mortality increases from 1.5% in those aged 50 to 59 years to 24% in those aged 80 to 89 years.

AF is a major public health problem because of the associated mortality, disability, and health care costs. The problem is amplified by the substantial nationwide undertreatment of patients who would benefit from anticoagulation for stroke prevention. According to one economic model, approximately 1.265 million patients with AF not receiving antithrombotic prophylaxis suffer 58,382 strokes annually with an associated total direct cost to Medicare of $4.8 billion.[5] Furthermore, early recognition and appropriate prophylaxis are hindered by the frequently

Financial Disclosure: The authors have no financial disclosures or relationships to report.
[a] The Mount Sinai Medical Center, Cardiovascular Institute, One Gustave Levy Place, Box 1030, New York, NY 10029-6574, USA; [b] National Center for Cardiovascular Research (CNIC), Melchor Fernandez Almagro 3, Madrid 28029, Spain
* Corresponding author. The Mount Sinai Medical Center, One Gustave Levy Place, Box 1030, New York, NY 10029-6574.
E-mail address: jose.castellano@mountsinai.org

asymptomatic nature of AF, occurring in at least one-third of patients. Consequently, earlier detection and more widespread recognition of patients likely to benefit from anticoagulation have the potential to reduce the rising burden of cardioembolic stroke in patients with AF.

PATHOPHYSIOLOGY OF THROMBUS FORMATION

Despite gaps in our knowledge, it is now clear that the pathogenesis of thrombus formation in AF is a multifactorial process that includes not only stasis in a poorly contractile left atrium, but also the presence of a prothrombotic or hypercoagulable state.[6] As reflected in Virchow triad, thrombogenesis in patients with AF occurs as a result of endocardial damage, blood stasis, and abnormal regulation of blood constituents responsible for clot formation and fibrinolysis (**Fig. 1**).

Prothrombotic Atrial Anatomy

The left atrial appendage (LAA) is by far the most common site of intra-atrial thrombus formation, both in patients with AF and in the presence of sinus rhythm. Among patients with AF presenting with stroke, LAA thrombus can be seen in approximately 23%.[7] The morphology of the LAA, a frequently long, narrow, and hooked extension of the left atrium, creates an anatomic substrate for blood stasis and thrombus formation. Interestingly, the shape of the LAA is highly variable between patients, and more complex lobular structures have been associated with a higher likelihood of thromboembolism in patients with AF, independent of other established stroke risk factors.[8]

Changes in the structure of the LAA can also be a consequence of AF. A wrinkled appearance attributable to edema and fibrinous transformation, as well as small areas of endothelial denudation and thrombotic aggregation, has been reported in patients with AF and stroke.[9] Further work has demonstrated the presence of myocytic

hypertrophy and/or necrosis, as well as a mononuclear cell infiltrate, within the LAA in patients with AF. There is also mounting evidence that AF predisposes to alterations in collagen degradation products and impaired extracellular matrix degradation, which is also affected as a consequence of various AF-related comorbidities (most notably hypertension).[10] Such alteration of the extracellular matrix has been shown to induce fibrosis and infiltration of the endocardium and may be an additional factor associated intra-atrial thrombus formation. These structural changes could account, at least in part, for the delay in return of atrial systole after successful cardioversion or ablation. Such changes highlight the residual risk for thrombus formation and the importance of anticoagulation even after restoration of sinus rhythm.[11]

Abnormal Blood Stasis

Stasis in the setting of AF occurs not only because of loss of atrial systole but also in relation to left atrial dilatation. Atrial dilatation is a crucial risk factor for thrombogenesis, as indicated by the finding that atrial size corrected for body surface area is an independent risk factor for stroke.[12] Abnormal stasis in the left atrium and LAA can be visualized on transesophageal echocardiogram with spontaneous echo contrast (SEC), which is thought to reflect an increased interaction between fibrinogen and erythrocytes, and its presence is related to the relative concentrations of each, with more fibrinogen needed to induce the same SEC effect at lower hematocrit levels. SEC highly depends on flow rate and therefore is more likely to occur in patients in AF. Importantly, SEC can also be seen after restoration of sinus rhythm, occurring in up to 37% of such patients at 3 months.[13] Thus, the presence of an increased LA size and SEC demonstrable on echocardiography further illustrates the imperative to consider the residual risk of thrombus formation after sinus rhythm restoration.

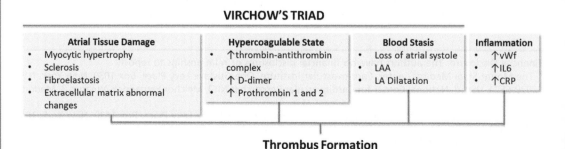

Fig. 1. Pathophysiological mechanisms underlying thrombus formation in AF.

Abnormal Blood Constituents

The main intravascular promoters of thrombogenesis are platelets and the various proteins of the coagulation cascade. In patients with AF, abnormal changes occur in these promoters, as well as in other blood constituents such as inflammatory cytokines and growth factors, resulting in activation of coagulation cascade and abnormal fibrinolytic activity. Over 20 years ago Gustafsson and colleagues[14] demonstrated the presence of hemostatic abnormalities in the plasma of patients with nonvalvular AF and associated these abnormalities with stroke. Another seminal report found elevated D-dimer levels, a marker of thrombogenesis, in patients with AF but not in controls in sinus rhythm; the presence of associated organic heart disease in this study was not associated with significant differences in fibrin D-dimer levels, attributing the hypercoagulable state to AF independent of its risk factors.[15] Interestingly, the high D-dimer levels associated with AF have been shown to be reduced by both anticoagulation[16] and cardioversion to sinus rhythm.[17]

Further indicators of increased thrombin generation in patients with AF, and particularly in patients with AF-related stroke, include increased levels of prothrombin fragments 1 and 2, thrombin-antithrombin III complex, and von Willebrand factor (vWF).[18] The presence of SEC on transesophageal echocardiography in patients with AF has been shown to correlate with higher concentrations of thrombin-antithrombin III complex, D-dimer, and vWF, which in turn has been associated with the presence of intracardiac thrombus.[19] Elevated concentrations of vWF, a well-established index of endothelial damage and dysfunction, independently predicts the presence of LAA thrombus in patients with AF.[20] Moreover, increased expression of vWF in the endocardium has been associated with increased myocyte diameter and enlarged LA dimensions in mitral valve disease. The availability of these biomarkers may be of particular value in patients classed as moderate risk of AF-related stroke, in whom measurement of high vWF levels, for example, may reclassify such patients as high risk.

Although such thrombotic indices confirm the association of AF with a prothrombotic milieu, the origins of this coagulation activation require further exploration. Recent interest has been directed toward inflammation—reflected by inflammatory cytokines, such as interleukins and C-reactive protein, as well as the release of various growth factors—"driving" the prothrombotic state in AF.

Inflammation

Inflammation in patients with AF can result in endothelial dysfunction and may also be linked directly to AF initiation and thrombogenesis. Increasing evidence has supported a link between inflammation and the initiation and perpetuation of AF.[21] In addition, changes in systemic inflammation have been linked to prothrombotic indices in AF. Although the precise mechanisms are not yet elucidated, certain inflammatory markers such as interleukin-6 and high-sensitivity C-reactive protein (hs-CRP) are elevated in patients with AF and have been selected as possible mediators. Elevated hs-CRP levels consistently correlate with cardiovascular risk and have been shown to be predictive of mortality and vascular death in AF, but not stroke itself.[22] In addition, studies have also shown a stepwise increase in hs-CRP levels in patients with increasing burdens of AF (from sinus rhythm to paroxysmal and persistent arrhythmia).[23] Increased hs-CRP and interleukin-6 levels could provide a biologically plausible explanation linking inflammation and thrombogenesis in patients with AF because they have both been shown to stimulate tissue factor production from monocytes in vitro.[11]

RISK STRATIFICATION IN PATIENTS WITH NONVALVULAR AF

Traditionally, the CHADS$_2$ score (congestive heart failure, hypertension, age $\geq$75 years, diabetes mellitus, and prior stroke [2 points]) has been used to identify patients with AF who would benefit from anticoagulation (**Table 1**). US practice guidelines suggest the use of antithrombotics for patients with nonvalvular AF and a CHADS$_2$ scores $\geq$2, whereas those with CHADS$_2$ score of 0 are at low risk of thromboembolism and should be treated with aspirin or no antithrombotic therapy. For patients at intermediate risk (CHADS$_2$ score = 1), these guidelines recommend decisions regarding anticoagulation therapy be based on the patient's risk of bleeding, ability to sustain anticoagulation, and personal preference.[24]

The CHADS$_2$ model, however, is limited by its failure to account for the increase in risk with age as a continuous variable, and its exclusion of other previously underappreciated risk factors, and thus may have only minimal clinical utility in predicting ischemic stroke.[25] In the AnTicoagulation and Risk factors In Atrial fibrillation (ATRIA) study, which evaluated a cohort of 13,559 patients with AF not taking anticoagulation, patients with and without thromboembolism had highly overlapping risk distributions using the CHADS$_2$ score.[26] Furthermore,

Table 1 CHADS risk scoring system		
Risk Factor	**Points**	**Stroke Rate (95% CI)[a]**
Congestive heart failure	+1	Score of 0 1.9%
Hypertension	+1	Score of 1 2.8%
Age ≥75 y	+1	Score of 2 4.0%
Diabetes	+1	Score of 3 5.9%
Stroke/TIA	+2	Score of 4 8.5%
Maximum score 6		Score of 5 12.5%
		Score of 6 18.9

Abbreviations: CI, Confidence interval; TIA, transient ischemic attack.
[a] Per 100 patients-year without antithrombotic therapy.
Data from Fuster V, Rydén LE, Cannom DS, et al. 2011 ACCF/AHA/HRS focused updates incorporated into the ACC/AHA/ESC 2006 guidelines for the management of patients with atrial fibrillation: a report of the American College of Cardiology Foundation/American Heart Association Task Force on practice guidelines. Circulation 2011;123:e269–367.

Table 2 CHADS-VASC risk scoring system		
Risk Factor	**Points**	**Annual Risk Score for Stroke**
		Score of 0 0%
Congestive heart failure/LV dysfunction[a]	+1	Score of 1 1.3%
Hypertension	+1	Score of 2 2.2%
Age ≥75 y	+2	Score of 3 3.2%
Diabetes	+1	Score of 4 4.0%
Stroke/TIA/ thromboembolism	+2	Score of 5 6.7%
Vascular disease (MI, aortic plaque, PAD)[b]	+1	Score of 6 9.8%
Age 65–74	+1	Score of 7 9.6%
Sex category (female)	+1	Score of 8 6.7%
Maximum score 9		Score of 9 15.2%

Abbreviations: LV, left ventricular; MI, myocardial infarction; PAD, peripheral artery disease; TIA, transient ischemic attack.
[a] LV ejection fraction ≤40%.
[b] Including prior revascularization, amputation due to PAD, or angiographic evidence of PAD.
Data from Camm AJ, Lip GY, De Caterina R, et al, ESC Committee for Practice Guidelines (CPG). 2012 focused update of the ESC Guidelines for the management of atrial fibrillation: an update of the 2010 ESC Guidelines for the management of atrial fibrillation. Developed with the special contribution of the European Heart Rhythm Association. Eur Heart J 2012;33:2719–47.

a large proportion of patients fall into the intermediate risk category of CHADS$_2$, leaving management ambiguous.[27] As this model has at best modest ability to identify patients at truly low risk of stroke, its utility in determining which patients may safely avoid anticoagulation is inadequate.

To overcome some of these limitations, the CHA$_2$DS$_2$VASc score was developed and expands on CHADS$_2$ by assigning 1 point for age ≥65 years (and 2 points for age ≥75), and 1 point each for vascular disease (prior myocardial infarction, complex aortic plaque, or symptomatic peripheral arterial disease) and female gender (**Table 2**). This score is therefore more inclusive of various stroke risk factors and can better distinguish patients between low and intermediate risk for thromboembolism than the traditional CHADS$_2$ model.[4] In a large Danish registry of 73,538 patients, 1-year rates of thromboembolism for patients at lowest risk (score = 0) were 0.78 per 100 person-years using CHA$_2$DS$_2$VASc and 1.67 per 100 person-years using the CHADS$_2$ model. Furthermore, using CHA$_2$DS$_2$VASc, rates of thromboembolism were lowered with anticoagulation in all risk categories except those with a score of 0. In addition, among patients at intermediate risk based on CHADS$_2$ score = 1, 93% were reclassified to higher risk based on CHA$_2$DS$_2$-VASc.[28] Similarly, in a large Swedish registry, although warfarin appeared beneficial in patients across all CHADS$_2$ scores, a CHA$_2$DS$_2$VASc score = 0 identified a cohort of patients at very low stroke risk in whom anticoagulation was associated with no benefit or some degree of risk.[29] In the EuroHeart Survey, which followed a cohort of 1084 patients with AF who were not taking anticoagulation for 1 year, whereas nearly 62% of patients would have been assigned to the intermediate risk category using the CHADS$_2$ score, resulting in ambiguous treatment recommendations for this majority, only 15% of patients were assigned to the intermediate risk category using CHA$_2$DS$_2$VASc.[30] Although a low-risk CHADS$_2$ score may provide false reassurance, prompting clinicians to defer anticoagulation in patients who might actually benefit, the CHA$_2$DS$_2$-VASc score is clearly more effective in distinguishing patients in whom anticoagulation may be safely deferred.

The decision whether to use anticoagulation must balance an individual patient's stroke risk with their risk of significant hemorrhage on anticoagulation. As such, bleeding risk models have been developed to complement stroke risk assessment and assist in clinical decision-making. The HAS-BLED bleeding risk score assigns points for hypertension, abnormal renal or liver function, stroke, bleeding history or predisposition, labile international normalized ratio (INR), age greater than 65 years, and drug or alcohol use, and increasing HAS-BLED scores correlate with a stepwise increment in major bleeding.[27] Other easily applied bleeding risk scores are also available, including the ATRIA score (which identifies the clinical factors predictive of warfarin-associated major hemorrhage as anemia, severe renal disease, age ≥75, prior hemorrhage, and hypertension) and HEMORR$_2$AGES (Hepatic or Renal disease, Ethanol abuse, Malignancy, Older age [>65 years], Reduced platelet count or function, rebleeding risk [2 points], uncontrolled hypertension, Anemia, Genetic factor, Excessive fall risk, and Stroke).[31] Although the European practice guidelines support the use of HAS-BLED and advise caution and regular patient review when the score is ≥3,[4] these bleeding risk scores are all effective in identifying patients at elevated bleeding risk and may be useful to influence treatment decisions, particularly for patients at intermediate stroke risk (**Table 3**).

Complicating management is the reality that bleeding risk models include many of the same risk factors that also impose greater risk of thromboembolism (eg, increasing age, prior stroke, and hypertension). For instance, advancing age is a risk factor for both stroke and warfarin-associated hemorrhage, and the fear of hemorrhage in the elderly often influences clinicians to withhold anticoagulation. However, the risk of bleeding increases only modestly in comparison

to the age-related risk of stroke in patients with AF.[26,27] Singer and colleagues[32] found the net clinical benefit favoring anticoagulation to increase steadily with age and was highest for those 85 years or older, highlighting the importance of effective stroke prevention in the elderly despite elevated bleeding risk. In a large Swedish registry that estimated the overall net benefit of warfarin anticoagulation among patients with AF at various strata of stroke and bleeding risk (assessed using the CHADS$_2$, CHA$_2$DS$_2$VASc, and HAS-BLED scores), warfarin reduced the stroke risk to a greater extent than it increased risk of intracranial hemorrhage, resulting in a positive net benefit from treatment, in all patients with AF except those at lowest stroke risk as determined by a CHA$_2$DS$_2$-VASc = 0. In patients with high-risk scores using either CHA$_2$DS$_2$VASc or HAS-BLED, warfarin use was associated with the most substantial net benefit.[29] The focus of anticoagulation management in patients with AF can now shift toward identification of patients at truly low stroke risk who can be followed safely without anticoagulation. Appreciation of an elevated bleeding risk based on a HAS-BLED score ≥3 may be most clinically useful in patients at intermediate stroke risk, when deferring anticoagulation may be prudently considered. In all other patients, anticoagulation should be implemented more liberally, withholding treatment only in patients with no CHA$_2$DS$_2$VASc risk factors or those at "very-high" bleeding risk (ie, those with prior episodes of major bleeding or malignant hypertension). With the introduction of new oral anticoagulants (OAC) that carry lower risk of major bleeding and are more easily administered than warfarin, this strategy will contribute to less complex clinical decision-making and will

Table 3
Clinical characteristics comprising the HAS-BLED bleeding risk score

Clinical Characteristic	Points	HAS-BLED Score (Total Points)	Bleeds Per 100 Patients-Year
Hypertension	1	0	1.13
Abnormal renal and liver function (1 patient each)	1 or 2	1	1.02
Stroke	1	2	1.88
Bleeding	1	3	3.74
Labile INRs	1	4	8.70
Elderly	1	5	No data
Drugs or alcohol (1 patient each)	1 or 2		

Data from Camm AJ, Lip GY, De Caterina R, et al, ESC Committee for Practice Guidelines (CPG). 2012 focused update of the ESC Guidelines for the management of atrial fibrillation: an update of the 2010 ESC Guidelines for the management of atrial fibrillation. Developed with the special contribution of the European Heart Rhythm Association. Eur Heart J 2012;33:2719–47.

result in more patients with AF being offered antithrombotic therapy than are currently in the United States (**Fig. 2**).[33]

STROKE PREVENTION: THE EXPANDING ROLE FOR ANTICOAGULATION

Anticoagulation is the only therapy in AF management that has thus far been shown to reduce AF-related mortality. Available options for prevention of thromboembolism in patients with AF include anticoagulant and antiplatelet agents. Warfarin decreases the risk of stroke by 67% compared with placebo,[34] and even more when assessed by on-treatment analysis.[35] Aspirin decreases the risk by 20% compared with placebo, and warfarin reduces stroke by about 40% compared with aspirin.[36] Unfortunately, warfarin has several limitations, including a narrow therapeutic index, frequent food and drug interactions, and the need for regular monitoring of anticoagulation intensity. Disappointingly, the proportion of time INR was in the therapeutic range averaged 65% in clinical trials but only 56% in retrospective studies. There is certainly room for improvement, because an 11.9% improvement in time within therapeutic range is associated with prevention of one thromboembolic event per 100 patient-years.[37]

Dual-antiplatelet therapy (DAPT) with aspirin and clopidogrel has been evaluated as a potential alternative to vitamin K antagonist therapy (VKA). In the Atrial fibrillation Clopidogrel Trial with Irbesartan for prevention of Vascular Events (ACTIVE-W) study, the annual risk of the primary outcome (stroke, embolism, myocardial infarction, or vascular death) was lower in the VKA group (3.9 vs 5.6%, RR 1.44, P = .0003), whereas rates of major

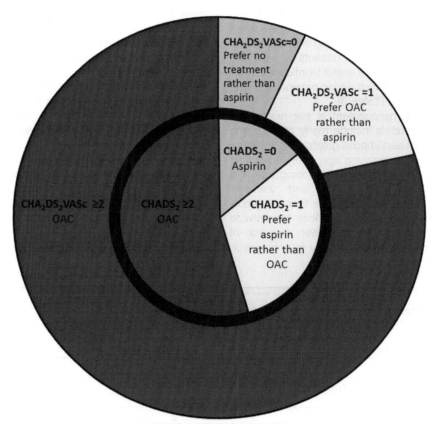

Fig. 2. Recommendations for prevention of stroke in patients with AF. The inner circle represents treatment recommendations based on the use of the $CHADS_2$ score, as in US Guidelines. The outer circle represents recommendations based on the CHA_2DS_2-VASc model, as outlined in the European guidelines, which advise anticoagulant therapy in a larger proportion of patients with AF. Bleeding risk assessment is recommended for patients at intermediate stroke risk (yellow-shaded area), with particular caution and regular patient review for those on warfarin therapy when the HAS-BLED score is ≥3. For patients at very high risk of bleeding (eg, those with malignant hypertension or prior episodes of major bleeding), conservative monitoring without treatment should be considered. OAC, oral anticoagulation. (*From* Fuster V, Chinitz JS. Net clinical benefit of warfarin: extending the reach of antithrombotic therapy for atrial fibrillation. Circulation 2012;125:2285–87; with permission.)

hemorrhage were similar and total adverse outcome was more frequent in patients randomized to DAPT.[38] Compared with aspirin alone in the ACTIVE-A trial, DAPT was associated with a 28% lower rate of stroke (2.4 vs 3.3%/y, $P<.001$), but a higher rate of major bleeding (2.0 vs 1.3%/y, $P<.001$).[39] Current US practice guidelines note that DAPT may be considered for patients with AF in whom anticoagulation with warfarin is considered unsuitable[24]; however, this strategy should not be expected to lower bleeding risk.

After more than 50 years, several novel OACs that do not require routine monitoring of anticoagulation intensity are now available as alternatives to VKA therapy. These new alternatives have additional benefits, such as fewer food and drug interactions, stable pharmacodynamics properties, and most notably, a lower incidence of intracranial hemorrhage. Dabigatran etexilate, an oral direct thrombin inhibitor, was compared with warfarin in the RE-LY trial and found that dabigatran 150 mg twice daily reduced the stroke rate by 34% with no increase in major bleeding. Furthermore, dabigatran reduced the rate of hemorrhagic stroke, and there was a trend toward reduced mortality ($P = .051$).[40] A lower dose of dabigatran (110 mg twice daily) yielded stroke rates noninferior to those with warfarin with lower rates of major hemorrhage, but this dose was not approved. Dabigatran is associated with a higher rate of gastrointestinal bleeding, and dyspepsia occurred in approximately 10% of patients treated with dabigatran in RE-LY. Its renal clearance results in drug accumulation in the setting of renal insufficiency resulting in FDA approval of the 75-mg twice daily dosing for patients with creatinine clearance (15–30 mL/min), although this dose has not been well studied.

Oral factor Xa inhibitors are the most recently approved OACs for prevention of AF-related thromboembolism. Rivaroxaban, dosed 20 mg once daily, was studied in the ROCKET-AF trial among 14,264 patients at high risk for thromboembolism (mean CHADS$_2$ score = 3.5) and proved noninferior to warfarin with similar rates of major bleeding.[41] Importantly, rivaroxaban was associated with fewer intracranial hemorrhages and fatal bleeding, and compared with the other novel agents has the advantage of once-daily dosing.

Apixaban, another oral factor Xa inhibitor, has perhaps garnered the most excitement of the novel agents and was the most recently approved for clinical use by the FDA in December 2012. After demonstrating superiority over aspirin with little difference in major bleeding in the AVERROES (Apixaban Versus Acetylsalicylic Acid [ASA] to Prevent Stroke in Atrial Fibrillation Patients Who Have Failed or Are Unsuitable for Vitamin K Antagonist Treatment) trial,[42] apixaban was compared with warfarin in the ARISTOTLE (Apixaban for Reduction in Stroke and Other Thromboembolic Events in Atrial Fibrillation) trial of 18,201 patients with AF and at least one risk factor for stroke (mean CHADS$_2$ score 2.1).[43] In this trial, Apixaban was superior to warfarin for prevention of stroke or systemic embolism and additionally demonstrated lower rates of major bleeding, a 58% relative risk reduction in intracranial hemorrhage, and unlike the other novel agents, achieved a statistically significant 11% relative risk reduction in all-cause mortality (**Table 4**).

ACHIEVEMENT OF SINUS RHYTHM AFTER AF ABLATION: WHAT IS THE RESIDUAL RISK OF STROKE?

Catheter ablation is an effective treatment strategy for the maintenance of sinus rhythm in patients with drug-refractory, symptomatic AF.[44] Its role in the reduction of stroke and mortality, however, remains less certain. Several large studies—most notably the AFFIRM (Atrial Fibrillation Follow-up Investigation of Rhythm Management) trial—have examined the effectiveness of a rate control versus a rhythm control strategy and have established that anti-arrhythmic drugs (AADs) offer no mortality or stroke reduction benefit above that of rate control.[45,46] There remains, though, a strong hemodynamic rationale for the maintenance of sinus rhythm—most notably lower left atrial filling pressure, lengthened diastolic filling time, and reduced atrioventricular valvular regurgitation—in addition to improvements in symptoms and quality of life.[47] Furthermore, on-treatment analysis of the AFFIRM data suggested a mortality benefit to rhythm control, but that this benefit might be attenuated by the frequently deleterious side effect profile of AADs.[48] Several studies have now shown that catheter ablation in patients with paroxysmal AF is more effective than AADs for the maintenance of sinus rhythm in patients who have previously failed AAD therapy,[49–52] leading to the hypothesis that effective catheter ablation might offer the benefits of maintaining sinus rhythm (perhaps including lower stroke rates) while avoiding the common adverse effects seen with AADs.

Several studies have now examined this theory. In 2006, Oral and colleagues[53] retrospectively evaluated stroke rate in 755 patients with paroxysmal or chronic AF who underwent catheter ablation. OAC was discontinued after 3 months in 79% of patients in sinus rhythm with a CHADS$_2$ score of 0, and in 68% of patients with a CHADS$_2$ score of 1 or more. None of these patients suffered a stroke during follow-up. Overall, the stroke rate in this cohort of patients compared favorably with

Table 4
Clinical trials of novel anticoagulants

	Dabigatran RE-LY n = 18,113	Rivaroxaban ROCKET-AF n = 14,264	Apixaban AVERROES n = 5600	Apixaban ARISTOTLE n = 18,201
Type	Noninferiority	Noninferiority	Superiority	Noninferiority
Study drugs	Dabigatran 150 mg bid Dabigatran 110 mg bid Warfarin (INR 2–3)	Rivaroxaban 20 mg qd Warfarin (INR 2–3)	Apixaban 5 mg bid Aspirin 81–324 mg qd	Apixaban 5 mg bid Warfarin (INR 2–3)
Other Doses	None. 75 mg bid (unstudied) was approved by FDA for CrCl 15–30 mL/min	15 mg qd in patients with CrCl 30–49 mL/min	2.5 mg bid in patients with 2 criteria: age $\geq$80 y, weight $\leq$60 kg, Cr $\geq$1.5 mg/dL	
Stroke risk	Moderate-high risk $CHADS_2 \geq 1$	Moderate-high risk $CHADS_2 \geq 2$	Moderate-high risk $CHADS_2 \geq 1$	Moderate-high risk $CHADS_2 \geq 1$
Primary efficacy outcome	9% reduction in stroke or systemic embolism for 110 mg, 34% reduction for 150 mg ($P<.001$ for both)	21% reduction in stroke or systemic embolism ($P<.001$)	55% reduction in stroke or systemic embolism ($P<.001$)	21% reduction in stroke or systemic embolism (noninferiority $P<.001$)
Safety outcome	20% reduction in major bleeding for 110 mg ($P = .003$), no difference for 150 mg	No difference in major and clinically relevant nonmajor bleeding ($P = .44$)	No difference in major bleeding ($P = .57$)	31% reduction in major bleeding ($P<.001$)

From Chinitz JS, Castellano JM, Kovacic JC, et al. Atrial fibrillation, stroke, and quality of life. Ann N Y Acad Sci 2012;1254:140–50; with permission.

patients from the Framingham cohort without any history of AF. Nademanee and colleagues[54] prospectively examined 674 high-risk AF patients (defined as age greater than 65 years old with at least 1 additional $CHADS_2$ risk factor) undergoing catheter ablation; at 836 ± 605 days, 81.4% of patients were in sinus rhythm. The 5-year survival rate was 92% versus 64% ($P<.0001$) and the annual stroke rate was 0.4% versus 2% ($P = .004$) for patients in sinus rhythm and recurrent AF, respectively. Sinus rhythm after the procedure was the most important independent predictor of survival, a finding consistent across several studies.[55–57] Recently, a study by Lin and colleagues[58] documented similarly low stroke rates in patients in this high-risk cohort.

Bunch and colleagues[55] prospectively examined 690 low-risk ($CHADS_2 \leq 1$) patients who were discharged after catheter ablation on either aspirin or warfarin, with treatment choice made on the basis of overall $CHADS_2$ score and patient characteristics and preferences. Patients in the warfarin group were on the whole at a higher risk for stroke than those in the aspirin group. There were no strokes in the aspirin group and 4 strokes in the warfarin group at 327 ± 368 days of follow-up. Bunch and colleagues concluded that low-risk patients can safely be discharged on aspirin therapy alone after successful catheter ablation.

Last, in a large, multicenter retrospective study of 3355 patients, Themistoclakis and colleagues[59–61] documented low rates of stroke in AF ablation patients who maintain sinus rhythm after ablation. Of the 2692 patients who discontinued OAC, the stroke rate at 28 ± 13 months was 0.07% in a group in which 13% had a $CHADS_2$ score of at least 2. Patients maintained on OAC had a stroke rate of 0.45% and a major hemorrhage rate of 2%, suggesting a benefit to OAC discontinuation in patients with documented after ablation sinus rhythm irrespective of $CHADS_2$ score.

Although a low stroke rate in a select group of patients has been documented consistently across these observational studies, they all suffer from a relatively short follow-up time and lack of randomization. Furthermore, differing AF ablation techniques, postablation monitoring, and OAC regimens were used, making firm conclusions regarding appropriate management difficult. With rare exception, the convention has been to maintain OAC for a minimum of 3 months after ablation, and indefinitely in those still with documented AF or who otherwise remain at "high risk" for stroke (a term still requiring better definition in this population). If OAC was stopped, patients were begun on either single or dual antiplatelet therapy. Whether ongoing antiplatelet therapy is necessary in this population is not currently known. Several studies reported an increased frequency of stroke in the "early" postprocedural phase while awaiting therapeutic anticoagulation levels, highlighting the attendant risk soon after ablation. How the novel OAC agents now on the market will change this risk paradigm remains to be seen.

Two ongoing studies seek to answer several of these critical and unresolved issues. The Catheter Ablation versus Anti-arrhythmic Drug Therapy for Atrial Fibrillation Trial (CABANA) trial (clinicaltrials. gov identifier NCT00911508), which is currently enrolling patients, is a prospective superiority trial examining stroke and mortality in subjects randomized to catheter ablation or optimal medical therapy. The Early Treatment of Atrial Fibrillation for Stroke Prevention Trial[43] (clinicaltrials.gov identifier NCT01288352) will examine a strategy of "early" rhythm control using catheter ablation and AADs versus current standard practice. The results of these 2 trials, in conjunction with data gathered in previous observational studies, should better define the role of catheter ablation in reducing stroke and mortality.

Until the results of these important trials are available, thorough discussions with informed patients and consideration of individual preferences remain important factors guiding after ablation anticoagulation management. As late and asymptomatic AF recurrences are not uncommon after ablation, thorough and prolonged monitoring for arrhythmia recurrence after ablation, and perhaps echocardiography to assess for significant residual left atrial dysfunction, is necessary before cessation of antithrombotic therapy can be considered. Recently published consensus recommendations from the Heart Rhythm Society and European Heart Rhythm Association still recommend continued anticoagulation in patients with CHADS$_2$ $\geq$2 after successful ablation, with more flexibility in patients at lower stroke risk.[44]

SUMMARY

AF is the most common arrhythmia in clinical practice and is associated with substantial morbidity and mortality, primarily because of thromboembolic stroke. Better understanding of the complex mechanisms behind thromboembolism in patients with AF, together with more inclusive risk stratification models, can help identify those patients at elevated risk for stroke or hemorrhage, and perhaps most importantly distinguish those at lowest stroke risk in whom anticoagulation can be safely deferred. The last decade has seen a tremendous advance in pharmacologic and interventional therapy for patients with AF, providing clinicians with new tools to individualize stroke prevention with improved safety profiles.

REFERENCES

1. Miyasaka Y, Barnes ME, Gersh BJ, et al. Secular trends in incidence of atrial fibrillation in Olmsted County, Minnesota, 1980 to 2000, and implications on the projections for future prevalence. Circulation 2006;114:119–25.

2. Verheugt FW. Novel oral anticoagulants to prevent stroke in atrial fibrillation. Nat Rev Cardiol 2010;7: 149–54.

3. Wolf PA, Abbott RD, Kannel WB. Atrial fibrillation: a major contributor to stroke in the elderly. The Framingham Study. Arch Intern Med 1987;147: 1561–4.

4. European Heart Rhythm Association, European Association for Cardio-Thoracic Surgery, Camm AJ, Kirchhof P, Lip GY, et al. Guidelines for the management of atrial fibrillation: the Task Force for the Management of Atrial Fibrillation of the European Society of Cardiology (ESC). Eur Heart J 2010;31: 2369–429.

5. Caro JJ. An economic model of stroke in atrial fibrillation: the cost of suboptimal oral anticoagulation. Am J Manag Care 2004;10:S451–8 [discussion: S458–61].

6. Lip GY. Does atrial fibrillation confer a hypercoagulable state? Lancet 1995;346:1313–4.

7. Stoddard MF, Dawkins PR, Prince CR, et al. Left atrial appendage thrombus is not uncommon in patients with acute atrial fibrillation and a recent embolic event: a transesophageal echocardiographic study. J Am Coll Cardiol 1995;25:452–9.

8. Di Biase L, Santangeli P, Anselmino M, et al. Does the left atrial appendage morphology correlate with the risk of stroke in patients with atrial fibrillation? Results from a multicenter study. J Am Coll Cardiol 2012;60:531–8.

9. Masawa N, Yoshida Y, Yamada T, et al. Diagnosis of cardiac thrombosis in patients with atrial fibrillation in the absence of macroscopically visible thrombi. Virchows Arch A Pathol Anat Histopathol 1993;422:67–71.

10. Marin F, Roldan V, Climent V, et al. Is thrombogenesis in atrial fibrillation related to matrix metalloproteinase-1 and its inhibitor, TIMP-1? Stroke 2003;34:1181–6.

11. Watson T, Shantsila E, Lip GY. Mechanisms of thrombogenesis in atrial fibrillation: Virchow's triad revisited. Lancet 2009;373:155–66.

12. Di Tullio MR, Sacco RL, Sciacca RR, et al. Left atrial size and the risk of ischemic stroke in an ethnically mixed population. Stroke 1999;30:2019–24.

13. Wang YC, Lin JL, Hwang JJ, et al. Left atrial dysfunction in patients with atrial fibrillation after successful rhythm control for > 3 months. Chest 2005;128:2551–6.

14. Gustafsson C, Blomback M, Britton M, et al. Coagulation factors and the increased risk of stroke in nonvalvular atrial fibrillation. Stroke 1990;21:47–51.

15. Kumagai K, Fukunami M, Ohmori M, et al. Increased intracardiovascular clotting in patients with chronic atrial fibrillation. J Am Coll Cardiol 1990;16:377–80.

16. Lip GY, Lowe GD, Rumley A, et al. Increased markers of thrombogenesis in chronic atrial fibrillation: effects of warfarin treatment. Br Heart J 1995;73:527–33.

17. Lip GY, Rumley A, Dunn FG, et al. Plasma fibrinogen and fibrin D-dimer in patients with atrial fibrillation: effects of cardioversion to sinus rhythm. Int J Cardiol 1995;51:245–51.

18. Asakura H, Hifumi S, Jokaji H, et al. Prothrombin fragment F1 + 2 and thrombin-antithrombin III complex are useful markers of the hypercoagulable state in atrial fibrillation. Blood Coagul Fibrinolysis 1992;3:469–73.

19. Soncini M, Casazza F, Mattioli R, et al. Hypercoagulability and chronic atrial fibrillation: the role of markers of thrombin generation. Minerva Med 1997;88:501–5.

20. Heppell RM, Berkin KE, McLenachan JM, et al. Haemostatic and haemodynamic abnormalities associated with left atrial thrombosis in nonrheumatic atrial fibrillation. Heart 1997;77:407–11.

21. Boos CJ, Anderson RA, Lip GY. Is atrial fibrillation an inflammatory disorder? Eur Heart J 2006;27:136–49.

22. Lip GY, Patel JV, Hughes E, et al. High-sensitivity C-reactive protein and soluble CD40 ligand as indices of inflammation and platelet activation in 880 patients with nonvalvular atrial fibrillation: relationship to stroke risk factors, stroke risk stratification schema, and prognosis. Stroke 2007;38:1229–37.

23. Conway DS, Buggins P, Hughes E, et al. Relationship of interleukin-6 and C-reactive protein to the prothrombotic state in chronic atrial fibrillation. J Am Coll Cardiol 2004;43:2075–82.

24. Fuster V, Ryden LE, Cannom DS, et al. 2011 ACCF/AHA/HRS focused updates incorporated into the ACC/AHA/ESC 2006 guidelines for the management of patients with atrial fibrillation: a report of the American College of Cardiology Foundation/American Heart Association Task Force on practice guidelines. Circulation 2011;123:e269–367.

25. Keogh C, Wallace E, Dillon C, et al. Validation of the CHADS2 clinical prediction rule to predict ischaemic stroke. A systematic review and meta-analysis. Thromb Haemost 2011;106:528–38.

26. Fang MC, Go AS, Chang Y, et al. Comparison of risk stratification schemes to predict thromboembolism in people with nonvalvular atrial fibrillation. J Am Coll Cardiol 2008;51:810–5.

27. Lip GY. Implications of the CHA(2)DS(2)-VASc and HAS-BLED Scores for thromboprophylaxis in atrial fibrillation. Am J Med 2011;124:111–4.

28. Olesen JB, Lip GY, Hansen ML, et al. Validation of risk stratification schemes for predicting stroke and thromboembolism in patients with atrial fibrillation: nationwide cohort study. BMJ 2011;342:d124.

29. Friberg L, Rosenqvist M, Lip GY. Net clinical benefit of warfarin in patients with atrial fibrillation: a report from the Swedish atrial fibrillation cohort study. Circulation 2012;125:2298–307.

30. Lip GY, Nieuwlaat R, Pisters R, et al. Refining clinical risk stratification for predicting stroke and thromboembolism in atrial fibrillation using a novel risk factor-based approach: the Euro Heart Survey on atrial fibrillation. Chest 2010;137:263–72.

31. Gage BF, Yan Y, Milligan PE, et al. Clinical classification schemes for predicting hemorrhage: results from the National Registry of Atrial Fibrillation (NRAF). Am Heart J 2006;151:713–9.

32. Singer DE, Chang Y, Fang MC, et al. The net clinical benefit of warfarin anticoagulation in atrial fibrillation. Ann Intern Med 2009;151:297–305.

33. Fuster V, Chinitz JS. Net clinical benefit of warfarin: extending the reach of antithrombotic therapy for atrial fibrillation. Circulation 2012;125:2285–7.

34. Cairns JA. Stroke prevention in atrial fibrillation trial. Circulation 1991;84:933–5.

35. Albers GW, Sherman DG, Gress DR, et al. Stroke prevention in nonvalvular atrial fibrillation: a review of prospective randomized trials. Ann Neurol 1991;30:511–8.

36. Hart RG, Halperin JL. Atrial fibrillation and thromboembolism: a decade of progress in stroke prevention. Ann Intern Med 1999;131:688–95.

37. Wan Y, Heneghan C, Perera R, et al. Anticoagulation control and prediction of adverse events in patients with atrial fibrillation: a systematic review. Circ Cardiovasc Qual Outcomes 2008;1:84–91.

38. ACTIVE Writing Group of the ACTIVE Investigators, Connolly S, Pogue J, et al. Clopidogrel plus aspirin versus oral anticoagulation for atrial fibrillation in the Atrial fibrillation Clopidogrel Trial with

Irbesartan for prevention of Vascular Events (ACTIVE W): a randomised controlled trial. Lancet 2006;367:1903–12.

39. ACTIVE Investigators, Connolly SJ, Pogue J, et al. Effect of clopidogrel added to aspirin in patients with atrial fibrillation. N Engl J Med 2009;360: 2066–78.

40. Connolly SJ, Ezekowitz MD, Yusuf S, et al. Dabigatran versus warfarin in patients with atrial fibrillation. N Engl J Med 2009;361:1139–51.

41. Patel MR, Mahaffey KW, Garg J, et al. Rivaroxaban versus warfarin in nonvalvular atrial fibrillation. N Engl J Med 2011;365:883–91.

42. Connolly SJ, Eikelboom J, Joyner C, et al. Apixaban in patients with atrial fibrillation. N Engl J Med 2011;364:806–17.

43. Granger CB, Alexander JH, McMurray JJ, et al. Apixaban versus warfarin in patients with atrial fibrillation. N Engl J Med 2011;365:981–92.

44. Calkins H, Kuck KH, Cappato R, et al. 2012 HRS/EHRA/ECAS Expert Consensus Statement on Catheter and Surgical Ablation of Atrial Fibrillation: recommendations for patient selection, procedural techniques, patient management and follow-up, definitions, endpoints, and research trial design. Europace 2012;14:528–606.

45. Carlsson J, Miketic S, Windeler J, et al. Randomized trial of rate-control versus rhythm-control in persistent atrial fibrillation: the Strategies of Treatment of Atrial Fibrillation (STAF) study. J Am Coll Cardiol 2003;41:1690–6.

46. Wyse DG, Waldo AL, DiMarco JP, et al. A comparison of rate control and rhythm control in patients with atrial fibrillation. N Engl J Med 2002;347:1825–33.

47. Dorian P, Jung W, Newman D, et al. The impairment of health-related quality of life in patients with intermittent atrial fibrillation: implications for the assessment of investigational therapy. J Am Coll Cardiol 2000;36:1303–9.

48. Corley SD, Epstein AE, DiMarco JP, et al. Relationships between sinus rhythm, treatment, and survival in the Atrial Fibrillation Follow-Up Investigation of Rhythm Management (AFFIRM) Study. Circulation 2004;109:1509–13.

49. Wazni OM, Marrouche NF, Martin DO, et al. Radiofrequency ablation vs antiarrhythmic drugs as first-line treatment of symptomatic atrial fibrillation: a randomized trial. JAMA 2005;293:2634–40.

50. Wilber DJ, Pappone C, Neuzil P, et al. Comparison of antiarrhythmic drug therapy and radiofrequency catheter ablation in patients with paroxysmal atrial fibrillation: a randomized controlled trial. JAMA 2010;303:333–40.

51. Pappone C, Augello G, Sala S, et al. A randomized trial of circumferential pulmonary vein ablation versus antiarrhythmic drug therapy in paroxysmal atrial fibrillation: the APAF Study. J Am Coll Cardiol 2006;48:2340–7.

52. Jais P, Cauchemez B, Macle L, et al. Catheter ablation versus antiarrhythmic drugs for atrial fibrillation: the A4 study. Circulation 2008;118:2498–505.

53. Oral H, Chugh A, Ozaydin M, et al. Risk of thromboembolic events after percutaneous left atrial radiofrequency ablation of atrial fibrillation. Circulation 2006;114:759–65.

54. Nademanee K, Schwab MC, Kosar EM, et al. Clinical outcomes of catheter substrate ablation for high-risk patients with atrial fibrillation. J Am Coll Cardiol 2008;51:843–9.

55. Bunch TJ, Crandall BG, Weiss JP, et al. Warfarin is not needed in low-risk patients following atrial fibrillation ablation procedures. J Cardiovasc Electrophysiol 2009;20:988–93.

56. Hunter RJ, McCready J, Diab I, et al. Maintenance of sinus rhythm with an ablation strategy in patients with atrial fibrillation is associated with a lower risk of stroke and death. Heart 2012;98:48–53.

57. Saad EB, d'Avila A, Costa IP, et al. Very low risk of thromboembolic events in patients undergoing successful catheter ablation of atrial fibrillation with a CHADS2 score </=3: a long-term outcome study. Circ Arrhythm Electrophysiol 2011;4:615–21.

58. Lin YJ, Chao TF, Tsao HM, et al. Successful catheter ablation reduces the risk of cardiovascular events in atrial fibrillation patients with CHA2DS2-VASc risk score of 1 and higher. Europace 2013; 15:676–84.

59. Themistoclakis S, Corrado A, Marchlinski FE, et al. The risk of thromboembolism and need for oral anticoagulation after successful atrial fibrillation ablation. J Am Coll Cardiol 2010;55:735–43.

60. Camm AJ, Lip GY, De Caterina R, et al. 2012 focused update of the ESC Guidelines for the management of atrial fibrillation: an update of the 2010 ESC Guidelines for the management of atrial fibrillation. Developed with the special contribution of the European Heart Rhythm Association. Eur Heart J 2012;33:2719–47.

61. Chinitz JS, Castellano JM, Kovacic JC, et al. Atrial fibrillation, stroke, and quality of life. Ann N Y Acad Sci 2012;1254:140–50.

The Role of Cardiac Imaging in Stroke Prevention

Francesco Santoro, MD[a], Luigi Di Biase, MD, PhD[a,b,c,d],
Pasquale Santangeli, MD[a,b], Riccardo Ieva, MD[a],
J. David Burkhardt, MD[b],
Andrea Natale, MD, FACC, FHRS[b,d,e,f,g,h],*

KEYWORDS

- Stroke prevention • Imaging • Atrial fibrillation • Thrombi • Left atrial appendage closure device
- Left ventricular dysfunction • Valve disease

KEY POINTS

- CHADS2 and CHA2DS2-VASc scores are the cornerstone of the management of anticoagulation therapy in patients with atrial fibrillation (AF), but moderate-risk or low-risk patients need a different stratification, in which instance cardiac imaging can be useful.
- Imaging tools available for AF management include transthoracic echocardiography (TTE), which identifies conditions that predispose patients to AF or its progression, and transesophageal echocardiography (TEE), which can detect left atrium or left atrial appendage (LAA) thrombi and their resolution, and evaluate valve disease.
- Cardiac computed tomography and magnetic resonance imaging (MRI) can both add further information about the LAA, such as size and morphology.
- Imaging tools, chiefly TEE, are useful for anatomic screening, device implantation guidance, and follow-up surveillance in LAA closure.
- Left ventricular systolic dysfunction, especially during acute myocardial infarction with segmental wall immobility, but also in chronic disease, could lead to formation of left ventricular thrombus. Early recognition through echocardiographic evaluation (TTE or TEE) or MRI can be useful.
- Potential links have been found between patients with a previous history of stroke/transient ischemic attack and native valve disease (especially with rheumatic mitral valve disease). Echocardiography through TEE or TTE is currently the best tool with which to study and identify valve abnormalities.

INTRODUCTION

Stroke is a global health problem, affecting 15 million individuals worldwide annually, of whom 5 million die and 5 million become permanently disabled.[1] Two recent systematic and comprehensive reviews of a large volume of data showed that the incidence rate of stroke has decreased by

The authors have nothing to disclose.

[a] Department of Cardiology, University of Foggia, viale L Pinto, 1, 71100, Foggia, Italy; [b] Texas Cardiac Arrhythmia Institute, Heart & Vascular Department, St. David's Medical Center, 3000 N. IH 35 Suite 720, 78705, Austin, TX, USA; [c] Division of Cardiology and Montefiore-Einstein Center for Heart and Vascular Care, Montefiore Medical Center, Albert Einstein College of Medicine, 111 East 210th Street, 10467, Bronx, New York, NY, USA; [d] Department of Biomedical Engineering, Cockrell School of Engineering, The University of Texas at Austin, 107 W. Dean Keeton, BME Building, 78712, Austin, TX, USA; [e] EP Services, California Pacific Medical Center, 2100 Webster Street, 94115, San Francisco, CA, USA; [f] Division of Cardiology, Stanford Arrhythmia Service, Stanford University, 300 Pasteur Drive, 94305, Stanford, CA, USA; [g] Division of Cardiovascular Medicine, Case Western Reserve University, University Hospitals of Cleveland, 11100 Euclid Avenue, 44106-5038 Cleveland, OH, USA; [h] Interventional Electrophysiology, Department of Cardiology, Scripps Clinic, 10666 N Torrey Pines Road, 92037, La Jolla, CA, USA

* Corresponding author. North I-35, Suite 720, Austin, TX 78705.

E-mail address: dr.natale@gmail.com

Card Electrophysiol Clin 6 (2014) 17–29
http://dx.doi.org/10.1016/j.ccep.2013.11.004
1877-9182/14/$ – see front matter © 2014 Elsevier Inc. All rights reserved

42% in high-income countries in the past 4 decades, thanks to appropriate prevention, but has increased by more than 100% in low-income and middle-income countries in the same time period.[2,3]

Patients who survive a previous minor stroke or transient ischemic attack (TIA) are at an increased risk of subsequent vascular events and stroke.[4] The rate of recurrent stroke after the initial one is estimated at 3% to 10% in 30 days, 5% to 14% in 1 year, and 20% to 40% in 5 years.[5] In comparison with the initial episode, the recurrent stroke tends to be more severe.[6] Therefore, prevention of secondary stroke is of paramount clinical and economic importance.[7] The major secondary measures of stroke prevention, as manifested in the most recent American Heart Association (AHA)/American Stroke Association guidelines,[8] include the control of modifiable risk factors (eg, hypertension, diabetes, cigarette smoking, alcohol consumption, unhealthy dietary habits, and obesity), drug intervention for atherosclerotic disease, antithrombotic treatments for cardioembolism, and the use of antiplatelet agents for noncardioembolic stroke.

There are several links between heart disease and stroke. Twenty percent of ischemic strokes are caused by cardiogenic cerebral embolism. The main sources of emboli are the left atrium (LA) and the left atrial appendage (LAA) during AF, acute or chronic left ventricular (LV) dysfunction, native valve disease, the presence of prosthetic valves (mitral and aortic), and, probably, complex aortic plaques. There is a history of nonvalvular AF in about one-half of cases, valvular heart disease in one-fourth, and LV mural thrombus in almost one-third.[9]

Cardiac imaging might help to stratify a patient's risk and provide appropriate treatment.

ATRIAL FIBRILLATION AND ASSESSMENT OF LEFT ATRIAL FUNCTION

Stroke is the most serious complication of AF, and occurs in 5% of non-anticoagulated patients every year. The risk of stroke in patients with AF increases substantially with age, from 1.5% in individuals aged 50 to 59 years to 23,5% for those aged 80 to 89 years.[10] In addition, AF-associated strokes confer the worst outcomes.[11] Moreover, 15% of patients with AF suffer silent cerebral infarcts,[12] the implications of which are not known, but which likely could be responsible for dementia and Alzheimer disease.

Stroke prevention in patients with AF is based on the use of anticoagulation with warfarin, which reduces the risk of stroke by 60%,[13] and more recently on the use of novel anticoagulants,[14] such as the direct thrombin inhibitor dabigatran[15] or the selective factor Xa inhibitors apixaban and rivaroxaban.

Two clinical scores (CHADS2[16] and CHA2DS2-VASc[17]) constitute the cornerstone of the management of anticoagulation therapy in AF patients. CHADS2 is an acronym for Congestive heart failure, Hypertension, Age older than 75, Diabetes mellitus, and prior Stroke. Each of these risk factors counts as 1 point except for history of stroke, which counts as 2 points. Patients with a score of 2 or higher have to be treated with oral anticoagulation therapy (OAC) while those with a score of 1 can be treated with aspirin or OAC. CHA2DS2-Vasc represents an evolution of the previous score by the inclusion additional "stroke risk modifier" factors. These additional risk factors, counting 1 point, include age 65 to 74, female gender, and vascular disease (previous myocardial infarction [MI], peripheral arterial disease, or aortic plaque); furthermore, "age 75 and above" also has extra weight, with 2 points. The therapeutic approach is the same as for CHADS2, considering 2 points as the cutoff for starting OAC while patients with 1 point can be treated with aspirin or OAC.

These scores are useful for defining AF high-risk patients for stroke, but moderate-risk or low-risk patients need a different stratification, for which cardiac imaging can be useful (**Table 1**).

Transthoracic Echocardiography

Transthoracic echocardiography (TTE) identifies conditions that predispose patients to AF (mitral valve disease [stenosis or insufficiency] and LV systolic dysfunction) or its progression as LA size or volume. This information can influence the subsequent management strategies; For example, increased LA volume is associated with a low probability of successful cardioversion for chronic AF and/or maintenance of normal sinus rhythm[18,19] and with AF recurrence after catheter ablation.[20] TTE should be performed in the emergency room in patients with AF to assess for signs of acute heart failure, compromised LV function and valvular function, and right ventricular pressure. TTE can provide useful information to guide clinical decision making, but cannot be used to exclude thrombus in the LAA.

Transesophageal Echocardiography

Transesophageal echocardiography (TEE) is probably the most useful imaging tool in the context of stroke prevention in AF patients. TEE can detect LA or LAA thrombi, and their resolution, with high sensitivity and specificity.[21] It can also provide accurate information about the LAA (such as its

Table 1
Imaging tools to predict stroke in patients with atrial fibrillation

TTE	TEE	CCT, MRI
Evaluation of LA size/volume	Detection of LA thrombus, sludge Spontaneous echo contrast	Accurate detection of LAA thrombi (through CCT)
Study of native valvular disease	Evaluation of LAA emptying velocity	Recognition of LAA morphology
Identification of depressed LV function	Detection of complex aortic plaques on descending aorta	Quantification of LA fibrosis (through MRI)
	Complete study of natural valve disease (stenosis or insufficiency)	

Abbreviations: CCT, cardiac computed tomography; LA, left atrium; LAA, left atrial appendage; MRI, magnetic resonance imaging; TEE, transesophageal echocardiography; TTE, transthoracic echocardiography.

emptying velocity) and identify native valve disease or complex aortic plaques in the descending aorta (**Figs. 1–3**).

Blood stasis in the LA is clearly shown by TEE, and ranges from spontaneous echo contrast (SEC) to sludge. SEC is defined as dynamic smoke-like echoes, with the characteristic swirling motion with optimal gain setting during the cardiac cycle.[22] It reflects a low flow state, increased erythrocyte aggregation, and the presence of fibrinogen. SEC is considered to predict thrombus formation, and in fact its presence is associated with an increased thromboembolic risk.[23] A recent study reported that SEC in chronic AF is associated with a poor atrial substrate and lesser sinus rhythm maintenance after catheter ablation.[24] Sludge is a dynamic gelatinous, precipitous echodensity, without a discrete mass, present throughout the cardiac cycle in the LA or LAA. Sludge represents thrombus in situ that is a stage farther along the continuum toward thrombus formation. Moreover, increasing grades of SEC are associated with

decreasing LAA blood velocity, highlighting the relation of LAA dysfunction to thrombus formation.[25] Anticoagulation cannot reverse this phenomenon because it does not change the underlying hemodynamic abnormalities.[22]

The combination of blood stasis, hypercoagulability, and endocardial function of the atria, often referred to as Virchow's triad, is a prerequisite for in vivo thrombus formation.[26] LA thrombus is composed of fibrin, red blood cells, and platelets. It represents the major source of cardioembolic stroke and has to be carefully monitored in AF patients. The presence of thrombus on TEE is associated with a poor outcome and with a risk of embolism and death, respectively, of up to 10.4% and 15.8% per year, even in patients receiving OAC.[27] TEE has a high sensitivity for thrombus detection, but can still miss thrombi 2 mm or smaller. In this context 3-dimensional (3D) TEE has not showed a clear superiority to 2-dimensional (2D) TEE, but may help to not misdiagnose pectinate musculature as thrombus.[28] Different imaging techniques for thrombus detection are discussed in this section.

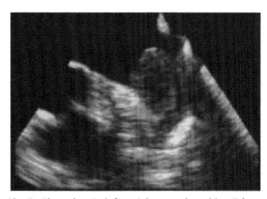

Fig. 1. Left atrial appendage, bilobed (detail from transesophageal echocardiography [TEE] 4-chamber view).

Fig. 2. Thrombus in left atrial appendage (detail from TEE 4-chamber view).

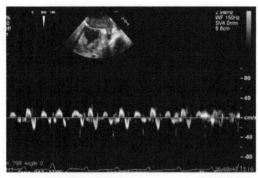

Fig. 3. Evaluation of low emptying velocities (about 20 mm/s) in left atrial appendage in a patient with atrial flutter (TEE 4-chamber view).

In AF patients without thrombus, the LAA passively empties with multiple small contractions that do not contribute to LV filling. The TEE, by evaluating the LAA emptying velocities, with pulsed-wave Doppler signal in this area, can also assess the mechanical function of the LAA. Low emptying velocities ($\leq$20 cm/s) correlate strongly with the presence of SEC and thrombus formation.[29] By contrast the LAA, during sinus rhythm, is a highly contractile muscular sac that obliterates its apex during the atrial systole with a characteristic pattern of emptying and a well-defined, pulsed-wave Doppler signal.[30] In the authors' clinical experience, TEE is performed 6 months after AF ablation to assess the contraction and flow velocity of the LAA. Only in cases with adequate LAA flow velocity is OAC discontinued. Emptying velocity higher than 40 cm/s is the cutoff for eventual suspension of OAC therapy.[31] In addition to an adequate LAA flow, the authors also confirm the presence of a consistent A wave as one of the two criteria for OAC discontinuation.

The assessment of LAA function is evaluated through its emptying velocities with pulsed-wave Doppler signal. Several imitations to this methodology should be considered. Age is an important risk factor; older patients have lower LAA emptying velocities.[32] Indeed in young patients, but not in the elderly, emptying velocities represent a risk factor for stroke.[33] Moreover, in patients with paroxysmal AF, during sinus rhythm the LAA may be stunned with low emptying velocity, introducing a determinant confounding factor. This LAA stunning has been observed and studied after AF electrical cardioversion,[34] and is typically related to AF duration.[35]

As shown in the SPAF III (Stroke Prevention in Atrial Fibrillation) trial,[36] the TEE is also useful to detect complex aortic plaques in the descending aorta, which are also associated with an increased thromboembolic risk. Indeed, with the introduction of CHA2DS2-Vasc score, aortic plaques were included in the group of vascular diseases that increase thromboembolic risk. This finding shows that stroke has multifactorial causes, especially in elderly patients with AF.

Puwanant and colleagues[37] clarified the appropriate indications for TEE. On comparing the findings of TEE in AF patients with the CHADS2 score, they discovered that the prevalence of LA/LAA thrombus/sludge significantly increased with an increasing CHADS2 score, and with a left ventricular ejection fraction (LVEF) of 35% or less or a history of congestive heart failure. These investigators stated that under these conditions TEE is needed to assess stroke risk, whereas it does not provide useful information in patients with a CHADS2 score of 0 when the therapeutic anticoagulation has been maintained.

Computed Tomography and Magnetic Resonance Imaging

Computed tomography (CT) and magnetic resonance imaging (MRI) have been used to provide the 3D anatomy before AF catheter ablation and to detect postprocedural complications. As their routine use has increased, further insights have been added. Cardiac computed tomography (CCT) provides accurate means to detect and exclude LAA thrombus with sensitivity and specificity of 96% and 92%, respectively,[38] implying that there is still a false-positive rate of 8%. Recently Sawit and colleagues[39] showed that delayed CCT at 1 minute improved the specificity (100%) and positive predictive value (100%) of CCT for detection of LAA thrombus in comparison with TEE. CCT is also able to differentiate thrombus from pseudothrombus, because these appear as filling defects on initial CCT.

CCT and MRI can both add further information about the LAA regarding its size and morphology. LAA size is associated with increased thromboembolic risk, especially in patients with nonvalvular AF.[40,41] A recent study by Di Biase and colleagues[42] investigated the relationship between LAA morphology and the risk of stroke. Patients with chicken-wing LAA morphology (48% of their population) were less likely to have an embolic event even after being controlled for comorbidities and CHADS2 score. This finding was confirmed by comparison with the remaining population. Compared with chicken-wing LAA, patients with cactus LAA were 4.08 times, windsock LAA 4.5 times, and cauliflower LAA 8.0 times more likely to have had a stroke/TIA. These data were subsequently confirmed by Kimura and colleagues[43] who emphasized that cauliflower LAA was significantly more common in patients with stroke.

Daccarett and colleagues[44] found that AF patients who have suffered an ischemic stroke have significantly higher levels of LA fibrosis as quantified by delayed-enhancement MRI. These investigators suggested that LA fibrosis, a variable of structural atrial remodeling, could be a valuable tool for clinicians to use in conjunction with the CHADS2 score. However, reliable detection of LA fibrosis by MRI has yet to be confirmed.

CARDIOVASCULAR RISK FACTORS AND STROKE RISK

Two studies, the Atrial Fibrillation Follow-up Investigation of Rhythm Management study[45] and the Rate Control versus Electrical Cardioversion for Persistent Atrial Fibrillation Study,[46] demonstrated that patients in the rhythm control group were still at risk for embolic events, especially those who withdrew from anticoagulation therapy or had inadequate anticoagulation. These findings imply that several stroke risk factors persisted in these patients even though they had good rhythm control. It is desirable to identify such patients who are particularly at risk.

Some cardiovascular risk factors, such as hypertension and diabetes, are well-known independent stroke risk factors,[47,48] but can also have a role in both LA and LAA dysfunction.

Diabetes has been proved to confer biochemical and histologic abnormalities to LA myocardial tissue as a result of persistent oxidative stress.[49] Moreover, several animal studies have shown that chronic hypertension is associated with significant atrial electrical and structural remodeling, and development of atrial fibrosis with the presence of slow atrial conduction areas.[50,51]

The study of LA and LAA function through imaging techniques, combined with the knowledge of these risk factors, can provide a body of information with which to stratify a patient's stroke risk.

LA function can be evaluated in several ways, one of the most important of which is 2D echocardiography through speckle tracking, which facilitates comprehensive evaluation of LA contractile, reservoir, and conduit function. Early changes of LA dynamics can be present in patients with cardiovascular risk factors. Mondillo and colleagues[52] showed that in patients with hypertension and/or diabetes and normal LA size, LA deformation dynamics are impaired, especially when these 2 risk factors are combined. LA strain may precede changes in traditional 2D measures of LA function, and can be used as a predictor of AF recurrence after catheter ablation.[53]

Another echocardiographic parameter, whose changes can appear later than those found with 2D speckle tracking, is LA volume. This parameter may be a more sensitive index of LA remodeling than LA dimension, and may be a prognostic marker.[54,55] LA volume is strictly related to the severity of LV diastolic dysfunction, and provides an index of cardiovascular risk and disease burden.[56] A larger LA volume was also associated with a higher risk of AF in older patients.[57]

LAA function, evaluated through its emptying velocities with pulsed-wave Doppler signal during TEE, could also be impaired in patients with cardiovascular risk factors. Bilge and colleagues,[58] studying LAA function in 66 patients (40–55 years old) in sinus rhythm with or without hypertension, found that patients with untreated hypertension had an impairment of LAA function, caused by marked elevation of afterload imposed on the LA. Similarly diabetes, by causing an increase in peripheral vascular resistance, can have the same effect on LAA function.[30]

Poor LAA contraction and LAA dilation is associated with LAA thrombus formation in both sinus rhythm and AF.[30] An early recognition of low LAA emptying velocities without LAA dilation can be useful for risk stratification. Indeed, low LAA wall velocity is an independent predictor for long-term recurrence of cerebrovascular events.[59]

When at least 3 clinical risk factors are present (age $\geq$65 years, hypertension, diabetes mellitus, coronary artery disease, and prior stroke or TIA), there is a higher prevalence of lower LAA peak emptying velocity and LAA thrombus.[60] Furthermore, Illien and colleagues[61] reported in a population of 301 patients with AF that a history of hypertension, diabetes, age 65 years or older, and LVEF 45% or less were all significantly related to the TEE finding of a thrombogenic milieu, including presence of dense SEC and/or LAA peak emptying velocity of 25 cm/s or less.

Cardiovascular risk factors, combined or alone, when causing an impairment of LA and LAA function, can increase the risk of stroke. An early recognition of these changes through cardiac imaging could be crucial for timely prevention.

LEFT VENTRICULAR DYSFUNCTION

Several conditions, transient or chronic, are related to LV dysfunction such as MI and dilated cardiomyopathy. Global or segmental (especially apical) wall immobility could lead to LV thrombus formation and following cardioembolic stroke.

Myocardial Infarction

Within the first 2 weeks after anterior MI, without acute reperfusion therapy intracardiac thrombus occurs in about one-third of patients and in even more patients in the presence of a large infarct involving the LV apex.[62,63] In fact, anterior wall MI carries a higher risk for stroke than inferior wall MI (25% vs 5%). In the absence of anticoagulant therapy, clinically evident cerebral infarction occurs in approximately 10% of patients with LV thrombus following MI.[8]

TTE can easily detect LV wall and apical thrombi. If the patient does not offer an optimal transthoracic view, TEE is preferred. Several studies have echocardiographically detected LV thrombi and cerebral embolism during acute MI.[64,65] MRI is another potential imaging option, with higher sensitivity and specificity,[66] but its use in the acute phase is still debated. In all of these cases, oral or subcutaneous anticoagulation therapy is required. Patients with ischemic stroke or TIA in the setting of acute MI complicated by LV mural thrombus formation identified by echocardiography or other cardiac imaging techniques should be treated with OAC for at least 3 months.[8]

Another condition, mimicking MI, is takotsubo cardiomyopathy, an acute and reversible LV dysfunction characterized by basal hyperkinesis and apical ballooning. The reduced blood flow in the LV apex can predispose to LV thrombus, which occurs in nearly 2.5% of cases.[67]

Cardiomyopathies with Reduced Left Ventricular Ejection Fraction

The role of LVEF in stroke prevention is still not clear, although approximately 10% of patients with ischemic stroke have an LVEF lower than 30%.[68] The risk of stroke increases almost 3-fold by 5 years, especially if heart failure occurs.[69] As shown by the Survival and Ventricular Enlargement (SAVE) trial, the risk of stroke increases by 18% for every decrease of 5% in LVEF, and doubles when LVEF decreases from 35% to 28%.[70] Georgiadis and colleagues[71] reported that cerebrovascular reactivity is impaired and decreases linearly with decreasing LVEF; in fact, reduced regional cerebral blood flow seen in patients who had heart failure could be a stroke-predisposing factor.[72]

High-risk patients with low LVEF require a follow-up including cardiac imaging. Routine TTE without contrast can yield misleading results concerning LV thrombus, but has high sensitivity and specificity when a large protuberant thrombus is present (**Fig. 4**). TEE performance, when the

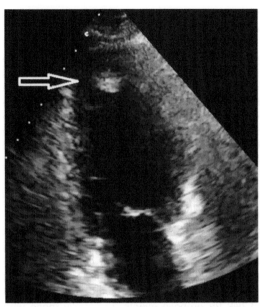

Fig. 4. Evidence of thrombus (*arrow*) in the apex of left ventricle during acute myocardial infarction (transthoracic echocardiography [TTE] 2-chamber view).

clinical indication is specifically for LV thrombus assessment, is an appropriate tool,[73] but delayed MRI has higher sensitivity in the detection of small and/or mural LV thrombi.[74]

When the detection of LV thrombus might influence treatment, clinicians should not rely on suboptimal TTE, and other imaging tests such as MRI should be considered. TTE and MRI could play complementary roles in further defining both the incidence and embolic potential of LV thrombi.[75]

Even if the importance of long-term anticoagulation therapy in patients with systolic dysfunction (LVEF <35%) and/or with a previous history of LV thrombus is not clear, prophylactic anticoagulation should be considered, especially if systolic dysfunction is combined with the presence of other comorbidities (ie, CHA2DS2-Vasc score risk factors).

VALVE EVALUATION
Native Valvular Heart Disease

Potential links have been found between patients with a previous history of stroke/TIA and native valve disease. Echocardiography is currently the best tool for studying and identifying this through TEE or TTE. According to the 2011 AHA Stroke Guidelines, patients with prior stroke/TIA and valve disease may require anticoagulation or antiplatelet therapy.[8] All possible valve diseases and their related risk for stroke are described in this section (**Table 2**).

Rheumatic mitral valve disease

Rheumatic mitral valve disease is the result of damage to the heart valves after repeated episodes of acute rheumatic fever. The valves become stretched and scarred and do not move normally, resulting in regurgitation and/or stenosis.[76] TTE is essential to confirm the diagnosis and monitor the heart valves to detect any progression of disease (**Figs. 5** and **6**).[77] The most common findings are pure mitral regurgitation (MR), followed by MR plus aortic regurgitation or MR plus mitral stenosis. On echocardiographic examination mitral valve leaflets in these patients are significantly thickened compared with normal leaflets.[78] These patients present with severe heart failure, pulmonary hypertension, and/or AF.

Rheumatic heart disease (RHD) represents pathologic features with a high risk for stroke. In patients with RHD and a history of stroke, the rate of recurrent embolism ranges from 30% to 65%.[79] Between 60% and 65% of these recurrences develop within the first year, most within 6 months of a prior stroke/TIA.[80,81] Long-term anticoagulant therapy can effectively reduce the risk of systemic embolism in these patients.[82] OAC therapy is reasonable in patients with prior stroke and rheumatic valve disease.[8]

Mitral annular calcification

Mitral annular calcification (MAC) is a common finding on echocardiographic examination. Calcification within the mitral annulus results from a degenerative process in the cardiovascular fibrous skeleton, which is reported to be accelerated by advanced age, systemic hypertension, hypercholesterolemia, diabetes mellitus, and chronic renal

failure,[83] and in young adults following radiotherapy.[84] The relative frequencies of calcific and thrombotic embolism are unknown,[85] but some data suggest that spicules of fibrocalcific material may embolize from the calcified mitral annulus.[86] In a variant of MAC known as caseous calcification, the rate of stroke events was 7% (**Fig. 7**).[87] Karas and colleagues[88] found that on TEE, MAC was significantly associated with proximal and distal complex aortic atheroma for evaluation of cerebral ischemia. These data confirm that MAC could be a predictor of stroke. Antiplatelet therapy may be considered in patients with prior stroke and MAC.

Aortic valve disease

Clinically symptomatic cerebral embolic events are uncommon in calcific aortic valve disease,[89] unless concomitant mitral valve disease, AF, or reduced LVEF are present. No randomized trials of selected patients with stroke and aortic valve disease exist, so recommendations are based on the evidence from larger antiplatelet trials of patients with stroke and TIA. Antiplatelet therapy may be reasonable in patients with ischemic stroke or TIA, and with native aortic valve disease even without AF.[8]

Strands

Strands are filiform fronds that occur at sites of valvular closure and can be detected by TEE. Strands originate as small thrombi on endocardial surfaces where the valve margins make contact, caused by wear and tear.[90] Several studies have associated them with stroke. Lee and colleagues[91] reported that 11 of 50 patients with presumed cerebral embolic events had filamentous strands on the mitral valve. Freedberg and colleagues[92] found that 10.6% of the patients with

Table 2		
Features of valve disease to evaluate during routine echocardiography in patients with previous history of stroke/transient ischemic attack, and correlation with therapy		
	Echocardiographic Features	**Therapeutic Approach**
Rheumatic valve disease	Mitral valve leaflets thickened compared with normal associated to moderate-severe stenosis and/or insufficiency	Anticoagulation is reasonable
Mitral annular calcification	Hyperechogenic area all over the mitral annulus	Antiplatelet therapy may be considered
Aortic calcification	Hyperechogenic area on the leaflets of the valve	Antiplatelet therapy may be reasonable
Strands	Filiform fronds that occur at sites of valvular closure	No trials showed benefits for antithrombotic or anticoagulation therapy

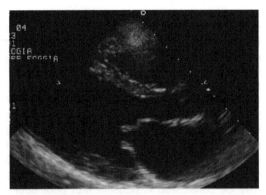

Fig. 5. Rheumatic mitral valve disease. Both anterior and posterior leaflets appear stretched and scarred (TTE parasternal long-axis view).

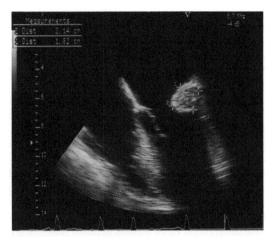

Fig. 7. Caseous calcification of the posterior mitral leaflet (TEE 4-chamber view).

embolic events had strands compared with 2.3% in those without such events. Tice and colleagues[93] reported that mitral valve strands were found in 6.3% of those undergoing TEE as a result of a recent cerebral ischemic event, compared with the 0.3% prevalence in patients referred for other indications. A randomized study that evaluated efficacy of antithrombotic therapies for stroke prevention failed to support an advantage of warfarin or aspirin for this purpose.[94]

Prosthetic Heart Valves

Patients with a mechanical prosthetic valve are at high risk for stroke and require treatment with oral anticoagulants.[95] Bioprosthetic valves, on the other hand, are associated with a lower rate of thromboembolism. In patients with bioprosthetic valves who have an otherwise unexplained ischemic stroke or TIA, OAC is suggested.[8]

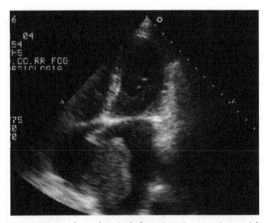

Fig. 6. Giant thrombus in left atrium in a patient with a severe mitral stenosis following rheumatic valve disease (TTE 4-chamber view).

CATHETER-BASED LEFT ATRIAL APPENDAGE OCCLUSION PROCEDURE: ROLE OF IMAGING

Different therapeutic approaches are currently being developed for stroke prevention in nonvalvular AF. The aim of these novel technologies is to offer an alternative to anticoagulation therapy in patients with a relative or absolute contraindication.

Isolation of the LAA from the body of the LA might reduce the risk of embolic events, and may be a treatment option for those patients who are not candidates for anticoagulation treatment.[96,97] There are several techniques for LAA closure: surgical, percutaneous, and, most recently, endoepicardial. Surgical LAA ligation or amputation might be considered in those patients undergoing mitral valve surgery or as an adjunct to a surgical maze procedure for the treatment of AF.[98]

Using a percutaneous approach, 3 devices have been developed: the WATCHMAN LAA system, the Amplatzer Cardiac Plug, and the WaveCrest device. These devices are delivered via a transseptal puncture approach generally under transesophageal and/or intracardiac echocardiographic guidance. The WATCHMAN device is the only one that has been proved not to be inferior to conventional warfarin therapy when comparing the primary efficacy end point of strokes (ischemic and hemorrhagic), cardiovascular or unexplained death, and systemic embolism.[99]

There is only one device for LAA closure using an endoepicardial approach, called the LARIAT. This system consists in snaring the LAA with an epicardial device, correctly positioned through connection of the epicardial and endocardial magnet-tipped guide wires.[100]

Except for surgical closure based on direct LAA visualization, the role of imaging in these novel techniques is crucial. Percutaneous LAA obliteration procedures rely heavily on TEE for anatomic screening, device implantation guidance, and follow-up surveillance. The Endoepicardial approach is based on a previous CCT to screen patients and assess the LAA morphology, size, and position, and TEE is used to exclude the presence of thrombus before the procedure, then to confirm closure at the end and during the follow-up.

For percutaneous devices, multiplanar TEE assessment is currently the main modality used to screen suitable candidates for device closure of the LAA. The main echocardiographic exclusion criterion is the presence of thrombus in the LAA. TEE is also used to assess the LAA morphology, ostial dimension, and maximum length of the dominant lobe to provide a series of baseline measurements for procedural planning. An assessment of the ostial dimensions of the LAA is performed to provisionally determine the size of the device required. Typically a device with a diameter larger than the LAA ostium is chosen to ensure sufficient anchoring for stable positioning. Device sizing is crucial to ensure device stability and optimum sealing of the LAA ostium, and to minimize the risk of leakage, which could provide a new source of future thromboembolism. The use of 3D TEE provides useful additive information with which to accurately define LAA orifice dimensions.[101]

During the procedures of both percutaneous or endoepicardial approaches, TEE and intracardiac echocardiography can be used in guiding the transseptal puncture, verifying the position of the delivery sheath, and aiding delivery and deployment of the device at the LAA ostium. To verify a correct positioning, the axis of the device has to be in alignment with the major axis of the LAA and no leaks must be detected at color-flow Doppler. A complete seal of the LAA orifice must be confirmed before release. The success of LAA occlusion can be determined periprocedurally using angiography and echocardiography.[102] A residual mild leak, between 1 and 3 mm diameter jet (through TEE), is considered an acceptable end point when assessing sealing of the percutaneous device.[103] This value is less than 1 mm diameter jet for the endoepicardial closure device. The same parameters can also be used to assess the success of occlusion at follow-up. Finally, screening at the end of the procedure and at discharge for any procedural complications, such as pericardial effusion, thrombus associated with implantation, or device migration or embolization (ie, with the first-generation WATCHMAN system[104]) should be performed.

Postprocedure echocardiographic follow-up is recommended at 1 month, 6 months, and annually, preferably with TEE. The main items to assess are: stability of the device, presence of thrombus. evidence of leak, and transmitral and pulmonary vein (PV) flow (particularly left upper PV).

SUMMARY

Cardiac imaging can provide several insights into stroke prevention. It can identify high-risk AF patients with low or moderate stroke risk according to CHADS2 and CHA2DS2-Vasc score. Cardiac imaging can be useful to show the presence of thrombi in transient or chronic LV dysfunction, in evaluating natural valve disease, and in handling new LAA closure devices. All of this information can help to provide the best management for patients, avoiding a catastrophic complication such as stroke.

REFERENCES

1. World Health Organization. Global burden of stroke. Available at: http://www.who.int/healthinfo/statistics/bod_cerebrovasculardiseasestroke.pdf.
2. Feigin VL, Lawes CM, Bennett DA, et al. Worldwide stroke incidence and early case fatality reported in 56 population-based studies: a systematic review. Lancet Neurol 2009;8:355–69.
3. Johnston SC, Mendis S, Mathers CD. Global variation in stroke burden and mortality: estimates from monitoring, surveillance, and modelling. Lancet Neurol 2009;8:345–54.
4. Talelli P, Greenwood RJ. Recurrent stroke: where do we stand with the secondary prevention of non-cardioembolic ischaemic strokes? Ther Adv Cardiovasc Dis 2008;2:387–405.
5. Petty GW, Brown RD Jr, Whisnant JP, et al. Survival and recurrence after first cerebral infarction: a population-based study in Rochester, Minnesota, 1975 through 1989. Neurology 1998;50:208–16.
6. Hardie K, Hankey GJ, Jamrozik K, et al. Ten-year risk of first recurrent stroke and disability after first-ever stroke in the Perth Community Stroke Study. Stroke 2004;35:731–5.
7. Phillips RA. A review of therapeutic strategies for risk reduction of recurrent stroke. Prog Cardiovasc Dis 2008;50:264–73.
8. Furie KL, Kasner SE, Adams RJ, et al. Guidelines for the prevention of stroke in patients with stroke or transient ischemic attack: a guideline for healthcare professionals from the American Heart Association/American Stroke Association. Stroke 2011;42:227–76.
9. Cardiogenic brain embolism: the second report of the Cerebral Embolism Task Force. Arch Neurol 1989;46:727–43.

10. Lin HJ, Wolf PA, Kelly-Hayes M, et al. Stroke severity in atrial fibrillation. The Framingham Study. Stroke 1996;27:1760–4.

11. Whitlock RP, Healey JS, Connolly SJ. Left atrial appendage occlusion does not eliminate the need for warfarin. Circulation 2009;120:1927–32.

12. Stewart S, Hart CL, Hole DJ, et al. Population prevalence, incidence, and predictors of atrial fibrillation in the Renfrew/Paisley study. Heart 2001;86:516–21.

13. Hart RG, Pearce LA, Aguilar MI. Meta-analysis: antithrombotic therapy to prevent stroke in patients who have nonvalvular atrial fibrillation. Ann Intern Med 2007;146:857–67.

14. Heidbuchel H, Verhamme P, Alings M, et al. European Heart Rhythm Association Practical Guide on the use of new oral anticoagulants in patients with non-valvular atrial fibrillation. Europace 2013;15(5):625–51.

15. Connolly SJ, Ezekowitz MD, Yusuf S, et al. Dabigatran versus warfarin in patients with atrial fibrillation. N Engl J Med 2009;361:1139–51.

16. Gage BF, Waterman AD, Shannon W, et al. Validation of clinical classification schemes for predicting stroke: results from the National Registry of Atrial Fibrillation. JAMA 2001;285(22):2864–70.

17. Camm AJ, Kirchhof P, Lip GY, et al. Guidelines for the management of atrial fibrillation: the Task Force for the Management of Atrial Fibrillation of the European Society of Cardiology (ESC). Eur Heart J 2010;31(19):2369–429.

18. Hoglund C, Rosenhamer G. Echocardiographic left atrial dimension as a predictor of maintaining sinus rhythm after conversion of atrial fibrillation. Acta Med Scand 1985;217:411–5.

19. Dittrich HC, Erickson JS, Schneiderman T, et al. Echocardiographic and clinical predictors for outcome of elective cardioversion of atrial fibrillation. Am J Cardiol 1989;63:193–7.

20. von Bary C, Dornia C, Eissnert C, et al. Predictive value of left atrial volume measured by non-invasive cardiac imaging in the treatment of paroxysmal atrial fibrillation. J Interv Card Electrophysiol 2012;34(2):181–8.

21. Klein AL, Murray RD, Grimm RA. Role of transesophageal echocardiography-guided cardioversion of patients with atrial fibrillation. J Am Coll Cardiol 2001;37:691–704.

22. Wazni OM, Tsao HM, Chen SA, et al. Cardiovascular imaging in the management of atrial fibrillation. J Am Coll Cardiol 2006;48(10):2077–84.

23. Leung DY, Black IW, Cranney GB, et al. Prognostic implications of left atrial spontaneous echo contrast in nonvalvular atrial fibrillation. J Am Coll Cardiol 1994;24(3):755–62.

24. Hartono B, Lo LW, Cheng CC, et al. A novel finding of the atrial substrate properties and long-term results of catheter ablation in chronic atrial fibrillation patients with left atrial spontaneous echo contrast. J Cardiovasc Electrophysiol 2012;23(3):239–46.

25. Fatkin D, Kelly RP, Feneley MP. Relations between left atrial appendage blood flow velocity, spontaneous echocardiographic contrast and thromboembolic risk in vivo. J Am Coll Cardiol 1994;23(4):961–9.

26. Yamashita T. Molecular basis of thromboembolism in association with atrial fibrillation. Circ J 2007;71(Suppl A):A40–4.

27. Leung DY, Davidson PM, Cranney GB, et al. Thromboembolic risks of left atrial thrombus detected by transesophageal echocardiogram. Am J Cardiol 1997;79:626–9.

28. Karakus G, Kodali V, Inamdar V, et al. Comparative assessment of left atrial appendage by transesophageal and combined two- and three-dimensional transthoracic echocardiography. Echocardiography 2008;25(8):918–24.

29. The Stroke Prevention in Atrial Fibrillation Investigators Committee on Echocardiography. Transesophageal echocardiographic correlates of thromboembolism in high-risk patients with nonvalvular atrial fibrillation. Ann Intern Med 1998;128:639–47.

30. Pollick C, Taylor D. Assessment of left atrial appendage function by transesophageal echocardiography. Implications for the development of thrombus. Circulation 1991;84(1):223–31.

31. Di Biase L, Burkhardt JD, Mohanty P, et al. Left atrial appendage: an underrecognized trigger site of atrial fibrillation. Circulation 2010;122(2):109–18.

32. Ilercil A, Kondapaneni J, Hla A, et al. Influence of age on left atrial appendage function in patients with nonvalvular atrial fibrillation. Clin Cardiol 2001;24(1):39–44.

33. Shinokawa N, Hirai T, Takashima S, et al. A transesophageal echocardiographic study on risk factors for stroke in elderly patients with atrial fibrillation: a comparison with younger patients. Chest 2001;120(3):840–6.

34. Fatkin D, Kuchar DL, Thorburn CW, et al. Transesophageal echocardiography before and during direct current cardioversion of atrial fibrillation: evidence for "atrial stunning" as a mechanism of thromboembolic complications. J Am Coll Cardiol 1994;23(2):307–16.

35. Manning WJ, Silverman DI, Katz SE, et al. Impaired left atrial mechanical function after cardioversion: relation to the duration of atrial fibrillation. J Am Coll Cardiol 1994;23(7):1535–40.

36. Zabalgoitia M, Halperin JL, Pearce LA, et al. Transesophageal echocardiographic correlates of clinical risk of thromboembolism in nonvalvular atrial fibrillation. Stroke Prevention in Atrial Fibrillation III Investigators. J Am Coll Cardiol 1998;31:1622–6.

37. Puwanant S, Varr BC, Shrestha K, et al. Role of the CHADS2 score in the evaluation of thromboembolic risk in patients with atrial fibrillation undergoing transesophageal echocardiography before pulmonary vein isolation. J Am Coll Cardiol 2009; 54(22):2032–9.

38. Romero J, Husain SA, Kelesidis I, et al. Detection of left atrial appendage thrombus by cardiac computed tomography in patients with atrial fibrillation: a meta-analysis. Circ Cardiovasc Imaging 2013;6(2):185–94.

39. Sawit ST, Garcia-Alvarez A, Suri B, et al. Usefulness of cardiac computed tomographic delayed contrast enhancement of the left atrial appendage before pulmonary vein ablation. Am J Cardiol 2012;109(5):677–84.

40. Ernst G, Stöllberger C, Abzieher F, et al. Morphology of the left atrial appendage. Anat Rec 1995;242:553–61.

41. Veinot JP, Harrity PJ, Gentile F, et al. Anatomy of the normal left atrial appendage: a quantitative study of age-related changes in 500 autopsy hearts: implications for echocardiographic examination. Circulation 1997;96:3112–5.

42. Di Biase L, Santangeli P, Anselmino M, et al. Does the left atrial appendage morphology correlate with the risk of stroke in patients with atrial fibrillation? Results from a multicenter study. J Am Coll Cardiol 2012;60(6):531–8.

43. Kimura T, Takatsuki S, Inagawa K, et al. Anatomical characteristics of the left atrial appendage in cardiogenic stroke with low CHADS2 scores. Heart Rhythm 2013;10(6):921–5.

44. Daccarett M, Badger TJ, Akoum N, et al. Association of left atrial fibrosis detected by delayed-enhancement magnetic resonance imaging and the risk of stroke in patients with atrial fibrillation. J Am Coll Cardiol 2011;57(7):831–8.

45. Wyse DG, Waldo AL, DiMarco JP, et al, The AFFIRM Investigators. A comparison of rate control and rhythm control in patients with atrial fibrillation. N Engl J Med 2002;347:1825–33.

46. Van Gelder IC, Hagens VE, Bosker HA, et al. A comparison of rate and rhythm control in patients with recurrent persistent atrial fibrillation. N Engl J Med 2002;347:1834–40.

47. Menotti A, Keys A, Blackburn H, et al. Twenty-year stroke mortality and prediction in twelve cohorts of the Seven Countries Study. Int J Epidemiol 1990; 19(2):309–15.

48. Tuomilehto J, Rastenyte D, Jousilahti P, et al. Diabetes mellitus as a risk factor for death from stroke. Prospective study of the middle-aged Finnish population. Stroke 1996;27(2):210–5.

49. Anderson EJ, Kypson AP, Rodriguez E, et al. Substrate-specific derangements in mitochondrial metabolism and redox balance in the atrium of the type 2 diabetic human heart. J Am Coll Cardiol 2009;54(20):1891–8.

50. Kistler PM, Sanders P, Dodic M, et al. Atrial electrical and structural abnormalities in an ovine model of chronic blood pressure elevation after prenatal corticosteroid exposure: implications for development of atrial fibrillation. Eur Heart J 2006;27(24): 3045–56.

51. Lau DH, Mackenzie L, Kelly DJ, et al. Hypertension and atrial fibrillation: evidence of progressive atrial remodeling with electrostructural correlate in a conscious chronically instrumented ovine model. Heart Rhythm 2010;7(9):1282–90.

52. Mondillo S, Cameli M, Caputo ML, et al. Early detection of left atrial strain abnormalities by speckle-tracking in hypertensive and diabetic patients with normal left atrial size. J Am Soc Echocardiogr 2011;24(8):898–908.

53. Hwang HJ, Choi EY, Rhee SJ, et al. Left atrial strain as predictor of successful outcomes in catheter ablation for atrial fibrillation: a two-dimensional myocardial imaging study. J Interv Card Electrophysiol 2009;26(2):127–32.

54. Pritchett AM, Mahoney DW, Jacobsen SJ, et al. Diastolic dysfunction and left atrial volume: a population-based study. J Am Coll Cardiol 2005; 45(1):87–92.

55. Poulsen MK, Dahl JS, Henriksen JE, et al. Left atrial volume index: relation to long-term clinical outcome in type 2 diabetes. J Am Coll Cardiol 2013. http://dx.doi.org/10.1016/j.jacc.2013.08.1622.

56. Tsang TS, Barnes ME, Gersh BJ, et al. Left atrial volume as a morphophysiologic expression of left ventricular diastolic dysfunction and relation to cardiovascular risk burden. Am J Cardiol 2002;90(12): 1284–9.

57. Tsang TS, Barnes ME, Bailey KR, et al. Left atrial volume: important risk marker of incident atrial fibrillation in 1655 older men and women. Mayo Clin Proc 2001;76(5):467–75.

58. Bilge M, Eryonucu B, Güler N, et al. Transesophageal echocardiography assessment of left atrial appendage function in untreated systemic hypertensive patients in sinus rhythm. J Am Soc Echocardiogr 2000;13(4):271–6.

59. Tamura H, Watanabe T, Nishiyama S, et al. Prognostic value of low left atrial appendage wall velocity in patients with ischemic stroke and atrial fibrillation. J Am Soc Echocardiogr 2012;25(5):576–83.

60. Wang YC, Lin JL, Hwang JJ, et al. Left atrial dysfunction in patients with atrial fibrillation after successful rhythm control for > 3 months. Chest 2005;128(4):2551–6.

61. Illien S, Maroto-Jarvinen S, Von der Recke G, et al. Atrial fibrillation: relation between clinical risk factors and transesophageal echocardiographic risk factors for thromboembolism. Heart 2003;89:165–8.

62. Fuster V, Halperin JL. Left ventricular thrombi and cerebral embolism. N Engl J Med 1989;320:392–4.

63. Natarajan D, Hotchandani RK, Nigam PD. Reduced incidence of left ventricular thrombi with intravenous streptokinase in acute anterior myocardial infarction: prospective evaluation by cross-sectional echocardiography. Int J Cardiol 1988; 20(2):201–7.

64. Nordrehaug JE, Johannessen KA, von der Lippe G. Usefulness of high-dose anticoagulants in preventing left ventricular thrombus in acute myocardial infarction. Am J Cardiol 1985;55: 1491–3.

65. Gueret P, Dubourg O, Ferrier A, et al. Effects of full-dose heparin anticoagulation on the development of left ventricular thrombosis in acute transmural myocardial infarction. J Am Coll Cardiol 1986;8: 419–26.

66. Delewi R, Nijveldt R, Hirsch A, et al. Left ventricular thrombus formation after acute myocardial infarction as assessed by cardiovascular magnetic resonance imaging. Eur J Radiol 2012;81(12): 3900–4.

67. Santoro F, Carapelle E, Cieza Ortiz SI, et al. Potential links between neurological disease and Tako-Tsubo cardiomyopathy: a literature review. Int J Cardiol 2013. http://dx.doi.org/10.1016/j.ijcard.2013.03.093.

68. Pullicino PM, Halperin JL, Thompson JL. Stroke in patients with heart failure and reduced left ventricular ejection fraction. Neurology 2000;54:288–94.

69. Witt BJ, Brown RD Jr, Jacobsen SJ, et al. Ischemic stroke after heart failure: a community-based study. Am Heart J 2006;152:102.

70. Loh E, Sutton MS, Wun CC, et al. Ventricular dysfunction and the risk of stroke after myocardial infarction. N Engl J Med 1997;336:251.

71. Georgiadis D, Sievert M, Cencetti S, et al. Cerebrovascular reactivity is impaired in patients with cardiac failure. Eur Heart J 2000;21:407.

72. Alves TC, Rays J, Fraguas R Jr, et al. Localized cerebral blood flow reductions in patients with heart failure: a study using 99mTc-HMPAO SPECT. J Neuroimaging 2005;15:150.

73. Weinsaft JW, Kim HW, Crowley AL, et al. LV thrombus detection by routine echocardiography: insights into performance characteristics using delayed enhancement CMR. JACC Cardiovasc Imaging 2011;4(7):702–12.

74. Weinsaft JW, Kim RJ, Ross M, et al. Contrast-enhanced anatomic imaging as compared to contrast-enhanced tissue characterization for detection of left ventricular thrombus. JACC Cardiovasc Imaging 2009;2(8):969–79.

75. Asinger RW, Herzog CA. Detecting LV thrombi: "T'ain't what you do (it's the way that you do it)". JACC Cardiovasc Imaging 2011;4(7):713–5.

76. Zhang W, Mondo C, Okello E, et al. Presenting features of newly diagnosed rheumatic heart disease patients in Mulago Hospital: a pilot study. Cardiovasc J Afr 2013;24(2):28–33.

77. Atatoa-Carr P, Lennon D, Wilson N, et al, New Zealand Rheumatic Fever Guidelines Writing Group. Rheumatic fever diagnosis, management, and secondary prevention: a New Zealand guideline. N Z Med J 2008;121(1271):59–69.

78. Ali SK, Eldaim IN, Osman SH, et al. Clinical and echocardiographic features of children with rheumatic heart disease and their serum cytokine profile. Pan Afr Med J 2012;13:36.

79. Coulshed N, Epstein EJ, McKendrick CS, et al. Systemic embolism in mitral valve disease. Br Heart J 1970;32:26–34.

80. Carter AB. Prognosis of cerebral embolism. Lancet 1965;2:514–9.

81. Wood P. Diseases of the heart and circulation. Philadelphia: JB Lippincott; 1956.

82. Fleming HA. Anticoagulants in rheumatic heart-disease. Lancet 1971;2:486.

83. Movahed MR, Saito Y, Ahmadi-Kashani M, et al. Mitral annulus calcification is associated with valvular and cardiac structural abnormalities. Cardiovasc Ultrasound 2007;5:14.

84. Santoro F, Ieva R, Lupo P, et al. Late calcification of the mitral-aortic junction causing transient complete atrio-ventricular block after mediastinal radiation of Hodgkin lymphoma: multimodal visualization. Int J Cardiol 2012;155(3):e49–50.

85. Fulkerson PK, Beaver BM, Auseon JC, et al. Calcification of the mitral annulus: etiology, clinical associations, complications and therapy. Am J Med 1979;66:967–77.

86. Ridolfi RL, Hutchins GM. Spontaneous calcific emboli from calcific mitral annulus fibrosus. Arch Pathol Lab Med 1976;100:117–20.

87. Deluca G, Correale M, Ieva R, et al. The incidence and clinical course of caseous calcification of the mitral annulus: a prospective echocardiographic study. J Am Soc Echocardiogr 2008;21(7):828–33.

88. Karas MG, Francescone S, Segal AZ, et al. Relation between mitral annular calcium and complex aortic atheroma in patients with cerebral ischemia referred for transesophageal echocardiography. Am J Cardiol 2007;99:1306–11.

89. Salem DN, Levine HJ, Pauker SG, et al. Antithrombotic therapy in valvular heart disease. Chest 1998; 114:590S.

90. Aziz F, Baciewicz FA Jr. Lambl's excrescences: review and recommendations. Tex Heart Inst J 2007; 34:366.

91. Lee RJ, Bartzokis T, Yeoh TK, et al. Enhanced detection of intracardiac sources of cerebral emboli by transesophageal echocardiography. Stroke 1991;22:734–9.

92. Freedberg RS, Goodkin GM, Perez JL, et al. Valve strands are strongly associated with systemic embolization: a transesophageal echocardiographic study. J Am Coll Cardiol 1995;26:1709–12.

93. Tice FD, Slivka AP, Walz ET, et al. Mitral valve strands in patients with focal cerebral ischemia. Stroke 1996;27:1183–6.

94. Homma S, Di Tullio MR, Sciacca RR, et al, PICSS Investigators. Effect of aspirin and warfarin therapy in stroke patients with valvular strands. Stroke 2004;35(6):1436–42.

95. Sullivan JM, Harken DE, Gorlin R. Pharmacologic control of thromboembolic complications of cardiac-valve replacement. N Engl J Med 1971; 284(25):1391–4.

96. Garcia-Fernandez MA, Perez-David E, Quiles J, et al. Role of left atrial appendage obliteration in stroke reduction in patients with mitral valve prosthesis: a transesophageal echocardiographic study. J Am Coll Cardiol 2003;42:1253–8.

97. Crystal E, Lamy A, Connolly SJ, et al, Left Atrial Appendage Occlusion Study. Left atrial appendage occlusion study (LAAOS): a randomized clinical trial of left atrial appendage occlusion during routine coronary artery bypass graft surgery for long-term stroke prevention. Am Heart J 2003; 145:174–8.

98. Bonow RO, Carabello BA, Chatterjee K, et al. 2008 Focused update incorporated into the ACC/AHA 2006 guidelines for the management of patients with valvular heart disease: a report of the American College of Cardiology/American Heart Association Task Force on Practice Guidelines (Writing Committee to Revise the 1998 Guidelines for the Management of Patients with Valvular Heart Disease): endorsed by the Society of Cardiovascular Anesthesiologists, Society for Cardiovascular Angiography and Interventions, and Society of Thoracic Surgeons. Circulation 2008;118:e523–661.

99. Holmes DR, Reddy VY, Turi ZG, et al. Percutaneous closure of the left atrial appendage versus warfarin therapy for prevention of stroke in patients with atrial fibrillation: a randomised non-inferiority trial. Lancet 2009;374:534–42.

100. Bartus K, Han FT, Bednarek J, et al. Percutaneous left atrial appendage suture ligation using the LARIAT device in patients with atrial fibrillation: initial clinical experience. J Am Coll Cardiol 2012. http://dx.doi.org/10.1016/j.jacc.2012.06.046.

101. Shah SJ, Bardo DM, Sugeng L, et al. Real-time three-dimensional transoesophageal echocardiography of the left atrial appendage: initial experience in the clinical setting. J Am Soc Echocardiogr 2008; 21:1352–8.

102. Ostermayer SH, Reisman M, Kramer PH, et al. Percutaneous left atrial appendage transcatheter occlusion (PLAATO system) to prevent stroke in high-risk patients with non-rheumatic atrial fibrillation: results from the international multi-center feasibility trials. J Am Coll Cardiol 2005;46:9–14.

103. Chue CD, de Giovanni J, Steeds RP. The role of echocardiography in percutaneous left atrial appendage occlusion. Eur J Echocardiogr 2011; 12(10):i3–10.

104. Sick PB, Schuler G, Hauptmann KE, et al. Initial worldwide experience with the WATCHMAN left atrial appendage system for stroke prevention in atrial fibrillation. J Am Coll Cardiol 2007;49: 1490–5.

Atrial Fibrillation and Stroke
A Neurologic Perspective

Siva K. Mulpuru, MD[a], Alejandro A. Rabinstein, MD[b],
Samuel J. Asirvatham, MD, FACC, FHRS[a,c,*]

KEYWORDS

- Atrial fibrillation • Dementia • Stroke • Ablation • Monitoring

KEY POINTS

- Atrial fibrillation is associated with long-term cognitive decline and stroke.
- Recognition of occult atrial fibrillation in patients with stroke, and appropriate use of risk stratification schemes for prevention of stroke and bleeding with anticoagulant therapy, are essential for optimal patient outcomes.
- Catheter-based ablation procedures are associated with silent cerebral events, and their role in long-term cognitive decline has to be carefully evaluated.

Atrial fibrillation (AF) is the most common supraventricular arrhythmia associated with reduced quality of life and increased risk of cerebrovascular disease. The prevalence of AF increases with age[1,2] and the presence of structural heart disease. There were 2.7 million Americans with AF in 2010, and there is a 25% chance of men and women more than 40 years of age developing AF in their lifetimes.[3] The prevalence of AF in the developed world is about 1% to 2% of the population. AF is associated with loss of effective atrial contractility, loss of atrioventricular synchrony, and stasis of blood with associated thrombus formation. Transient ischemic attacks and stroke caused by thromboembolism are the most severe complications from AF.

To provide a neurologic perspective, this article describes the pathogenesis of thrombus formation, associated risk factors for stroke with AF, various stroke risk stratification schemes, bleeding risk with anticoagulation therapy, and the current bleeding risk stratification schemes. Cognitive decline[4] is increasingly recognized as a long-term sequela of AF. It may be secondary to recurrent thromboembolism, microbleeds on anticoagulant therapy, or progression of vascular risk factors (hypertension, diabetes, atherosclerotic disease) associated with AF. The role of prolonged monitoring in detection of occult atrial fibrillation, and measures to reduce stroke in patients undergoing ablation procedures for AF are briefly explored.

EPIDEMIOLOGY OF AF

AF is uncommon in infants and children and occurs mostly in association with congenital heart disease. The risk of AF in young healthy adults is low, as shown in a screening study of Air Force personnel.[5] Several cross-sectional studies show the prevalence characteristics among subgroups of the US population. AF is more prevalent in elderly men and women (0.1% among patients less than 55 years of age and 9% among patients

Disclosures: Department of Internal Medicine, Mayo Clinic Career Development Grant to S.K. Mulpuru.
[a] Division of Cardiovascular Diseases, Department of Internal Medicine, Mayo Clinic, 200 First Street Southwest, Rochester, MN 55905, USA; [b] Department of Neurology, Mayo Clinic, 200 First Street, Rochester, MN 55905, USA; [c] Division of Pediatric Cardiology, Department of Pediatrics and Adolescent Medicine, Mayo Clinic, 200 First Street Southwest, Rochester, MN 55905, USA
* Corresponding author. Division of Cardiovascular Diseases, Department of Internal Medicine, Mayo Clinic College of Medicine, 200 First Street Southwest, Rochester, MN 55905.
E-mail address: asirvatham.samuel@mayo.edu

more than 80 years of age). AF is more common among men than among women across all subgroups and more common in white people than in black people.[1,6] As the population ages, the projected prevalence of AF for 2050 is about 7.56 million,[7] which will place a huge strain on the health care system.

The incidence of AF also increases with age (0.5 per 1000 person-years before age 50 years of age to 9.7 per 1000 patient years after age 70 years)[8] and the presence of other cardiovascular risk factors. The lifetime risk of developing AF from the Framingham Heart Study cohort was 26% for men and 23% for women.[9] Various risk factors associated with AF from population bases studies are listed in **Box 1**.

- AF is the most common supraventricular arrhythmia in the United States.
- The incidence and prevalence of AF increase with age.
- The lifetime risk of developing AF (from the Framingham Heart Study cohort) is 26% for men and 23% for women.

Box 1
Risk factors associated with AF

1. Hypertension
2. Coronary artery disease
3. Structural heart disease
   a. Valvular heart disease
   b. Heart failure and various cardiomyopathies
   c. Hypertrophic cardiomyopathy
   d. Congenital heart disease
   e. Myocarditis
4. Cardiopulmonary conditions
   a. Pulmonary embolism
   b. Chronic obstructive pulmonary disease
   c. Pericarditis
   d. Obstructive sleep apnea
5. Obesity
6. Diabetes
7. Metabolic syndrome
8. Hyperthyroidism
9. Chronic kidney disease
10. Cardiac and noncardiac surgery
11. Family history
12. Occurrence of other supraventricular arrhythmias.

CEREBROVASCULAR EVENTS AND AF

Strokes related to AF can involve any vascular territory and typically involve the cortex. However, cortical involvement is not necessary to suspect cardiac embolism. Some patients can have cardioembolic occlusion of a major intracranial vessel like the proximal middle cerebral artery causing infarction of subcortical structures but maintain adequate perfusion to the cortex through collateral flow. Although uncommon, the pattern of multiple acute brain infarctions in different vascular territories (anterior and posterior circulation or both hemispheres) indicates a proximal source of embolism. In these cases, the possibility of AF should be strongly considered. Patients with cardiac embolism from AF can present with severe deficits followed by rapid and complete or nearly complete spontaneous resolution (so-called spectacularly vanishing deficits). Recognition of this clinical presentation should prompt detailed evaluation of heart rhythm.

Patients with suspected cardiac embolism should be evaluated with electrocardiography, echocardiography (preferably transesophageal), and heart rhythm monitoring. Presence of AF, either persistent or paroxysmal, on electrocardiogram, cardiac telemetry, or Holter monitoring usually defines the stroke as cardioembolic and, in the absence of contraindications, is an indication to start long-term oral anticoagulation. However, even in patients with documented AF it is important to check the status of the blood vessels and exclude alternative mechanisms of stroke. A patient with a stroke in the right middle cerebral artery territory who has AF but also advanced stenosis of the right internal carotid artery with an ulcerated plaque needs carotid revascularization, not just anticoagulation. A patient with a small subcortical stroke or a pontine infarction with advanced basilar artery atherosclerosis may also have AF, but the stroke is less likely to be related to the arrhythmia, and the secondary stroke prevention treatment should address all possible causes of recurrent ischemia.

Strokes related to AF are associated with worse functional outcomes,[10] even after thrombolysis,[11] and are associated with higher rate of stroke recurrence in the absence of adequate anticoagulation.[12] Worse outcomes in strokes related to AF are probably caused by greater volumes of ischemic brain and greater risk of hemorrhagic conversion.[13] Thus, timely recognition of AF and initiation of anticoagulation in safe candidates are essential to avert the potentially serious consequences of ischemic cerebrovascular disease.

In addition, AF can cause early complications after a stroke. Patients with previously documented

AF on rate-controlling medications can develop rapid ventricular response after stroke, particularly if these medications are withheld. Thus, we recommend against withholding rate-controlling medications in patients with AF with stroke to minimize the risk of acute tachycardia, which may compromise cerebral perfusion and increases the use of intensive care resources.[14]

- Multiple acute cerebral infarcts should point to a central source of embolism.
- Patients with a suspicion for a central source of embolism should undergo rhythm monitoring to diagnose AF and transesophageal echocardiography to rule out a cardiac source of embolism.
- Strokes related to AF have worse outcomes because of greater volumes of ischemic tissue and higher risk of hemorrhagic conversion.
- AF is common after an acute stroke. Rate control medications should not be routinely withheld in patients after stroke with AF.

CRYPTOGENIC STROKES AND ROLE OF AF

Up to 30% to 40% of ischemic strokes have a negative work-up for an underlying cause and are classified as cryptogenic strokes.[15] AF is a well-established cause of ischemic strokes and is found in up to 25% of patients with first stroke.[16] Because patients can have paroxysmal AF, the diagnosis can be missed during brief periods of monitoring around the period of stroke. The risk of stroke in patients with short paroxysmal episodes of AF is similar to that in patients with continuous AF, and anticoagulation therapy reduces the stroke risk.[17]

In general, the yield of AF detection increases with the length of monitoring time.[18] Use of an extended loop recorder for 21 to 30 days can detect paroxysmal AF in up to 12% (95% confidence interval [CI], 8%–17%) of patients with cryptogenic stroke.[19] In a recent series of patients with cryptogenic stroke, monitoring with implantable loop recorders (ILRs) documented episodes of paroxysmal AF in 25% (95% CI, 14%–40%) of cases.[20] Most of the events were short (median of 6 minutes) and were only detected after extended monitoring (median duration of recording before the first AF episode was 48 days). Patients who had AF episodes detected on ILR were older, and had higher $CHADS_2$ (congestive heart failure, hypertension, age >75, diabetes, prior stroke) or CHADS-VASc (vascular disease, age 65–74 years, sex category) scores. They also had paroxysmal atrial complexes and evidence of interatrial conduction delay along with enlarged atria on echocardiography.

However, studies on paroxysmal AF detection with prolonged ambulatory monitoring have mostly been limited to case series of patients with cryptogenic stroke, and the question remains whether the finding of isolated, brief episodes of paroxysmal AF over many days of monitoring after a cryptogenic stroke is sufficient to consider that arrhythmia pathogenic and initiate anticoagulation. In the only study that compared prolonged ambulatory heart rhythm monitoring in patients with cryptogenic stroke with patients with stroke of established cause, the rate of paroxysmal AF detection was similar in both groups among patients 65 years or older (27% in the cryptogenic group vs 25% in the group with stroke of known cause; $P = .9$). Only among younger patients was there a strong trend for paroxysmal AF to be more commonly detected after a cryptogenic stroke (22% vs 3%; $P = .07$).[21] Therefore, the significance of finding brief episodes of paroxysmal AF through extended ambulatory monitoring in patients with cryptogenic stroke still needs to be defined, and the value of anticoagulation in these patients remains unclear. A controlled trial exploring the role of invasive high-quality monitoring versus noninvasive monitoring in patients with cryptogenic stroke (CRYSTAL-AF [Cryptogenic Stroke and underlying Atrial Fibrillation][22]) has completed enrollment and results will be available soon to guide monitoring in these patients. Ischemic strokes with a negative work-up are classified as cryptogenic strokes.

- Prolonged monitoring of rhythm can often detect AF in up to 25% of patients with cryptogenic stroke.
- Younger patients with cryptogenic strokes tend to have a higher prevalence of AF.
- The CRYSTAL-AF study, which will examine the role of prolonged invasive monitoring in patients with cryptogenic stroke, has completed enrollment and the results will be published soon.

PATHOGENESIS OF THROMBUS FORMATION AND STROKE

Thrombogenesis is multifactorial in patients with AF. Stasis of blood within a poorly contractile atrium along with underlying prothrombotic or hypercoagulable state provides a perfect milieu for thrombus formation. AF leads to structural changes in the tissue architecture. Endothelial damage, muscle hypertrophy or necrosis, and infiltration by mononuclear cells can happen with AF.[23] Altered renin-angiotensin-aldosterone system (RAAS) in AF leads to tissue changes and perpetuation of AF.[24]

Inflammation seems to play an important role in the prothrombotic state associated with AF. Endothelial damage and/or activation,[25] increased production of cytokines and chemokines, increased platelet activation,[26] and expression of fibrinogen[27] are associated with episodes of AF. Inflammatory markers are increased in patients with AF with associated spontaneous echocardiographic contrast in the left atrial appendage (LAA).[28] Inflammatory markers further increase platelet activation and sensitivity to tissue factor. Patients with AF have increased levels of collagen degradation products[29] and abnormal concentration of matrix metalloproteinase (MMPs)[30] and their inhibitors. Altered matrix can lead to perpetuation of AF because of conduction abnormalities, tissue infiltration, and fibrosis.

Inflammation seems to be a potent trigger of AF, and AF seems to sustain the prothrombotic and proinflammatory milieu. On endothelial activation, substances like the von Willebrand factor and selectin-P are released onto the endothelial surface, which promotes attachment of leukocytes to the endothelium, thereby contributing to a prothrombotic state. The concentration of prothrombotic indices is increased in patients with AF with stroke[31] or AF with multiple risk factors.[32] Enhanced fibrinolysis with alterations in growth factors like vascular endothelial growth factor (VEGF)[33] lead to enhanced thrombogenesis.[34] Presence of complex aortic plaque, which is a risk factor for stroke, is seen in up to 57% of patients with AF. About 25% of these patients have complex plaques (pedunculated, mobile, >4 mm thick, ulcerated) reflecting coexisting vascular and atherosclerotic risk factors.[35] Ischemic strokes in patients with AF are considered to be predominantly caused by embolization of larger particles from the LA. AF-associated ischemic strokes are associated with more hemispheric events and worse outcomes compared with ischemic strokes secondary to emboli from carotid disease.[36]

- AF is associated with stasis of blood in the atrium.
- Inflammatory markers are increased and a prothrombotic state is created.
- Activation of inflammatory cells with alteration of renin-angiotensinogen system results in ultrastructural tissue changes.
- Complex aortic plaques are frequently seen in patients with AF and stroke.

STROKE RISK STRATIFICATION

Patients with AF and valvular heart disease are at a higher risk of stroke (7%–15% per year) and benefit from long-term anticoagulation therapy.[37] Anticoagulant therapy for primary prevention was evaluated in 5 primary stroke prevention trials in patients with nonvalvular AF.[38–42] Pooled analysis of the 5 trials suggested 4 main risk factors for stroke: age greater than 65 years, history of stroke or transient ischemic attack (TIA), diabetes, and hypertension. Patients with none of these risk factors had 1% annualized risk of stroke, and patients with any of the risk factors had 4% annualized risk of stroke.[43] Investigators from the SPAF III (stroke prevention in atrial fibrillation) trial identified 2 additional risk factors: women with age greater than 75 years, and clinical heart failure.[44]

A simple scoring system for clinical assessment of stroke risk was created by combining all these risk factors and it has gained wide recognition under the acronym CHADS2.[45] Risk factors, scoring, and associated stroke risk are shown in **Table 1**.[46] Long-term anticoagulation therapy is beneficial in patients with CHADS2 score of 2 or more. Further risk stratification refinement of patients with low or moderate risk is made possible by the advent of the CHADS2-VASc scoring system.[47] This newer scoring system recognizes vascular disease (prior myocardial infarction, peripheral vascular disease, or aortic plaque) and female sex (if greater than 65 years of age) as risk factors. The scoring system with risk factors and associated risk is shown in **Tables 2** and **3**. Patients with scores of 2 or more benefit from anticoagulation therapy, and many with a score of zero do not even need antiplatelet agents.

Chronic renal dysfunction has recently been described as a predictor for stoke in patients with AF. As a result, the R_2CHADS_2 (renal dysfunction, congestive heart failure, hypertension, age >75, diabetes, prior stroke) scoring system was developed, which awards 2 points for creatinine clearance of less than 60 mL/min.[48] Several other echocardiographic parameters[49,50] (LA abnormality, reduced LAA emptying velocity, spontaneous echo contrast, thrombus, descending aortic plaque) are associated with higher risk of stroke. LAA morphology on computed tomography (CT) or magnetic resonance imaging (MRI) was recently correlated with stroke risk.[51] LAA with multiple small pockets (cauliflower or cactus) morphology on CT imaging is associated with higher risk of preprocedure-stroke or TIA.

- The CHADS2 scoring system identifies patients with high risk for stroke who would benefit from anticoagulation therapy.
- The CHADS2-VASc system further risk stratifies patients into low-risk and moderate-risk groups.

Table 1
Event rates by stroke risk factor, baseline CHADS2 score, and anticoagulation status in 11,526 adults with AF and no contraindications to warfarin therapy at baseline

Characteristics	Event Rate (per 100 Person-Years) (95% CI)		Crude Rate Ratio (95% CI)
	Taking Warfarin	Not Taking Warfarin	
Prior ischemic stroke	3.24 (2.39–4.41)	7.40 (5.24–10.43)	0.44 (0.28–0.69)
Diabetes mellitus	2.06 (1.55–2.73)	3.56 (2.77–4.58)	0.58 (0.40–0.84)
Hypertension	1.59 (1.32–1.91)	2.55 (2.18–2.98)	0.62 (0.49–0.79)
Congestive heart failure	1.22 (0.94–1.60)	3.54 (2.89–4.33)	0.35 (0.25–0.48)
Coronary heart disease	1.57 (1.22–2.02)	2.94 (2.40–3.61)	0.53 (0.39–0.74)
Age >75 y	1.43 (1.15–1.78)	3.22 (2.77–3.74)	0.45 (0.34–0.58)
None of the risk factors listed earlier	0.21 (0.07–0.65)	0.43 (0.24–0.79)	0.49 (0.14–1.74)
CHADS2 score (no. of patients)[a]			
0 (2557)	0.25 (0.11–0.55)	0.49 (0.30–0.78)	0.50 (0.20–1.28)
1 (3662)	0.72 (0.50–1.03)	1.52 (1.19–1.94)	0.47 (0.30–0.73)
2 (2955)	1.27 (0.94–1.72)	2.50 (1.98–3.15)	0.51 (0.35–0.75)
3 (1555)	2.20 (1.61–3.01)	5.27 (4.15–6.70)	0.42 (0.28–0.62)
4 (556)	2.35 (1.44–3.83)	6.02 (3.90–9.29)	0.39 (0.20–0.75)
5 or 6 (241)	4.60 (2.72–7.76)	6.88 (3.42–13.84)	0.67 (0.28–1.60)

[a] In the CHADS2 scoring system, 2 points are given for prior thromboembolism, and 1 point each for congestive heart failure, diagnosed hypertension, age 75 years or older, and diabetes mellitus. Number of patients represents those with that baseline score.

From Go AS, Hylek EM, Chang Y, et al. Anticoagulation therapy for stroke prevention in atrial fibrillation: how well do randomized trials translate into clinical practice? JAMA 2003;290:2688; with permission.

- Renal dysfunction, several echocardiographic parameters, and morphology of the appendage on CT scan correlate with stroke risk.

BLEEDING RISK STRATIFICATION

Long-term anticoagulation therapy for stoke prevention in patients with AF is associated with increased bleeding risk. The risk of major bleeding is associated with several preexisting risk factors and the degree of anticoagulation. Several recognized risk factors for bleeding are listed in **Box 2**. Several scoring systems (OBRI [Outpatient Bleeding Risk Index],[52] HEMORR2HAGES [hepatic or renal disease, ethanol abuse, malignancy, older age >75, reduced platelet count or function, rebleeding risk, hypertension, anemia, genetic factors, excessive fall risk, stroke],[53] HAS-BLED [hypertension, abnormal renal/liver function, stroke, bleeding history or predisposition, labile international normalized ratio, elderly, drugs/alcohol concomitantly],[54] ATRIA [the Anticoagulation and Risk Factors in Atrial Fibrillation] score[55]) were developed to estimate the risk of hemorrhage and can be used to provide an approximate risk/benefit ratio for patients treated with long-term anticoagulation therapy. The cumulative risk of hemorrhage over years of anticoagulation can be substantial

and increases as the patient ages (all hemorrhage risk stratification scores include age as one of the predictive variables).[56] Thus, serial reassessment of bleeding risk needs to be performed over time in chronically anticoagulated patients.

- Several risk stratification schemes are available to assess the bleeding risk in patients on anticoagulant therapy.
- The cumulative bleeding risk increases with age and serial assessments need to be performed.

DEMENTIA AND AF

A growing body of evidence suggests increased risk of cognitive impairment (objective memory impairment without measurable effect on activities of daily living) and dementia (severe impairment of memory and at least one other cognitive function causing limitation in the ability to perform activities of daily living) in patients with AF.[4,57–59] Dementia and AF share similar risk factors that include hypertension, heart failure, and diabetes. The prevalence of these risk factors for AF and dementia increases with age. Silent subclinical strokes may explain increased risk of dementia in patients with AF. Cerebral microbleeds detected on MRI

Table 2
Various risk factors included in the CHADS2-VASc scoring schema

(1) Risk Factors for Stroke and Thromboembolism in Nonvalvular AF

Previous stroke, TIA, or systemic embolism at age ≥75 y	Heart failure or moderate to severe LV systolic dysfunction (eg, LV EF ≤40%), hypertension, diabetes mellitus, female sex, age 65–74 y, vascular disease[a]

(2) Risk Factor–based Approach Expressed as a Point-based Scoring System, with the Acronym CHA$_2$DS$_2$-VASc (Note: Maximum Score is 9 Because Age May Contribute 0, 1, or 2 Points)

Risk Factor	Score
Congestive heart failure/LV dysfunction	1
Hypertension	1
Age ≥75 y	2
Diabetes mellitus	1
Stroke/TIA/thromboembolism	2
Vascular disease[a]	1
Age 65–74 y	1
Sex category (ie, female sex)	1
Maximum score	9

(3) Adjusted Stroke Rate According to CHA$_2$DS$_2$-VASc Score

CHAD$_2$S$_2$-VASc Score	Patients (n = 7329)	Adjusted Stroke Rate (%/year)[b]
0	1	0%
1	422	1.3%
2	1230	2.2%
3	1730	3.2%
4	1718	4.0%
5	1159	6.7%
6	679	9.8%
7	294	9.6%
8	82	6.7%
9	14	15.2%

Abbreviations: CHA$_2$DS$_2$-VASc, cardiac failure, hypertension, age ≥75 (doubled), diabetes, stroke (doubled)-vascular disease, age 65–74 and sex category (female); EF, ejection fraction (as documented by echocardiography, radionuclide ventriculography, cardiac catheterization, cardiac magnetic resonance imaging, and so forth); LV, left ventricular.

[a] Prior myocardial infarction, peripheral artery disease, aortic plaque. Rates of stroke in contemporary cohorts may vary from these estimates.

[b] Based on Lip GY, Frison L, Halperin J, et al. Identifying patients at high risk for stroke despite anticoagulation: a comparison of contemporary stroke risk stratification schemes in an anticoagulated atrial fibrillation cohort. Stroke 2010;41(12):2735.

From European Heart Rhythm Association, European Association for Cardio-Thoracic Surgery, Camm AJ, Kirchhof P, Lip GY, et al. Guidelines for the management of atrial fibrillation: the Task Force for the Management of Atrial Fibrillation of the European Society of Cardiology (ESC). Eur Heart J 2010;19:2382. http://dx.doi.org/10.1093/eurheartj/ehq278; with permission.

are manifestation of small vessel disease and may contribute to cognitive decline in patients with AF on anticoagulation therapy.[60] Beat-to-beat variability of brain perfusion,[61] reduced cardiac output with AF, proinflammatory state,[62] and development of periventricular white matter lesions[63] are other plausible explanations for this association.

The association of AF with dementia can be explained by the occurrence of strokes.[64] Overall there is more than 2-fold increased risk of cognitive impairment after a stroke. However, a recent meta-analysis confirms that there is an increased risk of dementia in patients with AF even without history of stroke.[4] The association was stronger for vascular dementia compared with Alzheimer dementia. Slow ventricular response (<50 beats per minute [bpm]) or fast ventricular response (>90 bpm) in AF is associated with increased risk

Table 3
Recommendations for stroke prevention therapy

Risk Category	CHA$_2$DS$_2$-VASc Score	Recommended Antithrombotic Therapy
One major risk factor or ≥2 clinically relevant nonmajor risk factors	≥2	OAC[a]
One clinically relevant nonmajor risk factor	1	Either OAC[a] or aspirin 75–325 mg daily (OAC is preferred rather than aspirin)
No risk factors	0	Either aspirin 75–325 mg daily or no antithrombotic therapy (no antithrombotic therapy is preferred rather than aspirin)

Abbreviations: INR, international normalized ratio; OAC, oral anticoagulation (such as a vitamin K antagonist [VKA] adjusted to an intensity range of INR 2.0–3.0 [target, 2.5]).

[a] OAC, such as a VKA, adjusted to an intensity range of INR 2.0 to 3.0 (target 2.5). New OAC drugs that may be viable alternatives to a VKA may be considered. For example, should both doses of dabigatran etexilate receive regulatory approval for stroke prevention in AF, the recommendations for thromboprophylaxis could evolve as follows considering stroke and bleeding risk stratification: (1) if oral anticoagulation is appropriate therapy, dabigatran may be considered as an alternative to adjusted dose VKA therapy. (1A) If a patient is at low risk of bleeding (eg, HAS-BLED [hypertension, abnormal renal/liver function, stroke, bleeding history or predisposition, labile international normalized ratio, elderly, drugs/alcohol concomitantly] score of 0–2), dabigatran 150 mg twice a day may be considered, in view of the improved efficacy in the prevention of stroke and systemic embolism (but lower rates of intracranial hemorrhage and similar rates of major bleeding events, when compared with warfarin); and (1B) If a patient has a measurable risk of bleeding (eg, HAS-BLED score of ≥3), dabigatran etexilate 110 mg twice a day may be considered, in view of a similar efficacy in the prevention of stroke and systemic embolism (but lower rates of intracranial hemorrhage and of major bleeding compared with VKA). (2) In patients with 1 clinically relevant nonmajor stroke risk factor, dabigatran 110 mg twice a day may be considered, in view of a similar efficacy with VKA in the prevention of stroke and systemic embolism but lower rates of intracranial hemorrhage and major bleeding compared with the VKA and (probably) aspirin. (3) Patients with no stroke risk factors (eg, CHA$_2$DS$_2$-VASc of 0) are clearly at such low risk that either aspirin 75 to 325 mg daily or no antithrombotic therapy is recommended. If possible, no antithrombotic therapy should be considered for such patients, rather than aspirin, given the limited data on the benefits of aspirin in this patient group (ie, lone AF) and the potential for adverse effects, especially bleeding.

From European Heart Rhythm Association, European Association for Cardio-Thoracic Surgery, Camm AJ, Kirchhof P, Lip GY, et al. Guidelines for the management of atrial fibrillation: the Task Force for the Management of Atrial Fibrillation of the European Society of Cardiology (ESC). Eur Heart J 2010;19:2384. http://dx.doi.org/10.1093/eurheartj/ehq278; with permission.

of dementia.[65] AF is also associated with smaller brain volume, with associated cognitive functional impairment, independently of the presence of cerebral infarcts.[66] Catheter-based ablation procedures for treatment of AF decreased the risk of dementia in a small series of patients, but these findings remain to be validated.[67] Future trials exploring dementia as an end point after catheter-based ablation of atrial fibrillation are necessary to clarify the causal relationship between the two disease states.

- Recent evidence suggests a clear link between AF and cognitive impairment.
- Cerebral infarcts, microbleeds secondary to anticoagulation therapy, inflammatory state associated with AF, and low cardiac output are plausible explanations for increased risk of dementia.
- The role of catheter-based ablation procedures to prevent development of cognitive impairment needs to be explored further.

DEVICE-DETECTED AF IN PATIENTS WITH STROKE RISK FACTORS

Several recent studies have assessed the incidence of AF with implanted devices (pacemakers and defibrillators). The prevalence of AF can be up to 31% in patients with multiple stroke risk factors.[68] Episodes lasting more than 5.5 hours are associated with higher risk of thromboembolism in the subsequent 30-day period.[69] Patients with higher virtual CHADS2 scores had more frequent episodes of AF lasting more than 6 hours, suggesting severity or rate of disease progression. Several recent studies have linked modest amounts of device-detected AF (up to 6 minutes) with subsequent risk of thromboembolism and stroke.[70–72] Even in patients with high stroke risk scores, few patients had AF occurring in more than 10% of the follow-up days, underscoring the importance of long-term monitoring. As newer anticoagulants with increased efficacy and decreased bleeding risk compared with warfarin become available, future clinical trials will be necessary to evaluate the benefit of oral anticoagulation in patients with short episodes of device-detected AF and fewer stroke risk factors.

STROKE ASSOCIATED WITH ABLATION PROCEDURES

Silent ischemic cerebral events are frequently seen in patients undergoing catheter-based ablation procedures for AF.[73] The incidence of these events is related to the type of catheter (irrigated radiofrequency [RF], nonirrigated RF, cryoballoon, multielectrode), energy source (RF, cryoenergy, duty cycled RF),[74] degree of anticoagulation, and appropriate sheath management to prevent air embolism during the procedures. Most of the lesions improve with 72 hours and are rarely associated with clinical neurologic deficits.

- Short episodes of device-detected AF are associated with increased risk of thromboembolism in large registry-based studies.
- Subclinical stroke and diffusion-weighted MRI abnormalities are common after AF ablation procedures.

SUMMARY

As the population ages and risk factors for AF become prevalent, AF will continue to be a major clinical problem. AF is associated with long-term cognitive decline and stroke. Recognition of occult AF in patients with stroke and appropriate use of risk stratification schemes for prevention of stroke and bleeding with anticoagulant therapy are essential for optimal patient outcomes. Catheter-based ablation procedures are associated with silent cerebral events and their role in long-term cognitive decline has to be carefully evaluated.

REFERENCES

1. Heeringa J, van der Kuip DA, Hofman A, et al. Prevalence, incidence and lifetime risk of atrial fibrillation: the Rotterdam study. Eur Heart J 2006; 27:949–53.
2. Feinberg WM, Blackshear JL, Laupacis A, et al. Prevalence, age distribution, and gender of patients with atrial fibrillation. Analysis and implications. Arch Intern Med 1995;155:469–73.
3. Roger VL, Go AS, Lloyd-Jones DM, et al. Heart disease and stroke statistics–2012 update: a report from the American Heart Association. Circulation 2012;125:e2–220.
4. Kalantarian S, Stern TA, Mansour M, et al. Cognitive impairment associated with atrial fibrillation: a meta-analysis. Ann Intern Med 2013;158:338–46.
5. Hiss RG, Lamb LE. Electrocardiographic findings in 122,043 individuals. Circulation 1962;25:947–61.
6. Go AS, Hylek EM, Phillips KA, et al. Prevalence of diagnosed atrial fibrillation in adults: national implications for rhythm management and stroke prevention: the Anticoagulation and Risk Factors in Atrial Fibrillation (ATRIA) study. JAMA 2001;285: 2370–5.
7. Naccarelli GV, Varker H, Lin J, et al. Increasing prevalence of atrial fibrillation and flutter in the United States. Am J Cardiol 2009;104:1534–9.
8. Krahn AD, Manfreda J, Tate RB, et al. The natural history of atrial fibrillation: incidence, risk factors, and prognosis in the Manitoba follow-up study. Am J Med 1995;98:476–84.
9. Lloyd-Jones DM, Wang TJ, Leip EP, et al. Lifetime risk for development of atrial fibrillation: the Framingham Heart Study. Circulation 2004;110: 1042–6.
10. Saposnik G, Gladstone D, Raptis R, et al. Atrial fibrillation in ischemic stroke: predicting response to thrombolysis and clinical outcomes. Stroke 2013;44:99–104.
11. Seet RC, Zhang Y, Wijdicks EF, et al. Relationship between chronic atrial fibrillation and worse outcomes in stroke patients after intravenous thrombolysis. Arch Neurol 2011;68:1454–8.
12. Connolly S, Pogue J, Hart R, et al. Clopidogrel plus aspirin versus oral anticoagulation for atrial fibrillation in the Atrial Fibrillation Clopidogrel Trial with

Irbesartan for Prevention of Vascular Events (ACTIVE W): a randomised controlled trial. Lancet 2006;367:1903–12.

13. Tu HT, Campbell BC, Christensen S, et al. Pathophysiological determinants of worse stroke outcome in atrial fibrillation. Cerebrovasc Dis 2010;30:389–95.

14. Seet RC, Zhang Y, Rabinstein AA, et al. Risk factors and consequences of atrial fibrillation with rapid ventricular response in patients with ischemic stroke treated with intravenous thrombolysis. J Stroke Cerebrovasc Dis 2013;22:161–5.

15. White H, Boden-Albala B, Wang C, et al. Ischemic stroke subtype incidence among whites, blacks, and Hispanics: the Northern Manhattan Study. Circulation 2005;111:1327–31.

16. Marini C, De Santis F, Sacco S, et al. Contribution of atrial fibrillation to incidence and outcome of ischemic stroke: results from a population-based study. Stroke 2005;36:1115–9.

17. Hohnloser SH, Pajitnev D, Pogue J, et al. Incidence of stroke in paroxysmal versus sustained atrial fibrillation in patients taking oral anticoagulation or combined antiplatelet therapy: an ACTIVE W substudy. J Am Coll Cardiol 2007;50:2156–61.

18. Seet RC, Friedman PA, Rabinstein AA. Prolonged rhythm monitoring for the detection of occult paroxysmal atrial fibrillation in ischemic stroke of unknown cause. Circulation 2011;124:477–86.

19. Flint AC, Banki NM, Ren X, et al. Detection of paroxysmal atrial fibrillation by 30-day event monitoring in cryptogenic ischemic stroke: the Stroke and Monitoring for PAF in Real Time (SMART) registry. Stroke 2012;43:2788–90.

20. Cotter PE, Martin PJ, Ring L, et al. Incidence of atrial fibrillation detected by implantable loop recorders in unexplained stroke. Neurology 2013; 80(17):1546–50.

21. Rabinstein AA, Fugate JE, Mandrekar J, et al. Paroxysmal atrial fibrillation in stroke: a case-control study. J Stroke Cerebrovasc Dis 2013; 22(8):1405–11.

22. Sinha AM, Diener HC, Morillo CA, et al. Cryptogenic stroke and underlying atrial fibrillation (CRYSTAL AF): design and rationale. Am Heart J 2010;160:36–41.e1.

23. Frustaci A, Chimenti C, Bellocci F, et al. Histological substrate of atrial biopsies in patients with lone atrial fibrillation. Circulation 1997;96:1180–4.

24. Choudhury A, Varughese GI, Lip GY. Targeting the renin-angiotensin-aldosterone-system in atrial fibrillation: a shift from electrical to structural therapy? Expert Opin Pharmacother 2005;6: 2193–207.

25. Raviele A, Ronco F. Endothelial dysfunction and atrial fibrillation: what is the relationship? J Cardiovasc Electrophysiol 2011;22:383–4.

26. Akar JG, Jeske W, Wilber DJ. Acute onset human atrial fibrillation is associated with local cardiac platelet activation and endothelial dysfunction. J Am Coll Cardiol 2008;51:1790–3.

27. Kaski JC, Arrebola-Moreno AL. Inflammation and thrombosis in atrial fibrillation. Rev Esp Cardiol 2011;64:551–3 [in Spanish].

28. Tousoulis D, Zisimos K, Antoniades C, et al. Oxidative stress and inflammatory process in patients with atrial fibrillation: the role of left atrium distension. Int J Cardiol 2009;136:258–62.

29. Tziakas DN, Chalikias GK, Papanas N, et al. Circulating levels of collagen type I degradation marker depend on the type of atrial fibrillation. Europace 2007;9:589–96.

30. Marin F, Roldan V, Climent V, et al. Is thrombogenesis in atrial fibrillation related to matrix metalloproteinase-1 and its inhibitor, TIMP-1? Stroke 2003;34:1181–6.

31. Inoue H, Nozawa T, Okumura K, et al. Prothrombotic activity is increased in patients with nonvalvular atrial fibrillation and risk factors for embolism. Chest 2004;126:687–92.

32. Varughese GI, Patel JV, Tomson J, et al. The prothrombotic risk of diabetes mellitus in atrial fibrillation and heart failure. J Thromb Haemost 2005;3: 2811–3.

33. Chung NA, Belgore F, Li-Saw-Hee FL, et al. Is the hypercoagulable state in atrial fibrillation mediated by vascular endothelial growth factor? Stroke 2002; 33:2187–91.

34. Furui H, Taniguchi N, Yamauchi K, et al. Effects of treadmill exercise on platelet function, blood coagulability and fibrinolytic activity in patients with atrial fibrillation. Jpn Heart J 1987;28: 177–84.

35. Blackshear JL, Pearce LA, Hart RG, et al. Aortic plaque in atrial fibrillation: prevalence, predictors, and thromboembolic implications. Stroke 1999;30: 834–40.

36. Anderson DC, Kappelle LJ, Eliasziw M, et al. Occurrence of hemispheric and retinal ischemia in atrial fibrillation compared with carotid stenosis. Stroke 2002;33:1963–7.

37. Carabello BA. Modern management of mitral stenosis. Circulation 2005;112:432–7.

38. The effect of low-dose warfarin on the risk of stroke in patients with nonrheumatic atrial fibrillation. The Boston Area Anticoagulation Trial for Atrial Fibrillation Investigators. N Engl J Med 1990;323: 1505–11.

39. Ezekowitz MD, Bridgers SL, James KE, et al. Warfarin in the prevention of stroke associated with nonrheumatic atrial fibrillation. Veterans Affairs Stroke Prevention in Nonrheumatic Atrial Fibrillation Investigators. N Engl J Med 1992; 327:1406–12.

40. Petersen P, Boysen G, Godtfredsen J, et al. Placebo-controlled, randomised trial of warfarin and aspirin for prevention of thromboembolic complications in chronic atrial fibrillation. The Copenhagen AFASAK study. Lancet 1989;1:175–9.

41. Connolly SJ, Laupacis A, Gent M, et al. Canadian Atrial Fibrillation Anticoagulation (CAFA) study. J Am Coll Cardiol 1991;18:349–55.

42. Stroke prevention in atrial fibrillation study. Final results. Circulation 1991;84:527–39.

43. Risk factors for stroke and efficacy of antithrombotic therapy in atrial fibrillation. Analysis of pooled data from five randomized controlled trials. Arch Intern Med 1994;154:1449–57.

44. Adjusted-dose warfarin versus low-intensity, fixed-dose warfarin plus aspirin for high-risk patients with atrial fibrillation: stroke prevention in atrial fibrillation III randomised clinical trial. Lancet 1996;348:633–8.

45. Gage BF, van Walraven C, Pearce L, et al. Selecting patients with atrial fibrillation for anticoagulation: stroke risk stratification in patients taking aspirin. Circulation 2004;110:2287–92.

46. Go AS, Hylek EM, Chang Y, et al. Anticoagulation therapy for stroke prevention in atrial fibrillation: how well do randomized trials translate into clinical practice? JAMA 2003;290:2685–92.

47. Lip GY, Nieuwlaat R, Pisters R, et al. Refining clinical risk stratification for predicting stroke and thromboembolism in atrial fibrillation using a novel risk factor-based approach: the Euro Heart Survey on atrial fibrillation. Chest 2010;137:263–72.

48. Piccini JP, Stevens SR, Chang Y, et al. Renal dysfunction as a predictor of stroke and systemic embolism in patients with nonvalvular atrial fibrillation: validation of the R(2)CHADS(2) index in the ROCKET AF (rivaroxaban once-daily, oral, direct factor Xa inhibition compared with vitamin K antagonism for prevention of stroke and embolism trial in atrial fibrillation) and ATRIA (Anticoagulation and Risk Factors in Atrial Fibrillation) study cohorts. Circulation 2013;127:224–32.

49. Zabalgoitia M, Halperin JL, Pearce LA, et al. Transesophageal echocardiographic correlates of clinical risk of thromboembolism in nonvalvular atrial fibrillation. Stroke Prevention in Atrial Fibrillation III Investigators. J Am Coll Cardiol 1998;31:1622–6.

50. Transesophageal echocardiographic correlates of thromboembolism in high-risk patients with nonvalvular atrial fibrillation. The Stroke Prevention in Atrial Fibrillation Investigators Committee on Echocardiography. Ann Intern Med 1998;128:639–47.

51. Di Biase L, Santangeli P, Anselmino M, et al. Does the left atrial appendage morphology correlate with the risk of stroke in patients with atrial fibrillation? Results from a multicenter study. J Am Coll Cardiol 2012;60:531–8.

52. Beyth RJ, Quinn LM, Landefeld CS. Prospective evaluation of an index for predicting the risk of major bleeding in outpatients treated with warfarin. Am J Med 1998;105:91–9.

53. Gage BF, Yan Y, Milligan PE, et al. Clinical classification schemes for predicting hemorrhage: results from the national registry of atrial fibrillation (NRAF). Am Heart J 2006;151:713–9.

54. Pisters R, Lane DA, Nieuwlaat R, et al. A novel user-friendly score (HAS-BLED) to assess 1-year risk of major bleeding in patients with atrial fibrillation: the Euro Heart Survey. Chest 2010;138:1093–100.

55. Fang MC, Go AS, Chang Y, et al. A new risk scheme to predict warfarin-associated hemorrhage: the ATRIA (Anticoagulation and Risk Factors in Atrial Fibrillation) study. J Am Coll Cardiol 2011; 58:395–401.

56. Seet RC, Rabinstein AA, Christianson TJ, et al. Bleeding complications associated with warfarin treatment in ischemic stroke patients with atrial fibrillation: a population-based cohort study. J Stroke Cerebrovasc Dis 2013;22:561–9.

57. Bunch TJ, Weiss JP, Crandall BG, et al. Atrial fibrillation is independently associated with senile, vascular, and Alzheimer's dementia. Heart Rhythm 2010;7:433–7.

58. Dublin S, Anderson ML, Haneuse SJ, et al. Atrial fibrillation and risk of dementia: a prospective cohort study. J Am Geriatr Soc 2011;59:1369–75.

59. Santangeli P, Di Biase L, Bai R, et al. Atrial fibrillation and the risk of incident dementia: a meta-analysis. Heart Rhythm 2012;9:1761–8.

60. Gregoire SM, Smith K, Jager HR, et al. Cerebral microbleeds and long-term cognitive outcome: longitudinal cohort study of stroke clinic patients. Cerebrovasc Dis 2012;33:430–5.

61. Lavy S, Stern S, Melamed E, et al. Effect of chronic atrial fibrillation on regional cerebral blood flow. Stroke 1980;11:35–8.

62. Anderson JL, Allen Maycock CA, Lappe DL, et al. Frequency of elevation of C-reactive protein in atrial fibrillation. Am J Cardiol 2004;94:1255–9.

63. de Leeuw FE, de Groot JC, Oudkerk M, et al. Atrial fibrillation and the risk of cerebral white matter lesions. Neurology 2000;54:1795–801.

64. Kwok CS, Loke YK, Hale R, et al. Atrial fibrillation and incidence of dementia: a systematic review and meta-analysis. Neurology 2011;76:914–22.

65. Cacciatore F, Testa G, Langellotto A, et al. Role of ventricular rate response on dementia in cognitively impaired elderly subjects with atrial fibrillation: a 10-year study. Dement Geriatr Cogn Disord 2012;34:143–8.

66. Stefansdottir H, Arnar DO, Aspelund T, et al. Atrial fibrillation is associated with reduced brain volume and cognitive function independent of cerebral infarcts. Stroke 2013;44:1020–5.

67. Bunch TJ, Crandall BG, Weiss JP, et al. Patients treated with catheter ablation for atrial fibrillation have long-term rates of death, stroke, and dementia similar to patients without atrial fibrillation. J Cardiovasc Electrophysiol 2011;22:839–45.

68. Ziegler PD, Glotzer TV, Daoud EG, et al. Detection of previously undiagnosed atrial fibrillation in patients with stroke risk factors and usefulness of continuous monitoring in primary stroke prevention. Am J Cardiol 2012;110:1309–14.

69. Glotzer TV, Daoud EG, Wyse DG, et al. The relationship between daily atrial tachyarrhythmia burden from implantable device diagnostics and stroke risk: the TRENDS study. Circ Arrhythm Electrophysiol 2009;2:474–80.

70. Glotzer TV, Hellkamp AS, Zimmerman J, et al. Atrial high rate episodes detected by pacemaker diagnostics predict death and stroke: report of the Atrial Diagnostics Ancillary Study of the Mode Selection Trial (MOST). Circulation 2003; 107:1614–9.

71. Healey JS, Connolly SJ, Gold MR, et al. Subclinical atrial fibrillation and the risk of stroke. N Engl J Med 2012;366:120–9.

72. Shanmugam N, Boerdlein A, Proff J, et al. Detection of atrial high-rate events by continuous home monitoring: clinical significance in the heart failure-cardiac resynchronization therapy population. Europace 2012;14:230–7.

73. Gaita F, Caponi D, Pianelli M, et al. Radiofrequency catheter ablation of atrial fibrillation: a cause of silent thromboembolism? Magnetic resonance imaging assessment of cerebral thromboembolism in patients undergoing ablation of atrial fibrillation. Circulation 2010;122:1667–73.

74. Gaita F, Leclercq JF, Schumacher B, et al. Incidence of silent cerebral thromboembolic lesions after atrial fibrillation ablation may change according to technology used: comparison of irrigated radiofrequency, multipolar nonirrigated catheter and cryoballoon. J Cardiovasc Electrophysiol 2011;22: 961–8.

Transesophageal Echocardiography in Atrial Fibrillation

Teerapat Yingchoncharoen, MD, Saurabh Jha, MD, MS,
Luke J. Burchill, MBBS, PhD, Allan L. Klein, MD, FASE*

KEYWORDS

- Transesophageal echocardiography • Atrial fibrillation • Stroke • Left atrial appendage

KEY POINTS

- Transesophageal echocardiography (TEE) plays an important role in atrial fibrillation (AF), mainly to detect the presence of left atrial appendage (LAA) thrombus.
- TEE has proven to be useful in direct current cardioversion guidance and is indispensable for AF ablation and LAA occlusion.
- With the increasing numbers of patients affected by AF, the use of TEE will grow and become an important screening modality for detecting LAA thrombus.
- The future direction includes broader multi-institutional use; the implementation of further strategies to risk stratify the patients; as well as the use of new oral anticoagulants and their cost-effectiveness in patients with AF undergoing direct current cardioversion, AF ablation, and LAA occlusion.

Videos of spontaneous echocardiographic contrast (SEC), sludge and thrombus accompany this article at http://www.cardiacep.theclinics.com

Atrial fibrillation (AF) is the most common pathologic supraventricular tachycardia,[1] with an overall prevalence of 0.4% to 1% in the general population, increasing with age.[2–4] The estimate of the prevalence of AF in the United States ranged from ~2.7 million to 6.1 million in 2010 and is expected to increase to between ~5.6 and 12 million in 2050.[2,5] The mean age of patients with AF is 66.8 years for men and 74.6 years for women.[6] Approximately 2% patients in AF are 60 to 69 years old and 5% are greater than or equal to 70 years old. It is more common in men than in women and in Caucasians than in African-Americans.[7–10] AF is associated with an increased long-term risk of stroke,[11] heart failure, and all-cause mortality, especially in women.[12] The age and gender-adjusted 30-day and 1-year mortality is 11% and 25% respectively.[13]

AF is characterized by chaotic contraction of the atrium resulting in loss of atrial mechanical function, which leads to impaired diastolic filling of the left ventricle and predisposes to blood stasis. The coupling of endocardial damage as well as abnormalities of coagulation, platelets and fibrinolysis fulfill Virchow's triad for thrombogenesis and is consistent with a prothrombotic or hypercoagulable state in this arrhythmia.[14] The most serious complication of AF is systemic thromboembolism. AF is associated with approximately 1 in 6 ischemic strokes.[7] Data from the

Funding Support: None.
Financial Disclosures and/or Conflict of Interest: The authors have nothing to disclose.
Department of Cardiovascular Medicine, Cleveland Clinic, 9500 Euclid Avenue, Desk J1-5, Cleveland, OH 44195, USA
* Corresponding author.
E-mail address: kleina@ccf.org

Framingham study indicated that AF alone is associated with a 3-fold to 4-fold increased risk of stroke after adjustment for other stroke risk factors.[7] An ischemic stroke may occur in patients with AF either as the initial presentation and despite appropriate antithrombotic prophylaxis. When intracardiac thrombus is identified in patients with nonvalvular AF, its location is the left atrial appendage (LAA) in more than 90% of the cases.[15]

Electrical cardioversion of patients with AF to normal sinus rhythm is performed frequently to relieve symptoms, improve cardiac performance, and possibly decrease cardioembolic risk. AF ablation has emerged as an established strategy for a restoration of sinus rhythm in patients with AF. LAA occlusion offers a theoretically appealing method to reduce the incidence of stroke. This article discusses the role of transesophageal echocardiography (TEE) in patient evaluation before cardioversion, AF ablation, and LAA occlusion.

LAA

The LAA is a small, actively contracting, fingerlike blind cul-de-sac, situated on the lateral aspect of the left atrium (LA). The mouth of the LAA is located between the left ventricle and the left upper pulmonary vein (PV), extending over the atrioventricular groove and the surface of the left ventricle toward the left circumflex artery in the anterior direction (**Fig. 1**).[16] It is variable in size (ranging from 0.77 to 19.27 cm),[17] shape, and orientation (the principal axis is markedly bent or spiral). The appendage communicates with the atrial chamber through a narrow oval-shaped orifice with a mean long diameter of 17.4 ± 4 mm and a short diameter of 10.9 ± 4.2 mm measured in heart specimens.[18] It is lined with endothelium and trabeculated by pectinate muscle. The embryology of LAA is distinct from the body of the LA. The LA is formed by the absorption of the primordial PV and its branches, resulting in the smooth-walled cavity. In contrast, the trabecular LAA is the remnant of the original primordial LA, which develops during the third week of gestation.[19] The multiple small tunnels created by pectinate muscles and the narrow apex of the LAA are the two anatomic factors that lead to thrombus formation when LAA systolic function is impaired.[20] An autopsy study of 500 normal human hearts noted that 80% of the LAAs had multiple lobes and the presence of 2 lobes was most common, found in 54% of cases, followed by 3 lobes (23%), 1 lobe (20%), and 4 lobes (3%).[21]

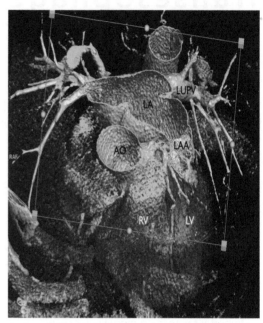

Fig. 1. Anatomic correlation of LAA and other cardiac structures. Ao, aorta; LA, left atrium; LUPV, left upper pulmonary vein; LV, left ventricle; RV, right ventricle. (*Courtesy of* Paul Schoenhagen, MD, Cleveland Clinic, Cleveland, OH.)

The LAA is best visualized in the midesophageal window starting at 0° and often with slight flexion or withdrawal of the probe to a more cranial position.[22] It is critical to image the LAA from multiple imaging planes including 0°, 45°, 90°, and 120°. The complex shape and multilobed structure of the LAA are usually only noted at an angle beyond 100° (**Fig. 2**). Often the biplane feature during TEE is used to assess the LAA in perpendicular views simultaneously and this is especially important for assessing LAA thrombus.

LAA FLOW VELOCITY PATTERN

LAA flow velocities can be assessed with TEE using pulsed wave Doppler with the sample volume placed 1 cm within the LAA. In patients with sinus rhythm, the LAA flow is quadriphasic (**Fig. 3**A, B) with a distinct pattern of contraction, as described below.[23,24]

1. During atrial systole, LAA contraction and emptying flow or late diastolic emptying velocity is seen immediately after the P wave, which is the most important wave during sinus rhythm. It is a marker of LAA contractile function; correlates with LAA ejection fraction, LA size, and pressure; and is a significant predictor of thromboembolic risk. The average LAA contraction velocity is 50 to 60 cm/s.

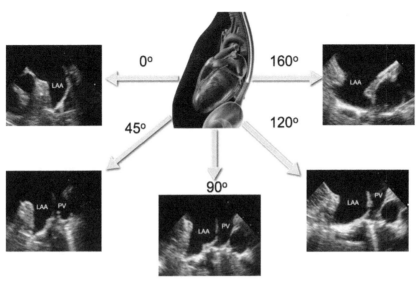

Fig. 2. Multiplane imaging of LAA at different angles from 0 to 160 degrees.

2. During early systole, LAA filling velocity is seen as a negative wave that occurs immediately after the LAA contraction. It is the result of the combined effect of LAA relaxation and elastic recoil. The average LAA filling velocity is 40 to 50 cm/s and correlates with LAA contraction velocity.

3. During the remainder of systole, systolic reflection waves are seen as low-velocity, multiple alternate inflow-outflow waves. They are usually detected in patients with a slow heart rate. Although the amplitude of these waves correlates with the LAA contraction and filling waves, their functional significance is unclear.

4. During left ventricular early diastole, early diastolic emptying velocity is seen as a low-velocity positive wave, immediately after mitral inflow E wave. The proposed mechanism underlying this wave includes a decrease in the

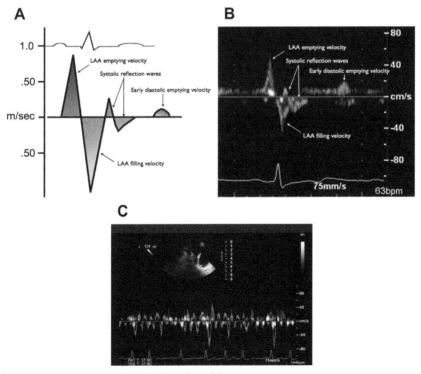

Fig. 3. LAA flow pattern in sinus rhythm (*A, B*) and AF (*C*).

LA pressure following the opening of the mitral valve, and also the external compression of LAA is caused by the distension of the LA. The average early diastolic emptying velocity is in the range of 20 to 40 cm/s and correlates with mitral E and PV diastolic velocities. Low LAA emptying velocities (<20 cm/s) is a marker of poor LAA mechanical function and correlates strongly with the presence of spontaneous echocardiographic contrast (SEC) and thrombus formation.[11] However, the results of LAA flow velocities to predict the immediate-term and long-term success of cardioversion have been inconsistent. LAA emptying velocities greater than 40 cm/s predict greater likelihood of sustained normal sinus rhythm for 1 year after cardioversion.[25]

Active LAA contraction is commonly observed in AF, with alternating positive and negative sawtooth–shaped flow signals of variable amplitude and regularity (see **Fig. 3**C).

INDICATIONS OF TEE IN AF

According to the 2011 American College of Cardiology Foundation (ACCF)/American Heart Association/Heart Rhythm Society (HRS) Guideline for Management of Atrial Fibrillation,[26] TEE is not part of the standard initial investigation of patients with AF. However, TEE could be used as an additional test in order to:

1. Detect sources and potential mechanisms of cardiogenic embolism
2. Stratify stroke risk
3. Guide cardioversion

TEE FOR ASSESSMENT OF SOURCES AND POTENTIAL MECHANISMS OF CARDIOGENIC EMBOLISM

Several TEE features have been associated with thromboembolism in patients with nonvalvular AF, including LA/LAA thrombus, LA/LAA SEC, reduced LAA flow velocity, and aortic atheromatous abnormalities.[27]

A multivariate analysis of clinical cohorts followed prospectively in clinical trials and other care settings revealed that TEE can identify thrombi in 15% to 20% of patients with AF who have clinical risk factors for ischemic stroke.[15] As mentioned, when intracardiac thrombus is identified in patients with nonvalvular AF, the location of the thrombus in more than 90% of cases is the LAA.[15]

The LAA thrombus must be differentiated from the pectinate muscles (**Table 1**), reverberation artifact originating from the Coumadin/warfarin ridge, septa between multiple lobes,[28] and severe SEC. The use of an ultrasonic contrast agent is an option for improving thrombus detection and differentiation of thrombus from artifact (**Fig. 4**). Three-dimensional TEE allows a more comprehensive assessment of multiple lobes of the LAA, which may be located in different planes (**Fig. 5**), and a more accurate estimation of LAA geometry and size.[29]

SEC, SLUDGE, AND THROMBUS

SEC is also known as smoke, a swirling haze of variable density, and reflects low blood flow velocity and nonlaminar flow.[30] It may be seen in up to 60% of patients with AF.[31] It is thought to be composed either of aggregated activated platelets and leukocytes[32] or fibrinogen-mediated erythrocyte aggregation.[33,34] Aspirin and warfarin therapy do not seem to affect the presence of LA SEC.[35] However, quantification of SEC in clinical practice is difficult and depends on image quality, gain settings, and operator experience. SEC is often graded as absent, mild or severe.[22]

Sludge is a dynamic, gelatinous, precipitous echodensity without a discrete mass and is present throughout the cardiac cycle. It is often difficult to differentiate sludge from thrombus. Sludge is thought to represent a stage beyond SEC in the continuum of thrombus formation (ie, thrombus in situ) and may have prognostic significance.[36]

Thrombus is typically a well-circumscribed and uniformly echodense intracavitary mass distinct from the underlying LA or the LAA endocardium and pectinate muscle that is present in more than 1 imaging plane. The presence of thrombus in patients with AF portends a poor prognosis because of the increased risk of thromboembolism and death,[25,37–39] and stands as an absolute contraindication to elective cardioversion and catheter ablation. TEE offers excellent visualization of the LA and LAA for thrombus with high sensitivity (92%–100%), specificity (98%–100%), and negative predictive value (98%–100%).[40–43] Despite its high accuracy, thrombi of <2 mm may be missed during TEE owing to the complex morphology of a multilobed LAA.[44] SEC, sludge, and thrombus are shown in **Fig. 6** and in Videos 1–3 (available online at http://www.cardiacep.theclinics.com).

AORTIC ATHEROMA AND OTHER SOURCES OF CARDIOGENIC EMBOLISM

Complex aortic atheroma or plaque identified by TEE is common and occurs in up to 57% of patients with AF, of whom about 25% have complex

Table 1
Differentiating features of LAA thrombus, artifacts, and pectinate muscles

Features	Thrombus	Reverberation Artifact	Pectinate Muscle
Example			
Location	Often at the tip of LAA and always confined to LAA lumen	2 times the object distance from the transducer	Confined to the body of the LAA
Motion with respect to LAA and heart movement	Independent	Fully dependent	Fully dependent
Echogenicity pattern compared with LAA walls	Different	Reverberations	Identical
Anatomic morphology	Varied but generally rounded	Consistent with object or structure causing artifact	Follow normal muscle anatomic orientation
LASEC	Often present	No relationship	No relationship

Abbreviation: LASEC, left atrial spontaneous echo contrast.
Adapted from Manning WJ. Role of echocardiography in the management of atrial fibrillation. In: Solomon SD, Bulwer BE, editors. Essential echocardiography: a practical handbook. Totowa (NJ): Springer; 2007. p. 311; with permission.

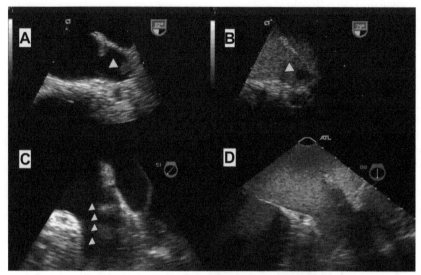

Fig. 4. Use of ultrasound contrast agent for LAA imaging. Contrast can improve the visualization of thrombus. In cases with suspected LAA thrombus (*A, arrowhead*), the persisting contrast free-area during administration of contrast indicated the presence of a thrombus (*B, arrowhead*). Contrast can also help distinguishing reverberation artifact from thrombus. In cases with reverberation artifact mimicking LAA thrombus (*C, arrowheads*), the capability of the contrast agent to completely opacify the LAA helps to exclude the LAA thrombus (*D*).

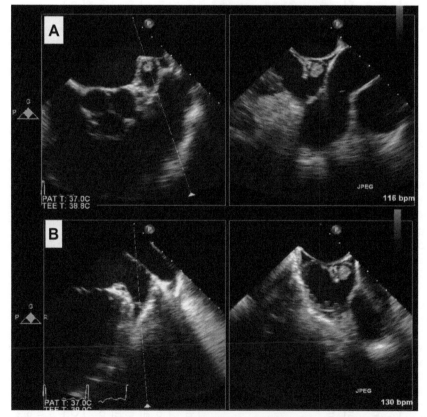

Fig. 5. Three-dimensional echocardiography using the biplane function showing a thrombus in the accessory lobe of the LAA (*A*). Conventional two-dimensional imaging of LAA at 60° (*B, left panel*) failed to detect the thrombus, which was located posteriorly in the accessory lobe (*B, right panel*).

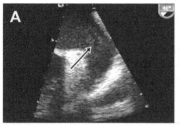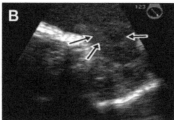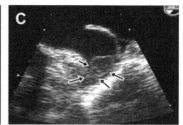

Fig. 6. SEC, sludge, and thrombus. Multiplane transesophageal echocardiographic images of the LAA (*arrows*) with smokelike echoes in SEC (*A*) (see Video 1, available online at http://www.cardiacep.theclinics.com), sludge (*B*) (see Video 2, available online at http://www.cardiacep.theclinics.com), and thrombus (*C*). (*From* Yarmohammadi H, Klosterman T, Grewal G, et al. Transesophageal echocardiography and cardioversion trends in patients with atrial fibrillation: a 10-year survey. J Am Soc Echocardiogr 2012;25:962–8; with permission.)

plaque (ie, thicker than 4 mm and with ulceration, pedunculation, or mobile elements).[45]

Complex plaque morphology has been linked to increased stroke risk.[46,47] The presence of mobile components superimposed on aortic plaque is strongly associated with brain embolization and is seen in elderly patients with stroke, with a range from 1.6% to 8.7%.[46–49]

Atrial septal defect and patent foramen ovale are not direct consequences of AF but can be identified accurately by TEE as alternative potential mechanisms for paradoxic systemic thromboembolism secondary to right-to-left shunting.

TEE-GUIDED DIRECT CURRENT CARDIOVERSION

Electrical cardioversion is the most effective method of restoring sinus rhythm and has an overall success rate of 75% to 93%. The likelihood of restoring sinus rhythm with cardioversion is inversely related to the chest wall impedance, duration of AF, LA size, and underlying heart disease.[50–52] In the absence of adequate anticoagulation, cardioversion is associated with a 5% to 7% risk of thromboembolic complications, which may be effectively reduced to <1% by therapeutic anticoagulation.[53–55] TEE is appropriate in the evaluation of patients with AF to facilitate clinical decision making with regards to anticoagulation and/or DCC according to the ACCF/American Society of Echocardiography 2011 Appropriateness Criteria for Echocardiography.[56] There are 7 appropriate indications and 4 inappropriate indications for TEE-guided direct current cardioversion (DCC) as shown by Grewal and colleagues[57] (**Box 1**). They found that most TEEs performed before DCC are appropriate (only 2.7% were deemed inappropriate), and congestive heart failure/hemodynamic compromise and being symptomatic were the most common indications. The prevalence of LA thrombus/sludge varied among indications for TEE. Temporal trends in

TEE-guided cardioversion between 1999 and 2008 at Cleveland Clinic show that the application of TEE-guided DCC has consistently increased (25% in 1999 vs 34% in 2008).[58]

When a rhythm-control strategy is chosen in patients with AF greater than or equal to 48 hours or of unknown duration, guidelines[59,60] recommend TEE to exclude LAA thrombus as an alternative to 3 weeks of effective preprocedural anticoagulation.

Box 1
Appropriate and inappropriate indications for TEE-guided DCC

Appropriate indications

1. Congestive heart failure/hemodynamic compromise

2. Symptomatic

3. Hospitalized and symptomatic

4. New-onset AF

5. High stroke risk

6. Subtherapeutic anticoagulation

7. Miscellaneous (eg, received TEE for a reason unrelated to AF such as an evaluation of valve function or endocarditis. The timing of the TEE coincidentally helped expedite DCC)

Inappropriate indications

1. Stable with therapeutic anticoagulation for greater than 3 weeks

2. AF for <48 hours

3. Permanent AF

4. Hospitalized but asymptomatic

Adapted from Grewal GK, Klosterman TB, Shrestha K, et al. Indications for TEE before cardioversion for atrial fibrillation: implications for appropriateness criteria. JACC Cardiovasc Imaging 2012;5:641–8; with permission.

The recommendation results from the findings in the landmark study entitled the Assessment of Cardioversion Using Transesophageal Echocardiography (ACUTE) Trial,[61] which was a large multicenter randomized, prospective trial of 1222 patients undergoing DCC for AF of greater than 48 hours. The trial assessed the usefulness of TEE-guided short-term anticoagulation strategy versus a conventional (3 weeks) therapeutic anticoagulation strategy (warfarin to an international normalized ratio [INR] of 2–3). Thrombus was found in 13.8% of patients who were in AF for more than 48 hours, which is comparable with other studies.[62] Both approaches were associated with comparably low risks of stroke (0.81% with the TEE approach and 0.5% with the conventional approach). After 8 weeks, there were no differences in the proportion of patients achieving successful cardioversion. However, the composite of major and minor bleeding occurred significantly less frequently in the TEE-guided arm than in the conventional arm (2.9% vs 5.5%; relative risk reduction, 0.53; P = .03), which was most likely related to the longer total duration of anticoagulation in the conventional group. The safety and efficacy of TEE-guided cardioversion with enoxaparin and unfractionated heparin were compared in the ACUTE II trial and the Anticoagulation in Cardioversion using Enoxaparin (ACE) trial. Ischemic stroke, bleeding, and death rates were not different between the patients scheduled for cardioversion of AF of more than 48 hours duration, but a TEE-guided enoxaparin strategy had a shorter duration of hospitalization.[63,64]

The new direct thrombin inhibitor, dabigatran, was recently evaluated in the substudy of the Randomized Evaluation of Long-Term Anticoagulation Therapy (RE-LY) trial, in which patients underwent cardioversion (13%–25% had precardioversion TEE) in a post-hoc analysis.[65] There was no difference in the prevalence of LAA thrombus or SEC in the 3 treatment arms (adjusted warfarin vs dabigatran 110 mg twice daily or 150 mg twice daily). The stroke and systemic embolism and bleeding rates within 30 days of cardioversion on the 2 doses of dabigatran were similar to those on warfarin with or without TEE-guidance. This finding may suggest that cardioversion can be performed on patients treated with dabigatran regardless of the use of TEE. Data from post-hoc analysis of the factor Xa inhibitor, rivaroxoban in the Efficacy and Safety Study of Rivaroxaban with Warfarin for the Prevention of Stroke and Non-Central Nervous System Systemic Embolism in Patients with Non-Valvular Atrial Fibrillation (ROCKET-AF) showed that there is no difference in the number of strokes or systemic embolisms (n = 3 in the warfarin group and n = 3 in the rivaroxaban group) over the median follow-up of 2.1 years in patients who underwent electrical cardioversion (n = 143), pharmacologic cardioversion (n = 142), or catheter ablation (n = 79).[66] Recent data from post-hoc analysis of the factor Xa inhibitor entitled Apixaban versus Warfarin in Patients with Atrial Fibrillation trial showed major cardiovascular events after cardioversion were rare and comparable between apixaban and warfarin.[67] The ongoing trial entitled Explore the Efficacy and Safety of Once-daily Oral Rivaroxaban for the Prevention of Cardiovascular Events in Subjects with Nonvalvular Atrial Fibrillation Scheduled for Cardioversion (X-VERT; ClinicalTrials.gov NCT01674647) is a prospective, randomized, open-label multicenter trial to compare the safety and efficacy of once-daily rivaroxaban versus warfarin in patients with nonvalvular AF.

Anticoagulation is required at least 4 weeks after cardioversion because of the variability of the return to fully coordinated atrial function (atrial stunning). Recovery of mechanical function may be delayed for several weeks depending in part on the duration of AF before cardioversion.[68,69] Pooled data from 32 studies of cardioversion of AF or atrial flutter suggest that 98% of clinical thromboembolic events occur within 10 days of cardioversion.[70] These data are not yet verified by prospective studies but support anticoagulation therapy for at least 4 weeks after cardioversion, or longer in patients who have thromboembolic risk factors. The anticoagulation strategies in patients who require cardioversion are summarized in **Table 2**.[71]

CHADS$_2$ SCORE AND PRE-DCC LA THROMBOGENIC MILIEU

The CHADS$_2$ score (congestive heart failure [1 point], hypertension [1 point], age >75 years [1 point], diabetes mellitus [1 point], and history of stroke transient ischemic attack or embolic event [2 points]), was shown to predict the short-term mortality in patients with AF receiving DCC. Yarmohammadi and colleagues[72] performed subgroup analysis of the ACUTE study with 541 patients who had a complete CHADS$_2$ score evaluation before DCC. The patients with a CHADS$_2$ score greater than or equal to 3 had a significantly higher all-cause mortality compared with patients with a CHADS$_2$ score less than 2 (4.3% vs 0.5%; P = .004). However, there is no clear trend in the incidence of LAA thrombus, stroke, or embolic events among patients with different CHADS$_2$ scores. The all-cause mortality difference most likely reflected the increasing burden of comorbidities with an increasing CHADS$_2$ score.

Table 2
Anticoagulation strategies in patients who require cardioversion

Length of Time in AF (h)	Elective Cardioversion	Timing and Anticoagulation Strategy
<48	Yes	Depends on the presence of risk factors for thromboembolism; may give AC in high-risk state (ie, recent postoperative mitral valve surgery)
<48	No	DCC may be performed without delay or need to start anticoagulation
>48 or unknown	Yes	A goal INR of 2.0–3.0 or possibly alternative anticoagulation with dabigatran, rivaroxaban, or apixaban for at least 3 wk before and 4 wk following DCC. Further prospective trials are needed to assess the role of these newer agents with TEE guided DCC
>48 or unknown	Yes	TEE can be performed while the patient is on IV heparin with a goal PTT ratio of 1.5–2.0 or enoxaparin and if no identifiable thrombus is present. DCC can safely be performed, followed by 4 wk of oral warfarin with goal INR of 2.0–3.0
>48 or unknown	Yes	If TEE shows a thrombus, then anticoagulation with warfarin with a goal INR of 2.0–3.0 for a period of 4–6 wk before a repeat TEE to assess for thrombus resolution. If no identifiable thrombus is visible on repeat TEE, then DCC should be followed by at least 4 wk of anticoagulation with INR of 2.0–3.0

Abbreviations: AC, anticoagulants; IV, intravenous; PTT, partial thromboplastin time.
Adapted from Zishiri ET, Callahan TD. Atrial fibrillation. In: Griffin BP, Callahan TD, Menon V, editors. Manual of cardiovascular medicine. 4th edition. Philadelphia: Lippincott Williams & Wilkins; 2013. p. 424–44; with permission.

AF ABLATION

Over the last 15 years, radiofrequency catheter ablation of the LA and PV isolation (PVI), as a potential curative treatment of AF, has rapidly evolved from an investigational procedure to a commonly performed procedure in many major hospitals throughout the world. The catheter ablation procedure was commonly recommended for patients with symptomatic AF refractory or intolerant to at least one class 1 or 3 antiarrhythmic drug. However, as per the recent consensus statement by the HRS task force released in 2012, a primary ablation procedure in patients with symptomatic AF can be considered even before a trial of antiarrhythmics and is given as a class IIa indication.[73] Restoration and maintenance of sinus rhythm by catheter ablation has been shown to significantly improve symptoms, exercise capacity, and quality of life, along with improvements in cardiac function.[26,74] Although the benefits of catheter ablation are profound, there is a potential risk of several immediate and delayed complications (some of which can be life threatening), which warrants careful patient selection and follow-up. Patients undergoing catheter ablation are usually evaluated with multimodality imaging and echocardiography, particularly TEE, which remains an integral part of the assessment. Transthoracic echocardiography (TTE) should be performed in all patients being considered as potential candidates for AF ablation to assess underlying causes and sequelae of long-standing AF as well as to precisely measure LA size, which is an important prognostic factor in predicting the risk of recurrence of atrial arrhythmias following AF ablation.[75] TEE can be performed as an alternative to detect baseline abnormalities in patients with poor transthoracic acoustic windows resulting from suboptimal images. The role of TEE in preprocedural planning, real-time intraprocedural guidance, and follow-up after catheter ablation is discussed below.

PREPROCEDURAL SCREENING AND ASSESSMENT WITH TEE

The prevalence of LA thrombus and sludge identified during TEE in patients referred for screening before AF ablation is 0.6% and 1.5% respectively.[76] The probability of identifying LA/LAA thrombus/sludge during precatheter ablation-screening TEE is directly related to the $CHADS_2$ score. Puwanant and colleagues[76] reviewed the pre-PVI TEE of 1058 patients and showed absence of thrombus or sludge in all 498 patients with a $CHADS_2$ score of 0. The HRS task force on catheter and surgical ablation of AF recommended that a screening TEE should be performed in all patients with AF more than 48 hours in duration or of an unknown duration if adequate systemic anticoagulation has not been maintained for at least 3 weeks before the ablation procedure.[73]

Several retrospective studies comparing cardiac computed tomography (CCT) with TEE have suggested a high negative predictive value of CCT to detect LA/LAA thrombus, making it a potential alternative tool for patients who cannot tolerate TEE.[77,78] In a meta-analysis by Romero and colleagues,[79] using pooled data from 19 studies and 2955 patients with AF who underwent TEE and CCT before electric cardioversion/PVI or after cardioembolic cerebrovascular accident, supported the role of CCT as a reliable alternative to TEE for detection of the LA/LAA thrombi. The mean sensitivity, specificity, positive predictive value, and negative predictive values for CCT were 96%, 92%, 41%, and 99%, respectively. The diagnostic accuracy of CCT was 94%, which was increased to 99% with the use of delayed contrast imaging.

Another important use of TEE in the preprocedural planning of an AF ablation is to provide information regarding the morphologic remodeling of the LA and PV anatomy. The most common pattern of PV anatomy is 2 separate right PVs and 2 separate left PVs. The vein draining the right middle lobe is usually a branch of the right superior PV. Variations in the PV anatomy are frequently observed, the most common being the supernumerary right PVs and a common ostium of the left PVs.[80] Although some of these variations are more frequently associated with AF, others may affect the success of the catheter ablation procedure, particularly if inadequately isolated. CCT and Cardiac Magnetic Resonance (CMR) are considered gold standard imaging modalities to define PV anatomy. Although TEE is not the first-line investigation to assess PV anatomy, it offers substantially lower costs and lack of radiation. In a study comparing different imaging modalities to assess PV anatomy, TEE identified 98% of the PVs with adequate Doppler measurements obtained. It was able to identify 83% of the PV ostia compared with computed tomography (CT); however, it underestimated the ostial diameters by 20%.[81] The identification of anatomic variations by TEE can sometimes become more challenging, but careful rotation of the probe should permit visualization of most of the veins. The left-sided PVs can be visualized at 110° with a counterclockwise rotation, whereas the right-sided veins can be seen at 45° to 60° with a clockwise rotation of the transducer.[82]

PROCEDURAL SCREENING

Intraoperative TEE provides direct visualization of the key anatomic structures and helps in various steps of the AF ablation, including transseptal puncture and optimization of catheter placement. Moreover, intraprocedural complications like thrombus formation, cardiac perforation/tamponade, mitral valve trauma, and early signs of PV stenosis can be identified promptly. In patients with chronic AF with significant LA dilatation, cardiac structures other than PVs, such as LA isthmus, coronary sinus, and LAA, may cause the initiation or perpetuation of AF. Real-time three-dimensional TEE can improve visualization of the normal anatomy and anatomic variants of left atrial segments that are potential targets for catheter ablation.[83]

Intraoperative TEE is limited by patient discomfort and the need to maintain the airway during prolonged procedures like AF ablation. Intracardiac echocardiography is frequently used by many centers and can help improve the safety and success of the ablation procedure.[84] Further details regarding the use of intracardiac echocardiography is beyond the scope of this article.

TEE FOLLOW-UP

One of the most serious complications of AF ablation is PV stenosis, which is caused by thermal injury to the PVs and is defined as a reduction of the diameter of a PV or PV branch. PV vein severity is categorized as mild, moderate, and severe based on reductions of less than 50%, 50% to 70%, and more than 70%, respectively.[73] There is a large variability in the reported incidence of PV after AF ablation, with different studies stating incidences from 0% to 38%.[73] Patients with PV stenosis often present with shortness of breath, cough, hemoptysis, chest pain, and recurrent pneumonia. With improvements in the understanding of the pathophysiology of PV stenosis, development of newer ablation techniques, avoidance of the ablation of the PV ostia, and use of intracardiac echocardiography, the incidence of PV stenosis after AF ablation has decreased.[73]

The diagnosis of PV stenosis is often reliably made by CCT and CMR. TEE is superior in providing functional data about PV flow, which may be important in making clinical diagnoses in patients with multiple comorbidities and nonspecific symptoms, as previously described. PV stenosis on TEE is suggested by a combination of anatomic narrowing, an increased pulsed Doppler flow velocity of more than 100 cm/s, and evidence of aliasing and spectral broadening on color Doppler.[85]

In a prospective single-blinded observational study, To and colleagues[82] compared the role of TEE and CT in the evaluation of the PVs before and after catheter PVI (Role of Transesophageal Echocardiography Compared to Computed Tomography in Evaluation of Pulmonary Vein Ablation for Atrial Fibrillation [ROTEA] study). Although no patients developed moderate or severe PV stenosis after PVI, there was a 30% to 50% reduction in the luminal diameter as detected by CT in 5% of patients. TEE underestimated PV ostial diameters, especially of inferior veins, compared with CT.[82] Severe spontaneous echo contrast and low LAA emptying velocities were noted in 10% of patients in sinus rhythm after PVI.

Assessment of the LA morphologic remodeling and mechanics, which can predict recurrence of atrial arrhythmias, is commonly done with TTE; however, TEE can also be used in patients with suboptimal TTE images.

PERCUTANEOUS CLOSURE DEVICES

Closure of the LAA to blood flow by transcatheter percutaneous implantation of an occluder device is an alternative strategy for reducing stroke risk in patients with nonvalvular AF who are unable to tolerate anticoagulants. The 2 LAA occlusion devices currently available are the WATCHMAN LAA closure device (Atritech Inc, Plymouth, MN; Boston Scientific, Natick, MA) and the Amplatzer cardiac plug (ACP) (St Jude Medical Inc, St. Paul, MN). Both systems use femoral venous access and transseptal puncture to deliver the device into the LA. The WATCHMAN device ranges from 21 to 33 mm and consists of a self-expanding nitinol frame that occludes the LAA lumen (**Fig. 7**A).[86] In the Watchman Left Atrial Appendage System for Embolic Protection in Patients With Atrial Fibrillation [PROTECT-AF] trial, a prospective, controlled, randomized study of patients with nonvalvular AF, the WATCHMAN occluder was noninferior to warfarin in reducing the risk of stroke, systemic emboli, or cardiovascular death.[87] Anticoagulation is indicated for 45 days after WATCHMAN implantation to allow for endothelialization,[88] although a recent nonrandomized study reported that aspirin and clopidogrel can be used in patients with an absolute contraindication to warfarin without a significant increase in stroke risk.[89]

The ACP device is a double-disc system that ranges from 16 to 30 mm and consists of a distal lobe that anchors the device in the lumen of the

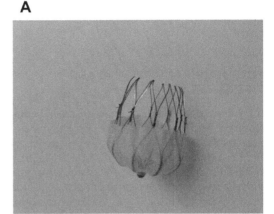

A

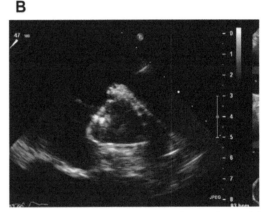

B

Fig. 7. (A) The WATCHMAN LAA occlusion device. (B) TEE image of the WATCHMAN LAA occlusion device.

LAA and a proximal disc that seals the ostium of the appendage (see **Fig. 7**B).[86] Anticoagulation is not required following deployment of the ACP occluder because dual antiplatelet therapy is effective in reducing stroke risk.[90] Friedman and colleagues[91] recently examined a novel percutaneous epicardial LAA ligation device (Aegis Medical, Vancouver, Canada) using electrical navigation and a remotely tightened suture in 4 canines. The procedure was performed successfully by single sheath puncture within the confines of the intact pericardial space. Singh and Holmes[92] also reported on a novel percutaneous pericardial snare and suture ligation device (LARIAT; SentreHeart, Palo Alto, CA) in a canine model. Nine of 10 canines underwent successful LAA closure without any leak.[93] Human studies are planned for both of these epicardial approaches.

The rate of serious adverse events after percutaneous LAA occlusion varies from 7% to 9%,[87,89,94] and such events include pericardial effusion (5%–7%), acute stroke (1%–2%), device embolization, transient myocardial ischemia, and femoral hematoma/pseudoaneurysm.[87,94,95]

Pericardial effusion and other complication rates have shown to decline with increased operator experience.[87]

PREPROCEDURAL SCREENING AND ASSESSMENT WITH TEE

TEE is the primary modality used to screen candidates for percutaneous device closure, the primary exclusion criterion being the presence of thrombus in the LAA. To guide device selection, multiplanar imaging is used to assess LAA size, shape, and lobularity. Key measurements include the dominant lobe length and the ostial diameter of the LAA, determined from multiple imaging planes including 0° (4-chamber), 45° (aortic valve), 90° (apical 2-chamber view), and 120° (long-axis view). To ensure proper anchoring and optimal closure of the LAA, devices are selected so that the diameter is larger than the ostium of the LAA. Since there is potential for device encroachment on the mitral valve and left upper PV, baseline assessment includes evaluation of mitral valve function, transmitral flow (peak E wave velocity), and PV flow.

PROCEDURAL SCREENING

TEE is used to guide transseptal puncture and verify the position of the delivery sheath before deployment of the occlusion device. Correct positioning is confirmed by good alignment of the occluder with the major axis of the LAA and by ensuring there is no interference with mitral leaflet excursion and PV flow. The WATCHMAN device should be centrally positioned and wedged in the LAA such that its orifice does not protrude out of the LAA ostium. With the ACP device, the distal anchoring lobe is deployed ~10 mm into the dominant lobe of the LAA. Without a landing zone of at least 10 mm, the ACP device cannot be used.

A complete seal of the LAA orifice must be confirmed before irretrievable release of the occluder. Color-flow Doppler is used to confirm successful occlusion, defined as grade 3 (mild/1-mm to 3-mm diameter jet) LAA leakage or better (**Table 3**).[96] Significant leakage suggests an undersized device and should prompt assessment for excessive device mobility predisposing to embolization. The location of the left circumflex artery between the LAA and anterior mitral valve leaflet raises the theoretic risk of coronary compression, which may manifest as new lateral ventricular dysfunction and/or mitral regurgitation.

Table 3
Echocardiographic color Doppler flow grading assessment of device sealing of the LAA at implantation, after the procedure, and at follow-up

Grade	Description
1	Severe leak with multiple jets of free flow
2	Moderate leak, >3-mm diameter jet
3	Mild leak, 1–3-mm diameter jet
4	Trace leak, <1-mm diameter jet
5	No leak

From Chue CD, de Giovanni J, Steeds RP. The role of echocardiography in percutaneous left atrial appendage occlusion. Eur J Echocardiogr 2011;12:i3–10; with permission.

TEE FOLLOW-UP

Echocardiographic surveillance is recommended at 1 and 6 months and then annually after the procedure.[96] The device is assessed for stability, leakage, and impingement of surrounding structures. Mitral valve function and PV flow are compared with baseline, along with LA dimensions. Device-related thrombus has been reported in up to 4% of patients following implantation of an LAA occluder.[89] Short-term anticoagulation is generally effective in resolving device-related thrombus, although this may not be a low-risk option for patients with a history of bleeding.[89,97] Recently there was a report of de-novo thrombus formation and latent ligation failure post LAA occluder deployment suggesting the need in follow-up of routine TEE and better anticoagulation rather than anti-platelets.[98] Although there is a theoretic risk of a residual atrial septal defect, most iatrogenic atrial septal defects caused by transseptal puncture close spontaneously and do not seem to be associated with an increased rate of stroke or embolization.[99]

SUMMARY

TEE plays an important role in AF, mainly to detect the presence of LAA thrombus. It has proved to be useful in DCC guidance and is indispensable for AF ablation and LAA occlusion. With the increasing numbers of patients affected by AF, the use of TEE will grow and become an important screening modality for LAA thrombus. The future direction includes broader multi-institutional use; the implementation of further tools to risk stratify the patients; and the use of a new spectrum of oral anticoagulants and their cost-effectiveness in patients with AF undergoing DCC, AF ablation, and LAA occlusion.

SUPPLEMENTARY DATA

Supplementary data related to this article can be found online at http://dx.doi.org/10.1016/j.ccep.2013.11.006.

REFERENCES

1. Link MS. Clinical practice. Evaluation and initial treatment of supraventricular tachycardia. N Engl J Med 2012;367:1438–48.

2. Go AS, Hylek EM, Phillips KA, et al. Prevalence of diagnosed atrial fibrillation in adults: national implications for rhythm management and stroke prevention: the AnTicoagulation and Risk Factors in Atrial Fibrillation (ATRIA) Study. JAMA 2001;285:2370–5.

3. Thom T, Haase N, Rosamond W, et al. Heart disease and stroke statistics–2006 update: a report from the American Heart Association Statistics Committee and Stroke Statistics Subcommittee. Circulation 2006;113:e85–151.

4. Feinberg WM, Blackshear JL, Laupacis A, et al. Prevalence, age distribution, and gender of patients with atrial fibrillation. Analysis and implications. Arch Intern Med 1995;155:469–73.

5. Miyasaka Y, Barnes ME, Gersh BJ, et al. Secular trends in incidence of atrial fibrillation in Olmsted County, Minnesota, 1980 to 2000, and implications on the projections for future prevalence. Circulation 2006;114:119–25.

6. Go AS, Mozaffarian D, Roger VL, et al. Executive summary: heart disease and stroke statistics–2013 update: a report from the American Heart Association. Circulation 2013;127:143–52.

7. Wolf PA, Abbott RD, Kannel WB. Atrial fibrillation as an independent risk factor for stroke: the Framingham Study. Stroke 1991;22:983–8.

8. Lake FR, Cullen KJ, de Klerk NH, et al. Atrial fibrillation and mortality in an elderly population. Aust N Z J Med 1989;19:321–6.

9. Phillips SJ, Whisnant JP, O'Fallon WM, et al. Prevalence of cardiovascular disease and diabetes mellitus in residents of Rochester, Minnesota. Mayo Clin Proc 1990;65:344–59.

10. Furberg CD, Psaty BM, Manolio TA, et al. Prevalence of atrial fibrillation in elderly subjects (the Cardiovascular Health Study). Am J Cardiol 1994; 74:236–41.

11. Risk factors for stroke and efficacy of antithrombotic therapy in atrial fibrillation. Analysis of pooled data from five randomized controlled trials. Arch Intern Med 1994;154:1449–57.

12. Stewart S, Hart CL, Hole DJ, et al. A population-based study of the long-term risks associated with atrial fibrillation: 20-year follow-up of the Renfrew/Paisley study. Am J Med 2002;113: 359–64.

13. Piccini JP, Hammill BG, Sinner MF, et al. Incidence and prevalence of atrial fibrillation and associated mortality among Medicare beneficiaries, 1993-2007. Circ Cardiovasc Qual Outcomes 2012;5:85–93.

14. Watson T, Shantsila E, Lip GY. Mechanisms of thrombogenesis in atrial fibrillation: Virchow's triad revisited. Lancet 2009;373:155–66.

15. Blackshear JL, Odell JA. Appendage obliteration to reduce stroke in cardiac surgical patients with atrial fibrillation. Ann Thorac Surg 1996;61:755–9.

16. Syed TM, Halperin JL. Left atrial appendage closure for stroke prevention in atrial fibrillation: state of the art and current challenges. Nat Clin Pract Cardiovasc Med 2007;4:428–35.

17. Qamruddin S, Shinbane J, Shriki J, et al. Left atrial appendage: structure, function, imaging modalities and therapeutic options. Expert Rev Cardiovasc Ther 2010;8:65–75.

18. Su P, McCarthy KP, Ho SY. Occluding the left atrial appendage: anatomical considerations. Heart 2008;94:1166–70.

19. Moore K, Persaud TVN, Torchia M. Chapter 13: cardiovascular system. In: The developing human: clinically oriented embryology. 9th edition. Saunders; 2013.

20. Ussia GP, Mule M, Cammalleri V, et al. Percutaneous closure of left atrial appendage to prevent embolic events in high-risk patients with chronic atrial fibrillation. Catheter Cardiovasc Interv 2009; 74:217–22.

21. Veinot JP, Harrity PJ, Gentile F, et al. Anatomy of the normal left atrial appendage: a quantitative study of age-related changes in 500 autopsy hearts: implications for echocardiographic examination. Circulation 1997;96:3112–5.

22. Wheeler R, Masani ND. The role of echocardiography in the management of atrial fibrillation. Eur J Echocardiogr 2011;12:i33–8.

23. Mugge A, Kuhn H, Nikutta P, et al. Assessment of left atrial appendage function by biplane transesophageal echocardiography in patients with non-rheumatic atrial fibrillation: identification of a subgroup of patients at increased embolic risk. J Am Coll Cardiol 1994;23:599–607.

24. Tabata T, Oki T, Fukuda N, et al. Influence of left atrial pressure on left atrial appendage flow velocity patterns in patients in sinus rhythm. J Am Soc Echocardiogr 1996;9:857–64.

25. Leung DY, Davidson PM, Cranney GB, et al. Thromboembolic risks of left atrial thrombus detected by transesophageal echocardiogram. Am J Cardiol 1997;79:626–9.

26. Wann LS, Curtis AB, January CT, et al. 2011 ACCF/AHA/HRS focused update on the management of patients with atrial fibrillation (updating the 2006 guideline): a report of the American College of Cardiology Foundation/American Heart Association

Task Force on Practice Guidelines. Circulation 2011;123:104–23.

27. Zabalgoitia M, Halperin JL, Pearce LA, et al. Transesophageal echocardiographic correlates of clinical risk of thromboembolism in nonvalvular atrial fibrillation. Stroke Prevention in Atrial Fibrillation III Investigators. J Am Coll Cardiol 1998;31:1622–6.

28. Mizuguchi KA, Burch TM, Bulwer BE, et al. Thrombus or bilobar left atrial appendage? Diagnosis by real-time three-dimensional transesophageal echocardiography. Anesth Analg 2009;108:70–2.

29. Providencia R, Trigo J, Paiva L, et al. The role of echocardiography in thromboembolic risk assessment of patients with nonvalvular atrial fibrillation. J Am Soc Echocardiogr 2013;26:801–12.

30. Black IW. Spontaneous echo contrast: where there's smoke there's fire. Echocardiography 2000;17:373–82.

31. Goldman ME, Pearce LA, Hart RG, et al. Pathophysiologic correlates of thromboembolism in nonvalvular atrial fibrillation: I. Reduced flow velocity in the left atrial appendage (The Stroke Prevention in Atrial Fibrillation [SPAF-III] study). J Am Soc Echocardiogr 1999;12:1080–7.

32. Zotz RJ, Muller M, Genth-Zotz S, et al. Spontaneous echo contrast caused by platelet and leukocyte aggregates? Stroke 2001;32:1127–33.

33. Mahony C, Ferguson J, Fischer PL. Red cell aggregation and the echogenicity of whole blood. Ultrasound Med Biol 1992;18:579–86.

34. Merino A, Hauptman P, Badimon L, et al. Echocardiographic "smoke" is produced by an interaction of erythrocytes and plasma proteins modulated by shear forces. J Am Coll Cardiol 1992;20:1661–8.

35. Black IW, Hopkins AP, Lee LC, et al. Left atrial spontaneous echo contrast: a clinical and echocardiographic analysis. J Am Coll Cardiol 1991;18:398–404.

36. Troughton RW, Asher CR, Klein AL. The role of echocardiography in atrial fibrillation and cardioversion. Heart 2003;89:1447–54.

37. Transesophageal echocardiographic correlates of thromboembolism in high-risk patients with nonvalvular atrial fibrillation. The Stroke Prevention in Atrial Fibrillation Investigators Committee on Echocardiography. Ann Intern Med 1998;128:639–47.

38. Bernhardt P, Schmidt H, Hammerstingl C, et al. Atrial thrombi–a prospective follow-up study over 3 years with transesophageal echocardiography and cranial magnetic resonance imaging. Echocardiography 2006;23:388–94.

39. Dawn B, Varma J, Singh P, et al. Cardiovascular death in patients with atrial fibrillation is better predicted by left atrial thrombus and spontaneous echocardiographic contrast as compared with clinical parameters. J Am Soc Echocardiogr 2005;18:199–205.

40. Aschenberg W, Schluter M, Kremer P, et al. Transesophageal two-dimensional echocardiography for the detection of left atrial appendage thrombus. J Am Coll Cardiol 1986;7:163–6.

41. Fatkin D, Scalia G, Jacobs N, et al. Accuracy of biplane transesophageal echocardiography in detecting left atrial thrombus. Am J Cardiol 1996;77:321–3.

42. Manning WJ, Weintraub RM, Waksmonski CA, et al. Accuracy of transesophageal echocardiography for identifying left atrial thrombi. A prospective, intraoperative study. Ann Intern Med 1995;123:817–22.

43. Olson JD, Goldenberg IF, Pedersen W, et al. Exclusion of atrial thrombus by transesophageal echocardiography. J Am Soc Echocardiogr 1992;5:52–6.

44. Halperin JL, Gomberg-Maitland M. Obliteration of the left atrial appendage for prevention of thromboembolism. J Am Coll Cardiol 2003;42:1259–61.

45. Blackshear JL, Pearce LA, Hart RG, et al. Aortic plaque in atrial fibrillation: prevalence, predictors, and thromboembolic implications. Stroke 1999;30:834–40.

46. Toyoda K, Yasaka M, Nagata S, et al. Aortogenic embolic stroke: a transesophageal echocardiographic approach. Stroke 1992;23:1056–61.

47. Vaduganathan P, Ewton A, Nagueh SF, et al. Pathologic correlates of aortic plaques, thrombi and mobile "aortic debris" imaged in vivo with transesophageal echocardiography. J Am Coll Cardiol 1997;30:357–63.

48. Jones EF, Kalman JM, Calafiore P, et al. Proximal aortic atheroma. An independent risk factor for cerebral ischemia. Stroke 1995;26:218–24.

49. Di Tullio MR, Sacco RL, Savoia MT, et al. Aortic atheroma morphology and the risk of ischemic stroke in a multiethnic population. Am Heart J 2000;139:329–36.

50. Dalzell GW, Anderson J, Adgey AA. Factors determining success and energy requirements for cardioversion of atrial fibrillation. Q J Med 1990;76:903–13.

51. Gallagher MM, Guo XH, Poloniecki JD, et al. Initial energy setting, outcome and efficiency in direct current cardioversion of atrial fibrillation and flutter. J Am Coll Cardiol 2001;38:1498–504.

52. Lundstrom T, Ryden L. Chronic atrial fibrillation. Long-term results of direct current conversion. Acta Med Scand 1988;223:53–9.

53. Klein AL, Murray RD, Grimm RA. Role of transesophageal echocardiography-guided cardioversion of patients with atrial fibrillation. J Am Coll Cardiol 2001;37:691–704.

54. Arnold AZ, Mick MJ, Mazurek RP, et al. Role of prophylactic anticoagulation for direct current cardioversion in patients with atrial fibrillation or atrial flutter. J Am Coll Cardiol 1992;19:851–5.

55. Weinberg DM, Mancini J. Anticoagulation for cardioversion of atrial fibrillation. Am J Cardiol 1989; 63:745–6.

56. American College of Cardiology Foundation Appropriate Use Criteria Task Force, American Society of Echocardiography, American Heart Association, et al. ACCF/ASE/AHA/ASNC/HFSA/HRS/SCAI/SCCM/SCCT/SCMR 2011 appropriate use criteria for echocardiography. A report of the American College of Cardiology Foundation Appropriate Use Criteria Task Force, American Society of Echocardiography, American Heart Association, American Society of Nuclear Cardiology, Heart Failure Society of America, Heart Rhythm Society, Society for Cardiovascular Angiography and Interventions, Society of Critical Care Medicine, Society of Cardiovascular Computed Tomography, and Society for Cardiovascular Magnetic Resonance Endorsed by the American College of Chest Physicians. J Am Coll Cardiol 2011;57:1126–66.

57. Grewal GK, Klosterman TB, Shrestha K, et al. Indications for TEE before cardioversion for atrial fibrillation: implications for appropriateness criteria. JACC Cardiovasc Imaging 2012;5:641–8.

58. Yarmohammadi H, Klosterman T, Grewal G, et al. Transesophageal echocardiography and cardioversion trends in patients with atrial fibrillation: a 10-year survey. J Am Soc Echocardiogr 2012; 25:962–8.

59. European Heart Rhythm Association, European Association for Cardio-Thoracic Surgery, Camm AJ, et al. Guidelines for the management of atrial fibrillation: the Task Force for the Management of Atrial Fibrillation of the European Society of Cardiology (ESC). Eur Heart J 2010;31:2369–429.

60. Wann LS, Curtis AB, Ellenbogen KA, et al. 2011 ACCF/AHA/HRS focused update on the management of patients with atrial fibrillation (update on Dabigatran): a report of the American College of Cardiology Foundation/American Heart Association Task Force on practice guidelines. Circulation 2011;123:1144–50.

61. Klein AL, Grimm RA, Murray RD, et al. Use of transesophageal echocardiography to guide cardioversion in patients with atrial fibrillation. N Engl J Med 2001;344:1411–20.

62. Wann LS, Curtis AB, Ellenbogen KA, et al. 2011 ACCF/AHA/HRS focused update on the management of patients with atrial fibrillation (update on dabigatran): a report of the American College of Cardiology Foundation/American Heart Association Task Force on Practice Guidelines. J Am Coll Cardiol 2011;57:1330–7.

63. Klein AL, Jasper SE, Katz WE, et al. The use of enoxaparin compared with unfractionated heparin for short-term antithrombotic therapy in atrial fibrillation patients undergoing transoesophageal echocardiography-guided cardioversion: Assessment of Cardioversion Using Transoesophageal Echocardiography (ACUTE) II randomized multicentre study. Eur Heart J 2006;27:2858–65.

64. Stellbrink C, Nixdorff U, Hofmann T, et al. Safety and efficacy of enoxaparin compared with unfractionated heparin and oral anticoagulants for prevention of thromboembolic complications in cardioversion of nonvalvular atrial fibrillation: the Anticoagulation in Cardioversion using Enoxaparin (ACE) trial. Circulation 2004;109:997–1003.

65. Nagarakanti R, Ezekowitz MD, Oldgren J, et al. Dabigatran versus warfarin in patients with atrial fibrillation: an analysis of patients undergoing cardioversion. Circulation 2011;123:131–6.

66. Piccini JP, Stevens SR, Lokhnygina Y, et al. Outcomes after cardioversion and atrial fibrillation ablation in patients treated with rivaroxaban and warfarin in the ROCKET AF trial. J Am Coll Cardiol 2013;61:1998–2006.

67. Flaker G, Lopez RG, Al-Khatib SM, et al. Efficacy and safety of Apixaban in patients following cardioversion for atrial fibrillation: Insights from the ARISTOTLE trial. J Am Coll Cardiol 2013 (Epub ahead of print).

68. Manning WJ, Silverman DI, Katz SE, et al. Temporal dependence of the return of atrial mechanical function on the mode of cardioversion of atrial fibrillation to sinus rhythm. Am J Cardiol 1995;75:624–6.

69. Grimm RA, Leung DY, Black IW, et al. Left atrial appendage "stunning" after spontaneous conversion of atrial fibrillation demonstrated by transesophageal Doppler echocardiography. Am Heart J 1995;130:174–6.

70. Berger M, Schweitzer P. Timing of thromboembolic events after electrical cardioversion of atrial fibrillation or flutter: a retrospective analysis. Am J Cardiol 1998;82:1545–7 A8.

71. Zishiri ET, Callahan TD. Atrial fibrillation. In: Griffin BP, Callahan TD, Menon V, et al, editors. Manual of cardiovascular medicine. 4th edition. Philadelphia: Lippincott Williams & Wilkins; 2013. p. 424–44.

72. Yarmohammadi H, Varr BC, Puwanant S, et al. Role of CHADS2 score in evaluation of thromboembolic risk and mortality in patients with atrial fibrillation undergoing direct current cardioversion (from the ACUTE trial substudy). Am J Cardiol 2012;110: 222–6.

73. Calkins H, Kuck KH, Cappato R, et al. 2012 HRS/EHRA/ECAS expert consensus statement on catheter and surgical ablation of atrial fibrillation: recommendations for patient selection, procedural techniques, patient management and follow-up, definitions, endpoints, and research trial design: a report of the Heart Rhythm Society (HRS) Task

Force on Catheter and Surgical Ablation of Atrial Fibrillation. Developed in partnership with the European Heart Rhythm Association (EHRA), a registered branch of the European Society of Cardiology (ESC) and the European Cardiac Arrhythmia Society (ECAS); and in collaboration with the American College of Cardiology (ACC), American Heart Association (AHA), the Asia Pacific Heart Rhythm Society (APHRS), and the Society of Thoracic Surgeons (STS). Endorsed by the governing bodies of the American College of Cardiology Foundation, the American Heart Association, the European Cardiac Arrhythmia Society, the European Heart Rhythm Association, the Society of Thoracic Surgeons, the Asia Pacific Heart Rhythm Society, and the Heart Rhythm Society. Heart Rhythm 2012;9:632–96.e21.

74. Hsu LF, Jais P, Sanders P, et al. Catheter ablation for atrial fibrillation in congestive heart failure. N Engl J Med 2004;351:2373–83.

75. Themistoclakis S, Schweikert RA, Saliba WI, et al. Clinical predictors and relationship between early and late atrial tachyarrhythmias after pulmonary vein antrum isolation. Heart Rhythm 2008;5: 679–85.

76. Puwanant S, Varr BC, Shrestha K, et al. Role of the CHADS2 score in the evaluation of thromboembolic risk in patients with atrial fibrillation undergoing transesophageal echocardiography before pulmonary vein isolation. J Am Coll Cardiol 2009; 54:2032–9.

77. Jaber WA, White RD, Kuzmiak SA, et al. Comparison of ability to identify left atrial thrombus by three-dimensional tomography versus transesophageal echocardiography in patients with atrial fibrillation. Am J Cardiol 2004;93:486–9.

78. Kim YY, Klein AL, Halliburton SS, et al. Left atrial appendage filling defects identified by multidetector computed tomography in patients undergoing radiofrequency pulmonary vein antral isolation: a comparison with transesophageal echocardiography. Am Heart J 2007;154:1199–205.

79. Romero J, Husain SA, Kelesidis I, et al. Detection of left atrial appendage thrombus by cardiac computed tomography in patients with atrial fibrillation: a meta-analysis. Circ Cardiovasc Imaging 2013;6:185–94.

80. Marom EM, Herndon JE, Kim YH, et al. Variations in pulmonary venous drainage to the left atrium: implications for radiofrequency ablation. Radiology 2004;230:824–9.

81. Wood MA, Wittkamp M, Henry D, et al. A comparison of pulmonary vein ostial anatomy by computerized tomography, echocardiography, and venography in patients with atrial fibrillation having radiofrequency catheter ablation. Am J Cardiol 2004;93:49–53.

82. To AC, Gabriel RS, Park M, et al. Role of transesophageal echocardiography compared to computed tomography in evaluation of pulmonary vein ablation for atrial fibrillation (ROTEA study). J Am Soc Echocardiogr 2011;24:1046–55.

83. Faletra FF, Ho SY, Regoli F, et al. Real-time three dimensional transoesophageal echocardiography in imaging key anatomical structures of the left atrium: potential role during atrial fibrillation ablation. Heart 2013;99:133–42.

84. Ruisi CP, Brysiewicz N, Asnes JD, et al. Use of intracardiac echocardiography during atrial fibrillation ablation. Pacing Clin Electrophysiol 2013;36: 781–8.

85. Sigurdsson G, Troughton RW, Xu XF, et al. Detection of pulmonary vein stenosis by transesophageal echocardiography: comparison with multidetector computed tomography. Am Heart J 2007;153:800–6.

86. Chue CD, de Giovanni J, Steeds RP. The role of echocardiography in percutaneous left atrial appendage occlusion. Eur J Echocardiogr 2011; 12:i3–10.

87. Holmes DR, Reddy VY, Turi ZG, et al. Percutaneous closure of the left atrial appendage versus warfarin therapy for prevention of stroke in patients with atrial fibrillation: a randomised non-inferiority trial. Lancet 2009;374:534–42.

88. Sick PB, Schuler G, Hauptmann KE, et al. Initial worldwide experience with the WATCHMAN left atrial appendage system for stroke prevention in atrial fibrillation. J Am Coll Cardiol 2007;49:1490–5.

89. Reddy VY, Mobius-Winkler S, Miller MA, et al. Left atrial appendage closure with the Watchman device in patients with a contraindication for oral anticoagulation: the ASAP study (ASA Plavix Feasibility Study With Watchman Left Atrial Appendage Closure Technology). J Am Coll Cardiol 2013;61: 2551–6.

90. Meier B, Palacios I, Windecker S, et al. Transcatheter left atrial appendage occlusion with Amplatzer devices to obviate anticoagulation in patients with atrial fibrillation. Catheter Cardiovasc Interv 2003; 60:417–22.

91. Friedman PA, Asirvatham SJ, Dalegrave C, et al. Percutaneous epicardial left atrial appendage closure: preliminary results of an electrogram guided approach. J Cardiovasc Electrophysiol 2009;20:908–15.

92. Singh IM, Holmes DR Jr. Left atrial appendage closure. Curr Cardiol Rep 2010;12:413–21.

93. Lee RJ, Bartus K, Yakubov SJ. Catheter-based left atrial appendage (LAA) ligation for the prevention of embolic events arising from the LAA: initial experience in a canine model. Circ Cardiovasc Interv 2010;3:224–9.

94. Whitlock RP, Healey JS, Connolly SJ. Left atrial appendage occlusion does not eliminate the

need for warfarin. Circulation 2009;120:1927–32 [discussion: 32].

95. Park JW, Bethencourt A, Sievert H, et al. Left atrial appendage closure with Amplatzer cardiac plug in atrial fibrillation: initial European experience. Catheter Cardiovasc Interv 2011;77:700–6.

96. Block PC, Burstein S, Casale PN, et al. Percutaneous left atrial appendage occlusion for patients in atrial fibrillation suboptimal for warfarin therapy: 5-year results of the PLAATO (Percutaneous Left Atrial Appendage Transcatheter Occlusion) Study. JACC Cardiovasc Interv 2009;2:594–600.

97. Cruz-Gonzalez I, Martin Moreiras J, Garcia E. Thrombus formation after left atrial appendage exclusion using an Amplatzer cardiac plug device. Catheter Cardiovasc Interv 2011;78:970–3.

98. Gray J, Rubenson D. De-novo thrombus formation and latent ligation failure following LAA exclusion. JACC Cardiovasc Imaging 2013;6:1218–9.

99. Singh SM, Douglas PS, Reddy VY. The incidence and long-term clinical outcome of iatrogenic atrial septal defects secondary to transseptal catheterization with a 12F transseptal sheath. Circ Arrhythm Electrophysiol 2011;4:166–71.

Drug Therapies for Stroke Prevention in Atrial Fibrillation
An Historical Perspective

Albert L. Waldo, MD

KEYWORDS

• Stroke prevention • Atrial fibrillation • Oral anticoagulants

KEY POINTS

In patients with atrial fibrillation:

- Increasing age is a major stroke risk, but the elderly, who need stroke prophylaxis therapy the most, are less likely to receive anticoagulant therapy.
- Aspirin is of questionable use for stroke prophylaxis.
- The new oral anticoagulants are largely an upgrade from warfarin therapy for stroke prophylaxis, but well managed warfarin therapy remains an acceptable and inexpensive treatment option.

INTRODUCTION

In a letter to *The Lancet* on June 10, 1972,[1] C. Miller Fisher, a neurologist at the Massachusetts General Hospital in Boston, wrote the following:

Sir, Your editorial (May 6, p. 1002) on the electrical conversion of atrial fibrillation provides an opportunity to comment on the long-term management of the many patients who remain in fibrillation. In our cerebrovascular studies, we have been struck by the number of patients in atrial fibrillation who have a severe stroke as the first manifestation of embolism. In the past year, 11 such patients, all over the age of 60, have been admitted to the Massachusetts General Hospital, and of these, 8 had otherwise been in relatively good health. 7 were diagnosed as having arteriosclerotic heart-disease, 4 rheumatic. It is our impression from this experience that all patients with chronic atrial fibrillation should be considered for longer-term prophylactic anticoagulant therapy before the first embolus. It is, of course, realised that the total number of those in fibrillation from whom these patients were selected is unknown, but this may not be important, since anticoagulant therapy reduces embolism and, when carefully regulated, is safe, particularly when compared with the prospect of a major stroke and a fate almost worse than death itself.

Thus, not so long ago, not only was the association of atrial fibrillation with stroke not well appreciated, but also neither was the prospect of long-term anticoagulation for stroke prevention. Not so long ago, the association of atrial fibrillation with embolic stroke, and the possibility of its prevention with oral anticoagulation, was only an idea. It was even believed that atrial fibrillation was only a marker for stroke, rather than a cause. It took a study from Framingham[2] to put that notion to rest. The Framingham group compared the incidence of strokes in patients in their 60s, 70s, and 80s who did not have atrial fibrillation with those who did. As expected, the incidence of stroke in patients without atrial fibrillation increased with each decade, but in each decade,

Supported in part by: The Jennie Zoline, Blue Dot, Glenstone and CMJ Amelior Foundations.
Division of Cardiovascular Medicine, University Hospitals Case Medical Center, 11100 Euclid Avenue, MS LKS 5038, Room 3080, Cleveland, OH 44106, USA
E-mail address: albert.waldo@case.edu

Card Electrophysiol Clin 6 (2014) 61–78
http://dx.doi.org/10.1016/j.ccep.2013.11.005
1877-9182/14/$ – see front matter © 2014 Elsevier Inc. All rights reserved.

there were always about 5 times more strokes in people with than without atrial fibrillation (**Table 1**). That study made it clear that atrial fibrillation was not simply a marker, but rather a cause of embolic stroke. However, it has also been known for many years that not all strokes in patients with atrial fibrillation are caused by clots that embolize from the left atrium.[3]

The Establishment of Warfarin Therapy for Stroke Prevention in Atrial Fibrillation

This review most often refers to warfarin rather than vitamin K antagonists (VKAs). That decision is because many of the studies cited used warfarin rather than other VKAs. In some studies, the type of VKA used was optional, but data on warfarin are applicable to all VKAs.

The efficacy of warfarin for stroke prevention in atrial fibrillation was shown by 5 intention-to-treat trials performed in the late 1980s and into the 1990s. They were the AFASAK (Copenhagen Atrial Fibrillation, Aspirin, Anti-Koagulation) trial,[4] the SPAF I (Stroke Prevention in Atrial Fibrillation I) trial,[5] the BAATAF (Boston Area Anticoagulation Trial for Atrial Fibrillation) trial,[6] the CAFA (Canadian Atrial Fibrillation Anticoagulation) trial,[7] and the SPINAF (Stroke Prevention in Nonvalvular Atrial Fibrillation) trial.[8] They were all prospective, randomized, placebo-controlled trials of warfarin versus placebo for the prevention of thromboembolic complications associated with atrial fibrillation. Some of these studies included randomization to an aspirin arm. All reported significant efficacy of warfarin over placebo except CAFA.[7] That study was stopped early before completion of its planned recruitment of 630 patients because of the publication of 2 other positive studies of similar design and objective. Thus, although the study showed efficacy for warfarin compared with placebo (**Fig. 1**), the confidence intervals (CIs) were wide because the

study randomized only 187 patients to warfarin and 191 patients to placebo. Nevertheless, when the data were pooled from these 5 studies,[9] they showed a risk reduction of 68% ($P = .001$; 95% CI, 50–79). When an on-treatment analysis of these studies was performed, there was an 83% risk reduction ($P<.001$; 95% CI, 69–90).[10] This factor essentially means that if warfarin is given to a patient with atrial fibrillation and an international normalized ratio (INR) in the therapeutic range (2–3) is maintained, the patient's risk for stroke is reduced to the same level as the risk that would be present if they were in sinus rhythm.

Most of those studies were performed in an era before the INR became a standard for measuring the adequacy of anticoagulation when using a VKA. Use of the INR was an important milestone, especially because a therapeutic range, with a target INR of 2.5, was established.[11,12] It also became clear that when the INR decreased to less than 2, there was a steep increase in the odds ratio for stroke, such that an INR of 1.7 doubled the risk of stroke, and an INR of 1.5 more than tripled the risk of stroke (**Fig. 2**). Moreover, these studies also showed that the risk of bleeding was flat from an INR of 1.5 to an INR of about 3.5 (**Fig. 2**). Thus, decreasing the INR to less than 2 does not decrease the risk of bleeding, but does increase the risk of stroke. The lessons learned were that it was important to maintain an INR in the therapeutic range to minimize the occurrence of embolic strokes, and that there was a critical and relatively safe range for this. The reason the target was 2.5 (ie, in the middle of the range) was that there are many uncertainties associated with administration of warfarin, in considerable part because of its interaction with numerous drugs (>100 were listed in the 2004 *Physicians' Desk Reference*) and foods so that the INR could be expected to vary over time.

Table 1
Data from the atrial fibrillation and stroke Framingham study with a 30-year follow-up

Age Group (y)	Previous Atrial Fibrillation (%)	Stroke per 1000 py$_O$	Stroke per 1000 py$_{AF}$	Incidence Density Ratio	Pop. AR (%)[a]
60–69	1.8	4.5	21.2	4.7	7.3
70–79	4.7	9.0	48.9	5.4	16.5
80–89	10.2	14.3	71.4	5.0	30.8

Abbreviations: Pop. AR, population attributable risk; py$_{AF}$, patient years with atrial fibrillation; py$_O$, patient years, no atrial fibrillation; (y), years.
[a] Adjusted for blood pressure.
Data from Wolf PA, Abbott RD, Kannell WB. Atrial fibrillation: a major contributor to stroke in the elderly. The Framingham Study. Arch Intern Med 1987;147:1561–4.

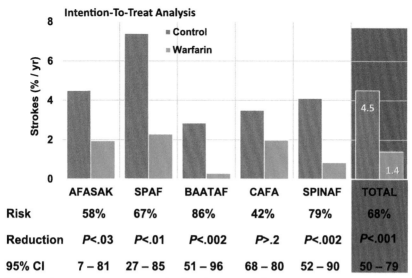

Fig. 1. Warfarin for stroke prevention in AF. Stroke data from 5 trials (AFASAK, SPAF, BAATAF, CAFA, and SPINAF) of warfarin versus placebo in patients with atrial fibrillation. See text for discussion. CI, confidence interval. (*From* Atrial Fibrillation Investigators. Risk factors for stroke and efficacy of antithrombotic therapy in atrial fibrillation. Analysis of pooled data from 5 randomized controlled trials. Arch Intern Med 1994;154:1449–57; with permission.)

Risk Factors for Stroke in Patients with Atrial Fibrillation

The Atrial Fibrillation Investigators' (AFI) analysis of the first 5 studies showed that not all patients with atrial fibrillation have the same risk for stroke.[9] AFI showed that stroke risk may be stratified by several factors, including a previous thromboembolic stroke or transient ischemic attack, hypertension, diabetes, congestive heart failure, poor left ventricular function, and age 65 years or older.

The stroke risk was further stratified into mild, moderate, and severe categories. Other risks, such as coronary artery disease, peripheral vascular disease, gender, thyrotoxicosis, rheumatic mitral valve disease, and hypertrophic cardiomyopathy were also important risk markers to consider.

A meta-analysis of data from several clinical trials[13] indicated that paroxysmal atrial fibrillation carried the same risk for stroke as persistent or

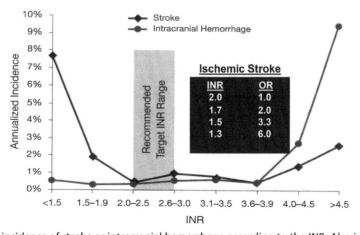

Fig. 2. Annualized incidence of stroke or intracranial hemorrhage according to the INR. Also included is the odds ratio (OR) for ischemic stroke based on the INR in patients who have atrial fibrillation. See text for discussion. INR, International Normalized Ratio; OR, odds ratio. (*Data from* Hylek EM, Skates SJ, Sheehan MA, et al. An analysis of the lowest effective intensity of prophylactic anticoagulation for patients with nonrheumatic atrial fibrillation. N Engl J Med 1996;335:540–6; and Hylek EM, Go AS, Chang Y, et al. Effect of intensity of oral anticoagulation on stroke severity and mortality in atrial fibrillation. N Engl J Med 2003;349:1019–26.)

permanent atrial fibrillation. However, patients younger than 65 years with lone atrial fibrillation (ie, atrial fibrillation in the absence of structural heart disease) have a very low risk for stroke, such that when weighing the benefits and risks of oral anticoagulation therapy per se, there was no benefit to treatment with oral anticoagulation. The opposite was true in the presence of risk factors for stroke.

To translate these risks derived from group data to the individual, several stroke risk stratification schemes are available. The $CHADS_2$ (**Fig. 3**) is a scheme that has been widely used for many years, and, until recently, was recommended for use by most guidelines on the treatment of atrial fibrillation.[14] Recently, the CHA_2DS_2 VASc stroke risk stratification score[15] has taken prominence, ostensibly because it is more accurate at identifying those at the low range of risk who probably do not need prophylactic oral anticoagulation. Nevertheless, the c-statistic for each of these stroke risk schemes is modest at best.[16,17] In a study published in 2007, the c-statistic for several stroke risk schemes ranged from 0.56 to 0.69. The c-statistic for $CHADS_2$ was 0.58. The best, still modest, was for the Framingham scheme,[16] at 0.69 (**Table 2**). The Framingham stroke risk stratification scheme[17] (**Fig. 4**) provides a 5-year risk of stroke, and emphasizes the importance of increasing age, higher systolic blood pressures, and being female (**Fig. 4**), but a copy of its scoring scheme is generally required for handy reference to apply it properly. This necessity is because the scheme assigns points relative to risk, and varies considerably depending on age and systolic blood pressure, among other variables, so that it is not easily remembered. So, too, for the latest, the ATRIA (Anticoagulation and Risk Factors in Atrial Fibrillation) stroke risk scheme (**Table 3**).[18] It, too, emphasizes increasing age as a risk, and, in terms of more recently calculated c-statistics,[18] has the best c-statistic (0.73), compared with $CHADS_2$ (0.69) and CHA_2DS_2 VASc (0.70), although still modest.

Underuse of Oral Anticoagulants

Although VKAs have clearly been shown to be effective as prophylaxis for patients with atrial fibrillation at risk for stroke, many studies have reported its underuse, even in patients with clear indications and no contraindications for such prophylaxis. As shown in numerous studies, the use of warfarin for stroke prevention in patients with atrial fibrillation who are eligible for warfarin is 41% to 65%.[19–25]

VKA use has been associated with several well-recognized problems which contribute to its management difficulty and underuse. These problems

CHADS₂

Risk Factor	Score
Cardiac failure	1
HTN	1
Age ≥75 y	1
Diabetes	1
Stroke	2

CHA₂DS₂-VASc

Risk Factor	Score
Cardiac failure	1
HTN	1
Age ≥75 y	2
Diabetes	1
Stroke	2
Vascular disease (MI, PAD, aortic atherosclerosis)	1
Age 65-74 y	1
Sex category (female)	1

Total Score	Annual Risk of Stroke (%)	
0	1.9	0
1	2.8	1.3
2	4.0	2.2
3	CHADS₂ → 5.9	3.2
4	8.5	4.0
5	12.5	6.7 ← CHA₂DS₂-VASc
6	18.2	9.8
7		9.6
8		6.7
9		15.2

Fig. 3. Two stroke risk stratification schemes: $CHADS_2$ and CHA_2DS_2 VASc. Also listed is the annual risk of stroke in percent based on the possible scores for each of these risk stratification schemes. See text for discussion. (*Data from* Gage BF, Waterman AD, Shannon W, et al. Validation of clinical classification schemes for predicting stroke: results of the National Registry of Atrial Fibrillation. JAMA 2001;285:2864–70; and European Heart Rhythm Association, European Association for Cardio-Thoracic Surgery, Camm AJ, et al. Guidelines for the management of atrial fibrillation: the Task Force for the Management of Atrial Fibrillation of the European Society of Cardiology (ESC). Eur Heart J 2010;31:2369–429.)

Table 2
c-Statistic for several risk stratification schemes used to predict atrial fibrillation–related thromboembolism

Risk Score	c-Statistic
ATRIA	0.73[a]
AF investigators	0.56
SPAF	0.60
CHADS$_2$	0.58/0.69[a]
CHA$_2$DS$_2$VaSc	0.70[a]
Framingham	0.62
7th American College of Chest Physicians	0.56

Stroke risk scheme and associated c-statistic from 2 different studies.

[a] Full score *data from* Singer DE, Chang Y, Borowsky LH, et al. A new risk scheme to predict ischemic stroke and other thrombo-embolism in atrial fibrillation: the ATRIA study stroke risk score. J Am Heart Assoc 2013;2(3):e000250. http://dx.doi.org/10.1161/JAHA.113.000250. See text for discussion.

Data from Fang MC, Go AS, Chang Y, et al. For the ATRIA Study Group. Comparison of risk stratification schemes to predict thromboembolism in people with nonvalvular atrial fibrillation. J Am Coll Cardiol 2008;51:810–15.

include its delayed onset and offset of action (eg, it may take several weeks to establish a stable dose of VKA to achieve and maintain an INR in the therapeutic range); the dose response to VKAs is unpredictable, so that the appropriate dose varies widely from patient to patient; there are numerous drug-drug and drug-food interactions, which often confound management with VKAs; its well-recognized narrow therapeutic range requires INR monitoring, and necessitates VKA dose adjustments; it is metabolized by the CYP450 enzyme system; it has common genetic polymorphisms (especially 2C9), which affect dose requirements; it has slow reversibility; and its use is inconvenient for patients and physicians. For patients who do take a VKA, data have shown that less than two-thirds have an INR in the therapeutic range at any one time, and, most often, less than half of the patients have an INR in the therapeutic range at any given time.[26] The latter is important because, as indicated earlier, if the INR decreases to less than 2, there is a steep increase in the odds ratio for stroke.[11,12]

The National Anticoagulation Benchmark and Outcomes Report (NABOR)[19] was a study of patients discharged from academic medical centers,

Framingham Risk Score
Predicted 5-Year Risk of Stroke in AF

Step 1

Age, y	Points
55-59	0
60-62	1
63-66	2
67-71	3
72-74	4
75-77	5
78-81	6
82-85	7
86-90	8
91-93	9
>93	10

Step 2

Sex	Points
Men	0
Women	6

Step 3

Systolic blood pressure, mm Hg	Points
<120	0
120-139	1
140-159	2
160-179	3
>179	4

Step 4

Diabetes	Points
No	0
Yes	5

Step 5

Prior stroke or TIA	Points
No	0
Yes	6

Add up points from steps 1 through 5

Look up predicted 5-year-risk of stroke in table

Points	5-year risk, %
0-1	5
2-3	6
4	7
5	8
6-7	9
8	11
9	12
10	13
11	14
12	16
13	18
14	19
15	21
16	24
17	26
18	28
19	31
20	34
21	37
22	41
23	44
24	48
25	51
26	55
27	59
28	63
29	67
30	71
31	75

Fig. 4. The Framingham risk score for predicting the 5-year risk of stroke in patients who have atrial fibrillation. See text for discussion. (*From* Wang TJ, Massaro JM, Levy D, et al. A risk score for predicting stroke or death in individuals with new-onset atrial fibrillation in the community: the Framingham Heart Study. JAMA 2003;290:1052; with permission.)

Table 3
The ATRIA stroke risk model point scoring system for stroke risk in atrial fibrillation

Risk Factor	Without Previous Stroke		With Previous Stroke	
	Points	Hazard Ratio	Points	Hazard Ratio
Age				
≥85 y	6	6.38	9	11.92
75–84 y	5	3.79	7	7.61
65–74 y	3	2.10	7	7.89
<65 y	0	—	8	8.99
Female	1	1.52	1	—
Diabetes	1	1.40	1	—
CHF	1	1.27	1	—
Hypertension	1	1.24	1	—
Proteinuria	1	1.40	1	—
eGFR <45 or ESRD	1	1.33	1	—

Possible point scores range from 0 to 12 for those without a previous stroke, and from 7 to 15 with a previous stroke. See text for discussion.

Abbreviations: CHF, congestive heart failure; eGFR, estimated glomerular filtration rate; ESRD, end-stage renal disease; y, years.

Data from Singer DE, Chang Y, Borowsky LH, et al. A new risk scheme to predict ischemic stroke and other thromboembolism in atrial fibrillation: the ATRIA study stroke risk score. J Am Heart Assoc 2013;2:e000250. http://dx.doi.org/10.1161/JAHA.113.000250.

Veterans Administration hospitals, and community hospitals. One of its objectives was to assess characteristics, risk factors, and antithrombotic treatment of atrial fibrillation in patients enrolled in a national multicenter database. This study found that patients with paroxysmal atrial fibrillation were significantly less likely (P<.001) to receive warfarin than patients with persistent or permanent atrial fibrillation, despite the fact that, as indicated earlier, data show that there is no significant difference in the incidence of stroke between these groups.[13] Also, although fall risk is perceived as an important factor in lack of administration of warfarin, there was no difference in fall risk between those who received warfarin and those who did not (P = .15).[13]

Other remarkable data from the NABOR (National Anticoagulation Benchmark Outcomes Report) study, and confirmed by other studies,[27] concern the 20.7% of all study patients who had a previous cardiovascular accident, transient ischemic attack (TIA) or systemic embolic event. In this cohort with the highest expected annual stroke rate, only 61.2% of patients received warfarin; 20.9% received aspirin only, and 17.9% received no treatment. Receiving no treatment is bad enough, but receiving aspirin is not much better. As is known from EAFT (European Atrial Fibrillation Trial), in patients with a previous stroke, TIA, or systemic embolism, treatment only with aspirin was associated with a 10.5%

annual stroke risk, and no treatment with a 12.6% annual stroke risk.[28] Thus, the latter two groups of patients received either treatment not indicated (aspirin) by guidelines or no treatment at all.

There are also relevant lessons learned from the AFFIRM (Atrial Fibrillation Follow-up Investigation of Rhythm Management) trial.[29] When the AFFIRM trial started in 1995, it was considered that one of the benefits of sinus rhythm was that patients did not have to take an anticoagulant despite the presence of stroke risks. When the trial ended, 57% of the strokes in the rhythm control arm occurred in people who were not taking warfarin (**Table 4**). Another 22% of strokes occurred in patients whose INR was less than 2. This finding is where the dictum of once on an oral anticoagulant, always on an oral anticoagulant comes from. Even in the rate control arm, one-third of the strokes occurred in patients who were not taking warfarin (**Table 4**), a protocol violation. This was not the first time that a study had shown that patients who have indications for continued oral anticoagulation because of stroke risks in the presence of atrial fibrillation stop taking their anticoagulant. Another 36% of patients in the rate control arm who had a stroke had an INR that was less than 2 (ie, out of therapeutic range, another well-known difficulty with warfarin therapy). Of course, there may be legitimate reasons for stopping anticoagulation (eg, bleeding), which is one of the reasons why it

Table 4
Relationship of ischemic stroke to the INR in the presence or absence of atrial fibrillation from the AFFIRM trial

	Rate Control (n) (%)	Rhythm Control (n) (%)
Ischemic stroke	77 (5.5)[a]	80 (7.1)[a]
INR ≥2.0	24 (31)	17 (21)
INR <2.0	28 (36)	18 (22)
Not taking warfarin	25 (33)	45 (57)
AF at time of event	53 (69)	30 (37)

Abbreviations: AF, atrial fibrillation; INR, International Normalized Ratio.
[a] Event rates derived from Kaplan-Meier analysis, P = .79.
Data from Wyse DG, Waldo AL, DiMarco JP, et al. A comparison of rate control and rhythm control in patients with atrial fibrillation. N Engl J Med 2002;347:1825–33; and Sherman DG, Kim SG, Boop BS, et al. National Heart, Lung and Blood Institute AFFIRM Investigators. Occurrence and characteristics of stroke events in the Atrial Fibrillation Follow-up Investigation of Sinus Rhythm Management (AFFIRM) study. Arch Intern Med 2005; 165(10):1185–91.

is preferred to have patients in sinus rhythm if it can be achieved safely and effectively.

Underuse of VKAs in Elderly Patients

The underuse of anticoagulation in the elderly is of particular concern, because stroke risk increases with increasing age. As reported by Friberg and colleagues,[30] in the Swedish atrial fibrillation cohort study of 182,678 patients with nonvalvular atrial fibrillation, the hazard ratio for stroke from age 65 years to 74 years was 2.97, relatively high, but from 75 years of age or older, it is much higher, at 5.28. Similar data were seen in the ATRIA study.[17] Yet, although the stroke risk increases with age, the use of anticoagulation decreases with age.[31] The NABOR study reported that for patients aged 80 years or older, there was a significant decrease (P>.01) in administering warfarin compared with those younger than 80 years, which was associated with a high perceived or actual bleeding risk. Nevertheless, although the bleeding risk was recognized as being higher in those older than 75 years compared with those younger, it did not make a difference in the use of warfarin until patients became older than 80 years. For all patients in the same study, the perceived or actual bleeding risk was not different between those who did or did not receive warfarin (P = .22) until patients were older than age 80 years, when it was significantly less.

Several factors seem to be involved in this underuse. In addition to the many problems with warfarin use cited earlier, the greatest concern is the risk for bleeding, particularly intracranial bleeding, and particularly as a result of falls or frailty. Thus, although the risk of ischemic stroke increases as people grow older, so does the risk of bleeding.[32,33] This concern for bleeding led, at one point, to a class II recommendation from the American College of Cardiology (ACC)/American Heart Association (AHA)/European Society of Cardiology (ESC) in their 2001 Guidelines to aim for a lower INR, target 2.0, range 1.6 to 2.5, for the primary prevention of ischemic stroke and systemic embolism in patients older than 75 years who are considered at increased risk of bleeding complications, but have no frank contraindications to oral anticoagulant therapy, and have had no previous stroke.[34] This recommendation was surprising, because the risk of bleeding is flat from an INR of 1.5 to about 3.5 (**Fig. 2**).[33] So, such therapy would only expose the patient to increased risk for stroke without a decreased risk of bleeding. This guideline is no longer present. Also, because the base rate of ischemic stroke is considerably greater than the risk of intracranial bleeding, the risk of ischemic stroke in the absence of anticoagulant therapy is considerably greater than the risk of intracranial bleeding while receiving an oral anticoagulant.[30,35] With the new oral anticoagulants, the risk of intracranial bleeding has been shown to be significantly less than with VKAs (see the following sections).

DRUG THERAPY FOR STROKE PREVENTION
Warfarin (VKA) Therapy

Warfarin has some long-established advantages. It has a long half-life, an established therapeutic range, and once-daily dosing. An antidote is available. Assessment of compliance is available. Its role in cardioversion and atrial fibrillation ablation is understood. It is cheap. No dosage adjustment is necessary for patients with renal impairment. Dose-adjusted warfarin therapy reduces the stroke risk by about two-thirds. It is as or more effective than new oral anticoagulants when the time in therapeutic range is 72% or greater. It is believed to be better for use in patients with coronary artery disease. Its almost 60 years of use has shown its pluses and minuses.

The importance of time in therapeutic range is now well established.[36] An INR between 2 and 3 is the recommended range for achieving a satisfactory blood level of warfarin, the target being 2.5. The problem is that keeping patients consistently in the therapeutic range is difficult. In an analysis of 8 trials published since 2000 by Argarwal and colleagues,[26] the INR ranged from 55% of the time in the ROCKET AF trial to 68% of the time in the SPORTIF V (Stroke prevention using an oral thrombin inhibitor in atrial fibrillation V) trial. Analysis of the ACTIVE W (Atrial Fibrillation Clopidogrel Trial with Irbasartan for Prevention of Vascular Events) trial, which was stopped early because of the clear efficacy of warfarin over clopidogrel plus aspirin for stroke prevention in patients with atrial fibrillation, showed that the INR was in the therapeutic range for 65% or less of the time, the efficacy results comparing warfarin with clopidogrel and aspirin were not different.

ROLE OF ASPIRIN IN PATIENTS WITH ATRIAL FIBRILLATION AT RISK FOR STROKE

Among the several studies that have compared aspirin with warfarin, it is clear that warfarin is superior to aspirin in diminishing the risk of stroke.[37] The first study to examine this was AFASAK.[4] In the AFASAK trial, the incidence of thromboembolic complications and vascular mortality was significantly lower in the warfarin group than in the aspirin and placebo groups, and the last 2 groups did not differ significantly from each other. However, with regard to safety, there were more bleeding episodes with warfarin than with aspirin. Of the several studies that have compared aspirin with placebo, only SPAF I reported a relative risk reduction in stroke with use of aspirin.[38] That study is not only an outlier, but it has also driven the meta-analyses of the several trials with aspirin that indicate that aspirin is clearly inferior to warfarin, but significantly better than placebo. Underappreciated from the SPAF I trial data is the clear internal inconsistency between patients in group I (comparing warfarin, aspirin, and placebo in patients eligible for warfarin) and patients in group II (comparing aspirin with placebo in patients with a relative or absolute contraindication to warfarin). Analysis of the data from this trial is informative (**Fig. 5**). Comparing outcomes in patients randomized to aspirin versus placebo in group I, there was only 1 event (stroke) in patients receiving aspirin, versus 18 events in patients receiving placebo. This finding was highly statistically significant (P<.001; a risk reduction of 94%). However, in group II, there were 25 events in patients receiving aspirin versus 26 events in patients receiving placebo. This finding was not statistically significant (P = .75, risk reduction 8%). Thus, there was an internal inconsistency. When the data from both groups were combined, the data were significant (P = .02, risk reduction 42%), but this was driven by what seems to be the outlier data from

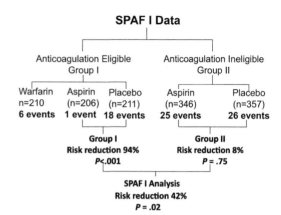

Fig. 5. Analysis of the data from the SPAF I trial in patients taking aspirin compared with patients taking placebo. The group I data also include data from patients taking warfarin. See text for discussion. (*Adapted from* The Stroke Prevention in Atrial Fibrillation Investigators. A differential effect of aspirin on prevention of stroke in atrial fibrillation. J Stroke Cerebrovasc Dis 1993;3:181–8.)

group I. Moreover, CIs of the combined data are necessarily extremely wide. It is also instructive to go back to the original publication of the SPAF I data[5] and, thereby, learn that in the warfarin-eligible group I patients, there were 6 strokes in the 210 patients receiving warfarin (ie, 6 times more strokes than in the 206 aspirin patients in group I) (**Fig. 5**). That finding emphasizes the outlier nature of outcome data for the patients taking aspirin in group I.

It is still further instructive to look at the SPAF III data.[39] When it was realized that it was no longer ethical to have a placebo arm, all SPAF I placebo patients were then randomized to warfarin versus aspirin (SPAF II).[40] The outlier aspirin patient data remained, affecting the conclusions of SPAF II. However, the SPAF investigators were concerned about the bleeding rate in the SPAF I and II trials. They used the prothrombin time ratio to monitor patients taking warfarin because the INR was not yet in standard use. When the INR became available, these investigators saw that the INR in these trials ranged from 2 to 4.5, apparently explaining the high bleeding rate.[40] The concern for bleeding, and the development of the AFI stroke risk schemes led to SPAF III.[39] The premise of SPAF III was that although warfarin was clearly effective in stroke prevention in atrial fibrillation, there was an important associated bleeding risk. Also, it was recognized that aspirin was not as effective as warfarin, but it was associated with less bleeding. The hope for SPAF III was that in patients with atrial fibrillation and stroke risk, aspirin could be combined with low-dose warfarin (target INR range of 1.2–1.5) to find if they could be as effective as warfarin alone with an INR between 2 and 3, target 2.5, but with less bleeding. The trial was stopped early because of the high stroke rate in patients in the combination low-dose warfarin-aspirin therapy arm. The stroke rate was 7.9%/y, the same rate as in the placebo arm in SPAF I. The SPAF III conclusion was that low-dose warfarin when combined with aspirin is not sufficient to prevent stroke or systemic embolism in high-risk patients with atrial fibrillation. Moreover, the major bleeding rate was identical in both groups. Low-risk patients who were not randomized to the main trial (ie, low-dose warfarin-aspirin vs standard-dose warfarin) were given only aspirin, and served as the nonrandomized aspirin-only low-stroke-risk study cohort. These were patients who had none of the high-risk AFI features (female, age >75 years, impaired left ventricular function, current systolic blood pressure greater than 160 mm Hg, or previous thromboembolism). When the SPAF III trial ended, simply a history of hypertension conferred a 3.6%/y risk of stroke in this aspirin-only low-risk cohort.[41]

It is instructive again to have a still closer look at the data from the SPAF trials. In the SPAF I and II trials, when the INRs were calculated later, they ranged from 2.0 to 4.5.[9,40] This finding was associated with a 4.2% annual rate of major hemorrhage and a 1.8% annual rate of intracranial hemorrhage. This finding, then, was the major source of concern over major bleeding with use of warfarin. However, when the SPAF III data are examined, in the patients who were randomized to the cohort with INR between 2 and 3, target 2.5, the annual rate of major hemorrhage per year was only 2.1%, and only 0.5% for intracranial hemorrhage, compared with those randomized to the aspirin–low-dose warfarin arm (INR 1.2–1.5), in whom there was a 2.4% annual hemorrhage rate per year and a 0.9% rate of intracranial hemorrhage per year.[39]

With subsequent studies, the data continued to mount about the lack of adequate efficacy for stroke prevention with use of aspirin. Hylek and colleagues[12] retrospectively studied the effects of the intensity of oral anticoagulation on stroke severity and mortality in a cohort of 13,559 patients with nonvalvular atrial fibrillation with 596 ischemic strokes. These investigators found that in patients with strokes on warfarin in whom the INR was 2 or greater, the severity and risk of death from stroke was reduced. When the INR was 2 or greater, there was only a 1% incidence of fatal in-hospital stroke, and only a 4% incidence of severe strokes with total dependence, whereas with aspirin use, there was a 6% rate of in-hospital

fatal strokes, and a 7% rate of severe strokes with total dependence. If the patient had a stroke while taking warfarin, but the INR was less than 2, the results were similar to those taking aspirin. In addition, comparing the 30-day total mortality, there was a 6% rate in the warfarin arm in the therapeutic range, and a 15% rate in the aspirin arm.

The BAFTA (Birmingham Atrial Fibrillation Treatment of the Aged) study[42] was a prospective, randomized, open-label trial comparing warfarin versus aspirin for stroke prevention in an elderly community population (everyone with atrial fibrillation was >75 years of age), with a blind assessment of end points. The BAFTA study was to determine the benefits and risks of oral anticoagulant versus aspirin therapy in reducing embolic stroke and systemic emboli in patients with atrial fibrillation without rheumatic heart disease. The primary aim was to compare the frequency of fatal and nonfatal disabling stroke (ischemic or hemorrhagic), intracranial hemorrhage, and other clinically significant arterial embolism in patients who had been randomly assigned to warfarin versus aspirin. In this aged population, as shown in **Table 5**, the stroke rate was 1.6% on warfarin, but 3.4% on aspirin ($P = .003$), and fatal strokes were not significantly different between the groups, although the rate was only 1% on warfarin versus 1.6% on aspirin. For disabling nonfatal strokes, the rate was 0.6%/y on warfarin versus 1.8%/y on aspirin ($P = .005$). Regarding the type of stroke, the rate of ischemic stroke was 0.8% on warfarin versus 2.5% on aspirin ($P = .0004$), but there was no difference in hemorrhagic stroke and no difference in intracranial hemorrhage (0.5% vs 0.4%; $P = .83$; 0.2% vs 0.1%, $P = .65$, respectively). There was also no difference in systemic embolism ($P = .36$). Thus, even in the elderly, there was no advantage of aspirin over conventional anticoagulation, in this case, warfarin. As commented by Garcia and Hylek[43] in their editorial accompanying publication of the article in *The Lancet*, "Mant and colleagues enrolled an unprecedented number of patients in an age group that has been largely under represented in randomized trials. BAFTA firmly establishes the superior efficacy of warfarin as a stroke prevention strategy in elderly patients with atrial fibrillation." Later, in a meta-analysis, van Walraven and colleagues[44] concluded that "as patients with atrial fibrillation age, the relative efficacy of antiplatelet therapy to prevent ischemic stroke appears to decrease, whereas it does not change for oral anticoagulation. Because stroke risk increases with age, the absolute benefit of oral anticoagulation increases as patients get older. These data provide more support for the use of oral anticoagulation in the

Table 5
The BAFTA study

	Warfarin (n = 488)		Aspirin (n = 485)		Warfarin vs Aspirin	
	n	Risk/y (%)	n	Risk/y (%)	RR (95% CI)	P
Stroke	21	1.6	44	3.4	0.46 (0.26–0.79)	.003
By severity						
Fatal	13	1.0	21	1.6	0.59 (0.27–1.24)	.14
Disabling nonfatal	8	0.6	23	1.8	0.33 (0.13–0.77)	.005
Type of stroke[a]						
Ischemic	10	0.8	32	2.5	0.30 (0.13–0.63)	.0004
Hemorrhagic	6	0.5	5	0.4	1.15 (0.29–4.77)	.83
Unknown	5	0.4	7	0.5	0.69 (0.17–2.51)	.53
Other ICH (subdural)[b]	2	0.2	1	0.1	1.92 (0.10–1113.3)	.65
Systemic embolism[c]	1	0.1	3	0.2	0.32 (0.01–3.99)	.36
Total number of events	24	1.8	48	3.8	0.48 (0.28–0.80)	.0027

This table presents the data on the primary events of warfarin versus aspirin for stroke prevention in an elderly community with atrial fibrillation. See text for discussion.

Abbreviations: ICH, intracranial hemorrhage; RR, relative risk.

[a] Type of stroke as determined by the end-point committee.
[b] Two of these were fatal (1 in each treatment group).
[c] Two of the systemic emboli were fatal (1 in each treatment group).

From Mant J, Hobbs FD, Fletcher K, et al. BAFTA Investigators. Midland Research Practices Network (MidReC). Warfarin versus aspirin for stroke prevention in an elderly community population with atrial fibrillation (the Birmingham Atrial Fibrillation Treatment of the Aged Study, BAFTA): a randomised controlled trial. Lancet 2007;370:497; with permission.

elderly, and for the fact that aspirin isn't of much, if any, use at all for prophylaxis against stroke."

Next came ACTIVE W, comparing the efficacy of clopidogrel plus aspirin versus VKAs in reducing the risk of vascular events in patients with atrial fibrillation.[36] The trial was stopped early because the primary end point of stroke, systemic embolism, myocardial infarction, and vascular death reached the point at which it was clear that VKA therapy was superior to the combination of clopidogrel plus aspirin. Looking at only the cumulative risk of stroke comparing clopidogrel plus aspirin versus VKA therapy, the relative risk of vascular events was 1.72 (P = .001) in favor of VKAs.

Then, there is the Japan Atrial Fibrillation Stroke Trial (JAST).[45] Because of the frequent hemorrhagic complications of oral anticoagulation therapy in Japanese patients, JAST examined the efficacy and safety of aspirin therapy in Japanese patients with nonvalvular atrial fibrillation at low risk in a prospective, randomized, multicenter trial. Patients with nonvalvular atrial fibrillation were randomized to aspirin (150–200 mg daily), or control (neither an antiplatelet agent nor an oral anticoagulant). The primary end points included cardiovascular death, symptomatic brain infarct, or TIA. After 426 patients were randomized to aspirin, and 445 to no therapy, the trial was stopped early

because there were 27 primary end points (3.1%/y; 95% CI, 2.1%–4.6%/y) with aspirin versus 23 (2.4%/y; 95% CI, 1.5%–3.5%/y) in controls, suggesting a low possibility of superiority of aspirin therapy for prevention of the primary end point. In addition, therapy with aspirin caused a marginally increased risk of major bleeding (7 patients; 1.6%) compared with controls (2 patients; 0.4%) (Fisher exact test P = .101). The study concluded that for stroke prevention in patients with nonvalvular atrial fibrillation, aspirin at 150 to 200 mg/d is neither effective nor safe.

Next came ACTIVE A,[46] a trial of aspirin versus the combination of aspirin and clopidogrel in patients ostensibly unsuitable for a VKA. There were fewer strokes in the aspirin-clopidogrel arm versus the aspirin arm (2.4%/y vs 3.3%/y, respectively; relative risk, 0.72); but there were more major bleeds with aspirin/clopidogrel versus aspirin (2.0%/y vs 1.3%/y, respectively; relative risk, 1.57). As observed by Go[47] in an accompanying editorial

...neither regimen studied in ACTIVE A was as effective as VKA therapy in prevention of ischemic stroke. And the rates of strokes in patients receiving clopidogrel and aspirin (2.4%) or aspirin alone (3.3%) were notably

higher than in patients at high risk for stroke who received high quality VKA therapy (approximately 1.1%–1.3%). These high stroke rates were seen despite the fact that nearly 40% of ACTIVE A patients had a $CHADS_2$ score of 0 or 1 (low predicted risk of stroke), and 34% had a $CHADS_2$ score of 2 (moderate predicted risk of stroke).

The AVERROES (Apixaban Versus Acetylsalicylic Acid [ASA] to prevent strokes in atrial fibrillation patients who have failed or are unsuitable for Vitamin K Antagonist Treatment) trial[48] of apixaban versus aspirin in patients unsuitable for warfarin is described later in the section on apixaban. However, the story is the same, putting the nail in the coffin for aspirin as either effective or safer prophylaxis against stroke in patients with atrial fibrillation at stroke risk.

Impact of the Aspirin Data on the Guidelines

Based on the preceding discussion, it should come as no surprise that the 2010 European Society of Cardiology Guidelines for the Management of Atrial Fibrillation[15] recommended that for a CHA_2DS_2-VASc score of 1, although oral anticoagulation or aspirin were options, they preferred oral anticoagulation. For a CHA_2DS_2-VASc score of 0, no therapy or aspirin were considered options, but no therapy was preferred. In their 2012 Focused Update,[49] it was recommended that because of poor efficacy and the risk of bleeding complications, aspirin or aspirin plus clopidogrel should be used for stroke prevention only in patients who refuse to take oral anticoagulants.

The Canadian Cardiovascular Society Guidelines[50] only list aspirin as an option with a $CHADS_2$ score = 0 if the patient either was female or had peripheral vascular disease. The guidelines indicate that most patients at intermediate risk for stroke ($CHADS_2$ = 1) should receive oral anticoagulant therapy, "…but aspirin is a reasonable alternative in some as indicated by risk-benefit" (risk benefit is not further defined).

The 2012 American College of Chest Physicians (ACCP) Guidelines of Antithrombotic Therapy for Atrial Fibrillation, Ninth Edition[51] indicate that for patients with atrial fibrillation, including those with paroxysmal atrial fibrillation at low risk of stroke ($CHADS_2$ score of 0), no therapy is suggested rather than antithrombotic therapy. For patients who do choose antithrombotic therapy, aspirin 75 mg to 325 mg once daily is suggested, rather than oral anticoagulation or combination therapy with aspirin and clopidogrel. For patients with atrial fibrillation, including those with paroxysmal atrial fibrillation at intermediate risk for stroke (a $CHADS_2$ score of 1), oral anticoagulation is recommended rather than no therapy. Furthermore, oral anticoagulation is suggested rather either than aspirin (75 mg–325 mg once daily) or combination therapy with aspirin and clopidogrel. For patients unsuitable or who choose not to take an oral anticoagulant (for reasons other than concerns about major bleeding), combination therapy with aspirin and clopidogrel is suggested rather than aspirin (75 mg–325 mg once daily). The ACCP 2012 Guidelines suggest that for a $CHADS_2$ score of 0, no therapy rather than antithrombotic therapy is recommended; for a $CHADS_2$ score of 1, oral anticoagulation rather than no therapy; and oral anticoagulation rather than either aspirin or aspirin plus clopidogrel is recommended. For a $CHADS_2$ score of 2 or greater, oral anticoagulation is recommended rather than no therapy, rather than aspirin, and rather than aspirin plus clopidogrel. The 2013 ACC/AHA/Heart Rhythm Society (HRS) Atrial Fibrillation Treatment Guidelines draft also largely eliminates aspirin therapy, but its publication must be awaited before its recommendations can be definitively reported.

The New Oral Anticoagulants (Dabigatran, Rivaroxaban, Apixaban, Edoxaban)

There are 4 new oral anticoagulants, 3 of which have been approved for use in patients. The 4 are dabigatran (Pradaxa), rivaroxaban (Xarelto), apixaban (Eliquis), and edoxaban (Lixiana). Potential advantages include: fast onset and offset of action; significantly less intracerebral bleeding; no routine coagulation monitoring required; predictable pharmacodynamics and pharmacokinetics; a broad therapeutic window; a short half-life; and minimal influence of comedications and food. Such characteristics clearly are an advantage over VKAs. Thus, the new agents hold promise of benefits to individual patients and to public health. They remove many, if not most, of the burdens associated with taking warfarin and have a significantly lower associated risk of intracranial hemorrhage. They also have the potential to replace poor-quality VKA anticoagulation and to attract patients with atrial fibrillation who have avoided warfarin therapy. Also, they have the potential to lead to greater persistence in taking oral anticoagulants. These factors can increase the proportion of patients with atrial fibrillation at intermediate to high risk for stroke who receive effective stroke prevention therapy.

However, there are some potential disadvantages as well. They include no validated tests to measure anticoagulation effects; there is no established therapeutic range; there is no antidote for most agents;

whom and how to switch from warfarin; compliance assessment is more difficult than with VKAs; the potential for long-term adverse effects and events is unknown; balancing cost against efficacy is unclear; and there is a lack of head-to-head studies comparing the new agents. The new anticoagulants should be used with care in patients with poor renal function. Factor Xa inhibitors are less dependent on renal excretion than dabigatran (for apixaban ~27%, rivaroxaban ~33%, edoxaban ~35%, and dabigatran ~80%). Because renal elimination is important for all these drugs, although monitoring of the INR is no longer necessary, monitoring of renal function at appropriate intervals (at least every 6 months) is indicated. They should be used with care in frail elderly patients; dosing in the elderly is poorly understood, and may involve changes in hepatic or renal function or tissue metabolism. All these drugs have interactions with *P*-glycoprotein inhibitors and inducers, and all but dabigatran have interactions with CYP3A4 enzyme inhibitors and inducers.

Although there have been no head-to-head studies of these new oral anticoagulants, some characteristics can be compared (**Table 6**). Dabigatran is a direct thrombin (factor IIa) inhibitor, whereas rivaroxaban, apixaban, and edoxaban are factor Xa inhibitors. Dabigatran and apixaban are administered twice daily (every 12 hours), whereas rivaroxaban and edoxaban are administered once daily. The dabigatran pill that is swallowed is a prodrug, dabigatran extilate, which is metabolized in the gut to dabigatran. Its oral bioavailability is only 6.5%. Bioavailability of the other 3 drugs is more than 40%. Rivoraxaban needs to be taken with a meal to maximize

absorption. The half-life of dabigatran is 12 to 17 hours, of rivaroxaban, 9 to 12 hours, of apixaban 8 to 15 hours, and of edoxaban 8 to 11 hours. The time to maximum inhibition by these drugs is 30 minutes to 2 hours for dabigatran, 1 to 4 hours for rivaroxaban and apixaban, and 1 to 2 hours for edoxaban. With this rapid onset of action, there is virtually never a need for bridging when using these new agents. Regarding dose adjustment, for dabigatran, the dose is 150 mg twice daily, except for patients with a creatinine clearance (CrCl) 15 to 30 mL/min, when it is 75 mg twice daily; for rivaroxaban, for patients with a CrCl greater than 50 mL/min, it is 20 mg once daily with the evening meal, except for patients with CrCl 15 to 50 mL/min, when it is 15 mg once daily with the evening meal; for apixaban, it is 5 mm twice daily, except that there is a dose adjustment to 2.5 mg twice daily if 2 of the following 3 are present: age 80 years or older, weight less than 60 kg; creatinine 5 mg/dL or greater. The results of the ENGAGE AF trial and presumed approval by the US Food and Drug Administration (FDA) for the dosing of edoxaban are awaited.

CLINICAL TRIALS WITH THE NEW ORAL ANTICOAGULANTS
Dabigatran

The major clinical trial with dabigatran in patients with nonvalvular fibrillation was RE-LY (Randomized evaluation of long-term anticoagulant therapy).[52] It was a noninferiority, randomized, open-label trial in patients with atrial fibrillation and 1 or more risk factors for stroke in the absence of a contraindication and with blinded adjudication

Table 6
New oral anticoagulants: comparison of selected data

	RE-LY	ROCKET AF	ARISTOTLE	ENGAGE AF-TIMI 48
Drug	Dabigatran	Rivaroxaban	Apixaban	Edoxaban
Dose studied (mg)	150, 110	20	5	60, 30
Dose frequency	Twice daily	Daily	Twice daily	Daily
Drug target	Factor IIa	Factor Xa	Factor Xa	Factor Xa
Subjects studied	18,113	14,264	18,206	21,105
Half-life (h)/time to maximum inhibition (h)	12–17/0.5–2	9–12/1–4	8–15/1–4	8–11/1–2
First efficacy end point	Stroke/SEE	Stroke/SEE	Stroke/SEE	Stroke/SEE
Dose adjustment (mg) for age, weight, or GFR	No	Yes 20 → 15	Yes 5 → 2.5	Yes 60 → 30 30 → 15
Mode of elimination (%)	Renal 80	Renal ~36	Renal ~27	Renal ~35

Abbreviations: GFR, glomerular filtration rate; SEE, systemic embolic event.
Data from Refs.[59–62]

of events. The primary efficacy outcome was systemic embolism. The primary safety outcome was major bleeding. In RE-LY, 18,113 patients with nonvalvular atrial fibrillation were randomized 2:1 to dabigatran versus warfarin. The randomization to dabigatran dose was blinded and divided into a dose of 150 mg twice daily, or a dose of 110 mg twice daily. To be eligible, patients had to have 1 or more of the following characteristics: a previous stroke or TIA; a left ventricular ejection fraction less than 40 or New York Heart Association heart failure class II: age 75 years or older: age 65 to 74 years with diabetes mellitus, hypertension, or coronary artery disease. The average time in therapeutic range of those who were assigned to warfarin was 64%. In terms of stroke, analysis of the data showed that the 150-mg dose of dabigatran was superior to warfarin (P<.001), but the 110-mg dose was only noninferior to warfarin (P<.001). In terms of major bleeding, the 110-mg dose was superior to warfarin (P = .003), but the 150-mg dose was only noninferior to warfarin. With regard to intracranial hemorrhage, both the 110-mg and 150-mg doses were superior to warfarin (P<.001 for both the 110-mg dose, and the 150-mg dose). The 110-mg dose was not approved by the FDA because they did not see any advantage to that dose, and believed that the superiority to warfarin of the 150-mg dose for ischemic stroke was too important. They were apparently not influenced by the significantly less major bleeding with the 110-mg dose compared with warfarin (0.003), although it was noninferior to warfarin for efficacy. However, the FDA, based on pharmacokinetic data, did recommend a dose of 75 mg every 12 hours in the presence of renal insufficiency (CrCl <30 mL/min).

In 2011, the ACC Foundation/AHA/HRS published their focused update of the guidelines on atrial fibrillation.[53] Of the new oral anticoagulants, only dabigatran had been approved by the FDA at that time. The guidelines indicated that

Dabigatran is useful as an alternative to warfarin for the prevention of stroke in patients with atrial fibrillation. Selection of patients with atrial fibrillation and one or more risk factors for stroke who could benefit from treatment with dabigatran as opposed to warfarin should consider individual clinical features, including the ability to comply with twice daily dosing, availability of an anticoagulation management program, patient preferences, cost, and other factors. Because of the twice daily dosing and greater risk of non-hemorrhagic adverse effects with

dabigatran, patients already taking warfarin with excellent INR control may have little to gain by switching to dabigatran.

The randomized, phase 2 study to evaluate the safety and pharmacokinetics of oral dabigatran etexilate in patients after heart valve replacement (RE-ALIGN)[54] was performed to validate a new regimen for the administration of dabigatran to prevent thromboembolic complications in patients with mechanical heart valves. The trial was terminated prematurely after the enrollment of 252 patients because of an excess of thromboembolic and bleeding events among patients in the dabigatran group. In the as-treated analysis, dose adjustment or discontinuation of dabigatran was required in 52 of 162 patients (32%). Ischemic or unspecified stroke occurred in 9 patients (5%) in the dabigatran group and in no patients in the warfarin group. Major bleeding occurred in 7 patients (4%) and 2 patients (2%), respectively. All patients with major bleeding had pericardial bleeding. The use of dabigatran in patients with mechanical heart valves was associated with increased rates of thromboembolic and bleeding complications, compared with warfarin, thus showing no benefit and an excess risk.

Rivaroxaban

ROCKET AF (Rivaroxaban once daily oral direct factor Xa inhibitor compared with vitamin K antagonism for prevention of stroke and embolism trial in AF) was the major clinical trial of rivaroxaban in patients with atrial fibrillation. The hypothesis of the ROCKET AF[55] trial was that the efficacy of rivaroxaban is noninferior to that of dose-adjusted warfarin for reducing the risk of stroke and non–central nervous system (CNS) systemic embolism in patients with nonvalvular atrial fibrillation. The primary efficacy end point was a composite of stroke and non-CNS systemic embolism. The principal safety end point was a composite of major and nonmajor clinically relevant bleeding. The ROCKET AF trial enrolled 14,264 patients with nonvalvular atrial fibrillation and moderate to high risk of stroke. The patients had to have the following risk factors: either a previous stroke, TIA, or non-CNS systemic embolism or at least 2 of the following: congestive heart failure or left ventricular ejection fraction 35% or less; hypertension; age 75 years or older, or diabetes. Patients were randomized in a double-blind, double-dummy fashion to rivaroxaban 20 mg once daily or 15 mg in the presence of a CrCl of 30 to less than 50 mL/min. Those randomized to warfarin were randomized for a target in the range of

2.0 to 3.0. Although enrollment of subjects without a previous stroke or TIA or systemic embolism and only 2 risk factors was to be capped at 10%, when the trial ended, it turned out to be 13%, with 87% having a CHADS$_2$ score of 3 or greater. The mean CHADS$_2$ score was 3.5 in both the rivaroxaban and warfarin randomized groups, and 55% of the patients had had a previous stroke or TIA.

When the trial ended, data analyzed on an intention-to-treat basis showed that in terms of stroke and non-CNS embolism, rivaroxaban was noninferior to warfarin. It just missed superiority (P = .117). The hazard ratio for the intention-to-treat analysis was 0.88, a 12% relative risk reduction. Had there been as many as 18,000 patients, as there were in RE-LY and ARISTOTLE, the P value may have been significant. However, a pre-specified on-treatment analysis did show superiority, with a hazard ratio of 0.79 (a 21% relative risk reduction, P = .015). There was significantly less intracranial hemorrhage in patients receiving rivaroxaban compared with warfarin, the hazard ratio being 0.41 (a relative risk reduction of 59%; P≤.001). However, the average time for patients on warfarin to be in therapeutic range in this trial was 55%, with the mean being 57.8%. With regard to major bleeding, there was no significant difference between warfarin and rivaroxaban, except that there was significantly more gastrointestinal bleeding with rivaroxaban than warfarin.

The labeling for the indication received from the FDA was that "rivaroxaban is indicated to reduce the risk of stroke and systemic embolism in patients with nonvalvular atrial fibrillation. There are limited data on the relative effectiveness of rivaroxaban compared to warfarin in reducing the risk of stroke and systemic embolism when warfarin therapy is well controlled." The reason for the lack of data was related to the relatively low amount of time in therapeutic range of the patients randomized to warfarin.

Apixaban

The major clinical trial of apixaban on stroke prevention in nonvalvular atrial fibrillation and patients was ARISTOTLE (Apixaban for reduction in stroke and other Thromboembolic events in atrial fibrillation trial).[56] It was a trial in 18,206 patients with atrial fibrillation or atrial flutter randomized in a double-blind, double-dummy fashion either to warfarin with an INR between 2 and 3, target 2.5, or apixaban 5 mg twice daily, but 2.5 mg twice daily if they had 2 of the following 3 characteristics: weight of 60 kg or less; age 80 years or older, a creatinine 1.5 mg/dL or greater. The hypothesis was that apixaban was noninferior to standard

therapy with warfarin in preventing stroke and systemic embolism in moderate-risk to high-risk patients (stroke and ≥1 additional risk factor). The primary efficacy end point was confirmed ischemic or hemorrhagic stroke or systemic embolism. The secondary efficacy end points were a composite of confirmed ischemic or hemorrhagic stroke, systemic embolism, and all-cause death. The primary safety end point was time to first occurrence of confirmed major bleeding. The treatment period was up to 4 years or until 448 primary outcome events had been observed. It was stratified by warfarin-naive status. For the primary outcome of stroke (ischemic or hemorrhagic) or systemic embolism, it not only met the inferiority criteria (P<.001) but also proved to be superior to warfarin (P = .01; hazard ratio, 0.79). With regard to the efficacy outcome, the superiority was all on the safety side, in that there was significantly less hemorrhagic stroke or conversion of ischemic stroke to hemorrhagic stroke (P<.001). There was no difference in ischemic stroke. In addition, for the secondary end point of all-cause death, apixaban was superior to warfarin (P = .046; hazard ratio, 0.89). Also for stroke, systemic embolism, or all-cause death, apixaban again was superior to warfarin (P = .019; hazard ratio, 0.89). In terms of the safety outcome of major bleeding, apixaban was superior to warfarin (P<.001; hazard ratio, 0.69; relative risk reduction, 31%).

AVERROES[48] was a double-blind study of patients with atrial fibrillation who were at increased risk for stroke, and for whom VKA therapy was unsuitable. Patients were randomized to receive apixaban, 5 mg twice daily, or aspirin, 81 to 324 mg daily, to determine whether apixaban was superior. The study was stopped early because of the clear superiority of apixaban over aspirin. The curves on the Kaplan-Meier graph for cumulative risk separated early, and continued to separate until the study was stopped because of clear efficacy of apixaban over aspirin. Apixaban was highly superior to aspirin for prevention of ischemic stroke (P = .001), but there was no difference in hemorrhagic stroke. There was no significant difference between apixaban and aspirin in major bleeding, clinically relevant nonmajor bleeding, fatal bleeding, or intracranial bleeding. The only significant difference was that there was more minor bleeding with apixaban that aspirin. As indicated earlier, this study, once again, showed that for patients with atrial fibrillation at risk for stroke, not only was oral anticoagulation superior to aspirin in efficacy but also there were no benefits to aspirin in bleeding, except for clinically relevant minor bleeding. Not only was apixaban superior in efficacy, there were no safety benefits of any consequence from aspirin. This finding, again, emphasizes the minimal, if any, effect of aspirin in stroke prevention in patients with atrial fibrillation.

Edoxaban

The major trial of edoxaban on stroke prevention in nonvalvular atrial fibrillation patients was the ENGAGE-AF-TIMI 48 (Effective Anticoagulation With Factor Xa Next Generation in Atrial Fibrillation–Thrombolysis in Myocardial Infarction 48) trial. This was a randomized double-blind, double-dummy trial, which compared 2 once-daily edoxaban dose regimens with warfarin in 21,205 patients with atrial fibrillation and moderate to high risk of stroke (CHADS$_2$ score $\geq$2) The hypothesis was that edoxaban would be noninferior to standard therapy with warfarin in preventing stroke and systemic embolism in these moderate-risk to high-risk CHADS$_2$ patients. Patients were enrolled to either warfarin with an INR in the range of 2 to 3, target 2.5, or to edoxaban either 60 mg once daily or 30 mg once daily. The primary efficacy end point was a composite of the primary end point of stroke and systemic embolic events. The secondary efficacy end points were a composite of clinical outcome of stroke, systemic embolic events, and all-cause mortality, also major bleeding events. The treatment period would be at least 2 years. Although the trial has finished, and the data locked, no data has yet been presented for the public at the time of this writing.

WHO IS NOT A CANDIDATE FOR THE NEW ORAL ANTICOAGULANTS?

Especially because the new oral anticoagulants are largely an upgrade from VKAs, consideration should be given to who is not or may not be a candidate for the new oral anticoagulants. They are patients who are stable on warfarin; whose CrCl is less than 30 mL/min and even 30 mL/min to 40 mL/min; who have severe hepatic dysfunction (because the new oral anticoagulants have significant liver metabolism); with mechanical heart valves or who are noncompliant with warfarin. Patients who are comfortable with their warfarin therapy, and whose time in therapeutic range is more than 75%, probably should be in no hurry to switch. They may forego a small absolute reduction in risk of intracranial hemorrhage, but they likely will benefit as more experience is gained with the new agents. For others, the case for the use of the new oral anticoagulants may be more compelling, particularly if out-of-pocket costs are acceptable.

RISKS AND BENEFITS OF COMBINING ASPIRIN WITH ANTICOAGULANT THERAPY IN PATIENTS WITH ATRIAL FIBRILLATION

The combination of an oral anticoagulant with 1 or 2 antiplatelet agents is an area of great importance, because many patients with coronary artery disease also have atrial fibrillation and associated risk for stroke. In the SPORTIF trials (ximelagatran vs warfarin), the addition of aspirin to either the warfarin or the ximelagatran arm was associated with no reduction in stroke or systemic embolism.[57] However, major bleeding occurred significantly more often with aspirin plus warfarin (3.9% per year) than with warfarin alone (2.3% per year; $P = .01$; aspirin plus ximelagatran, 2.0% per year) or ximelagatran alone (1.9% per year).[57] Aspirin combined with anticoagulant therapy was associated with no reduction in stroke or systemic embolism in patients with atrial fibrillation. However, aspirin combined with warfarin was associated with an incremental rate of major bleeding of 1.6% per year.

The APPRAISE 2 (Apixaban for prevention of acute ischemic events 2) trial[58] studied patients with acute coronary syndrome already on aspirin or aspirin plus clopidogrel. The study was a double-blind, placebo-controlled clinical trial comparing apixaban at a dose of 5 mg twice daily with placebo in addition to standard antiplatelet therapy in patients with a recent acute coronary syndrome and at least 2 additional risk factors for recurrent ischemic events. The trial was terminated prematurely after recruitment of 7,392 patients because of an increase in major bleeding events with apixaban in the absence of a counterbalancing reduction in recurrent ischemic events. This trial included more intracranial and fatal bleeding events with apixaban than with warfarin.

SUMMARY OF THE NEW ORAL ANTICOAGULANT TRIALS

The trials all showed noninferiority compared with adjusted dose warfarin with regard to all strokes and systemic emboli. Formal superiority was shown with the 150-mg dose of dabigatran, and with apixaban. The reduced rate of stroke observed with the use of all 3 agents largely reflects a reduction in the rate of hemorrhagic stroke, an unanticipated finding of considerable clinical importance. The rates of gastrointestinal hemorrhage were increased with the use of dabigatran (150-mg dose) and rivaroxaban, but were reduced with apixaban. There is ongoing controversy regarding a small increase in the rate of myocardial infarction with dabigatran.

CONCLUDING REMARKS

There is now a relative abundance of oral antico-agulants that are effective in minimizing stroke and systemic embolism in patients with atrial fibrillation at risk. All the agents have a high degree of efficacy and acceptable safety records. They all have their pluses and minuses in terms of selection of a drug. The choice should be made on an individual basis. Probably the most important thing is to make the choice in the first instance. All too often, patients with atrial fibrillation and stroke risks and no contraindications to oral anticoagulation fail to receive an anticoagulant. If they receive warfarin, all too often, they are not in the therapeutic range. The new oral anticoagulants offer a measure of improvement over many of the limits of warfarin. Again, there are many factors that may and should be considered in the selection of the oral anticoagulants. Once again, the important thing is to select one of them when indicated.

REFERENCES

1. Fisher CM. Treatment of chronic atrial fibrillation [letter to the editor]. Lancet 1972;299:1284.
2. Wolf PA, Abbott RD, Kannell WB. Atrial fibrillation: a major contributor to stroke in the elderly. The Framingham Study. Arch Intern Med 1987;147:1561–4.
3. Sherman DG, Kim SG, Boop BS, et al. Occurrence and characteristics of stroke events in the Atrial Fibrillation Follow-up Investigation of Sinus Rhythm Management (AFFIRM) study. Arch Intern Med 2005;165:1185–91.
4. Petersen P, Boysen G, Godtfredsen J, et al. Placebo-controlled, randomized trial of warfarin and aspirin for prevention of thromboembolic complications in chronic atrial fibrillation. The Copenhagen AFASAK study. Lancet 1989;1:175–9.
5. Stroke prevention in atrial fibrillation study. Final results. Circulation 1991;84:527–39.
6. Singer DE, Hughes RA, Gress DR, et al. The effect of aspirin on the risk of stroke in patients with non-rheumatic atrial fibrillation. The BAATAF Study. Am Heart J 1992;124:1567–73.
7. Connolly SJ, Laupacis A, Gent M, et al. Canadian Atrial Fibrillation Anticoagulation (CAFA) Study. J Am Coll Cardiol 1991;18:349–55.
8. Ezekowitz MD, Bridgers SL, James KE, et al. Warfarin in the prevention of stroke associated with non-rheumatic atrial fibrillation. Veterans Affairs Stroke Prevention in Non-Rheumatic Atrial Fibrillation Investigators. N Engl J Med 1992;327:1406–12.
9. Atrial Fibrillation Investigators. Risk factors for stroke and efficacy of antithrombotic therapy in atrial fibrillation. Analysis of pooled data from five randomized controlled trials. Arch Intern Med 1994;154:1449–57.
10. Albers GW, Sherman DG, Gress DR, et al. Stroke prevention in nonvalvular atrial fibrillation: a review of prospective randomized trials. Ann Neurol 1991;30:511–8.
11. Hylek EM, Skates SJ, Sheehan MA, et al. An analysis of the lowest effective intensity of prophylactic anticoagulation for patients with non-rheumatic atrial fibrillation. N Engl J Med 1996;335:540–6.
12. Hylek EM, Go AS, Chang Y, et al. Effect of intensity of oral anticoagulation on stroke severity and mortality in atrial fibrillation. N Engl J Med 2003;349:1019–26.
13. Hart RG, Pearce LA, Rothbart RM, et al. Stroke with intermittent atrial fibrillation: incidence and predictors during aspirin therapy. Stroke Prevention in Atrial Fibrillation Investigators. J Am Coll Cardiol 2000;35:183–7.
14. Gage BF, Waterman AD, Shannon W, et al. Validation of clinical classification schemes for predicting stroke: results of the National Registry of Atrial Fibrillation. JAMA 2001;285:2864–70.
15. European Heart Rhythm Association, European Association for Cardio-Thoracic Surgery, Camm AJ, et al. Guidelines for the management of atrial fibrillation: the Task Force for the Management of Atrial Fibrillation of the European Society of Cardiology (ESC). Eur Heart J 2010;31:2369–429.
16. Fang MC, Go AS, Chang Y, et al, For the ATRIA Study Group. Comparison of risk stratification schemes to predict thromboembolism in people with nonvalvular atrial fibrillation. J Am Coll Cardiol 2008;51:810–5.
17. Wang TJ, Massaro JM, Levy D, et al. A risk score for predicting stroke or death in individuals with new-onset atrial fibrillation in the community: the Framingham Heart Study. JAMA 2003;290:1049–56.
18. Singer DE, Chang Y, Borowsky LH, et al. A new risk scheme to predict ischemic stroke and other thromboembolism in atrial fibrillation: the ATRIA study stroke risk score. J Am Heart Assoc 2013;2(3):e000250. http://dx.doi.org/10.1161/JAHA.113.000250.
19. Waldo AL, Becker RC, Tapson VF, et al, NABOR Steering Committee. Hospitalized patients with atrial fibrillation and a high risk of stroke are not being provided with adequate anticoagulation. J Am Coll Cardiol 2005;46:1729–36.
20. Go AS, Hylek EM, Borowsky LH, et al. Warfarin use among ambulatory patients with nonvalvular atrial fibrillation: the anticoagulation and risk factors in the atrial fibrillation (ATRIA) study. Ann Intern Med 1999;131:927–34.

21. Hylek EM, C'Antonio J, Evans-Molina C, et al. Translating the results of randomized trials into clinical practice: the challenge of warfarin candidacy among hospitalized elderly patients with atrial fibrillation. Stroke 2006;37:1075–80.

22. Birman-Deych E, Radford MJ, Nilasena DS, et al. Use and effectiveness of warfarin in Medicare beneficiaries with atrial fibrillation. Stroke 2006;37:1070–4.

23. Walker AM, Bennett D. Epidemiology and outcomes in patients with atrial fibrillation in the United States. Heart Rhythm 2008;5:1365–72.

24. Williams CJ. Presentation at the American College of Cardiology 58th Annual Scientific Session, March 29–31, 2009.

25. Nieuwlaat R, Cappuci A, Lip GY, et al, Euro Heart Survey Investigators. Antithrombotic treatment in real-life atrial fibrillation patients: a report from the Euro Heart Survey on Atrial Fibrillation. Eur Heart J 2006;27:3018–26.

26. Agarwal S, Hachamovitch R, Menon V. Current trial-associated outcomes with warfarin in prevention of stroke in patients with nonvalvular atrial fibrillation: a meta-analysis. Arch Intern Med 2012;172:623–31.

27. Nieuwlaat R, Capucci A, Camm AJ, et al, European Heart Survey Investigators. Atrial fibrillation management: a prospective survey in ESC member countries: the Euro Heart Survey on Atrial Fibrillation. Eur Heart J 2005;26:2422–34.

28. European Atrial Fibrillation Trial Investigators. Secondary prevention in non-rheumatic atrial fibrillation after transient ischaemic attack or minor stroke. EAFT (European Atrial Fibrillation Trial) Study Group. Lancet 1993;342:1255–61.

29. Wyse DG, Waldo AL, DiMarco JP, et al. A comparison of rate control and rhythm control in patients with recurrent persistent atrial fibrillation. N Engl J Med 2002;347:1825–33.

30. Friberg L, Rosenqvist M, Lip GY. Evaluation of risk stratification schemes for ischaemic stroke and bleeding in 182 678 patients with atrial fibrillation: the Swedish Atrial Fibrillation Cohort study. Eur Heart J 2012;33:1500–10.

31. White RH, McBurnie MA, Manolio T, et al. Oral anticoagulation in patients with atrial fibrillation: adherence with guidelines in an elderly cohort. Am J Med 1999;106:165–71.

32. Fang MC, Go AS, Hylek EM, et al. Age and the risk of warfarin-associated hemorrhage: the anticoagulation and risk factors in atrial fibrillation study. J Am Geriatr Soc 2006;54:1231–6.

33. Fang MC, Chang Y, Hylek EM, et al. Advanced age, anticoagulation intensity, and risk for intracranial hemorrhage among patients taking warfarin for atrial fibrillation. Ann Intern Med 2004;141:745–52.

34. Fuster V, Rydén LE, Asinger RW, et al. ACC/AHA/ESC Guidelines for the management of patients with atrial fibrillation: executive summary. J Am Coll Cardiol 2001;38:1231–65.

35. Olesen JB, Lip GY, Lindhardsen J, et al. Risks of thromboembolism and bleeding with thromboprophylaxis in patients with atrial fibrillation: a net clinical benefit analysis using a 'real world' nationwide cohort study. Thromb Haemost 2011;106:739–49.

36. Connolly S, Pogue J, Hart R, et al. Clopidogrel plus aspirin versus oral anticoagulation for atrial fibrillation in the Atrial fibrillation Clopidogrel Trial with Irbersartan for Prevention of Vascular Events (ACTIVE W): a randomized controlled trial. Lancet 2006;367:1903–12.

37. Hart RG, Halperin JL, Pearce LA, et al, Stroke Prevention in Atrial Fibrillation Investigators. Lessons from the Stroke Prevention in Atrial Fibrillation trials. Ann Intern Med 2003;138:831–8.

38. The SPAF Investigators. A differential effect of aspirin on prevention of stroke in atrial fibrillation. J Stroke Cerebrovasc Dis 1993;3:181–8.

39. The SPAF III Investigators. Adjusted-dose warfarin versus low-intensity, fixed-dose warfarin plus aspirin for high-risk patients with atrial fibrillation: Stroke Prevention in Atrial Fibrillation III randomised clinical trial. Lancet 1996;348(9028):633–8.

40. The SPAF II Investigators. Warfarin versus aspirin for prevention of thromboembolism in atrial fibrillation: Stroke Prevention in Atrial Fibrillation II Study. Lancet 1994;343:687–91.

41. SPAF III Writing Committee: patients with nonvalvular atrial fibrillation at low risk for stroke during treatment with aspirin. SPAF III Study. JAMA 1998;279:1273–7.

42. Mant J, Hobbs FD, Fletcher K, et al, BAFTA investigators, Midland Research Practices Network (MidReC). Warfarin versus aspirin for stroke prevention in an elderly community population with atrial fibrillation (the Birmingham Atrial Fibrillation Treatment of the Aged Study, BAFTA): a randomised controlled trial. Lancet 2007;370:493–503.

43. Garcia D, Hylek E. Stroke prevention in elderly patients with atrial fibrillation. Lancet 2007;370:460–1.

44. van Walraven C, Hart RG, Connolly S, et al. Effect of age on stroke prevention therapy in patients with atrial fibrillation: the atrial fibrillation investigators. Stroke 2009;40:1410–6.

45. Sato H, Ishikawa K, Kitabatake A, et al. Low-dose aspirin for prevention of stroke in low-risk patients with atrial fibrillation: Japan Atrial Fibrillation Stroke Trial. Stroke 2006;37:447–51.

46. ACTIVE Investigators, Connolly SJ, Pogue J, et al. Effect of clopidogrel added to aspirin in patients with atrial fibrillation. N Engl J Med 2009;360:2066–78.

47. Go AS. The ACTIVE pursuit of stroke prevention in patients with atrial fibrillation. N Engl J Med 2009; 360:2127–9.
48. Connolly SJ, Eikelboom J, Joyner C, et al, AVER-ROES Steering Committee and Investigators. Apixaban in patients with atrial fibrillation. N Engl J Med 2011;364(9):806–17.
49. Lip GY. Recommendations for thromboprophylaxis in the 2012 focused update of the ESC guidelines on atrial fibrillation: a commentary. J Thromb Haemost 2013;11:615–26.
50. Skanes AL, Healey JS, Cairns JA, et al. Focused 2012 Update for the Canadian Cardiovascular Society Atrial Fibrillation Guidelines: recommendations for stroke prevention and rate/rhythm control. Am J Cardiol 2012;28:125–36.
51. You JJ, Singer DE, Howard PA, et al. Antithrombotic therapy for atrial fibrillation: antithrombotic therapy and prevention of thrombosis, 9th ed: American College of Chest Physicians Evidence-Based Clinical Practice Guidelines. Chest 2012;141: e531S–75S.
52. Connolly SJ, Ezekowitz MD, Yusuf S, et al, The RE-LY Steering Committee and Investigators. Dabigatran versus warfarin in patients with atrial fibrillation. N Engl J Med 2009;361:1139–51.
53. Wann LS, Curtis AB, Ellenbogen KA, et al. 2011 ACCF/AHA/HRS focused update on the management of patients with atrial fibrillation (update on dabigatran). A report of the American College of Cardiology Foundation/American Heart Association Task Force on Practice Guidelines. Heart Rhythm 2011;8(3):e1–8.
54. Eikelboom JW, Connolly SJ, Brueckmann M, et al, RE-ALIGN Investigators. Dabigatran versus warfarin in patients with mechanical heart valves. N Engl J Med 2013;369:1206–14.
55. Patel MR, Mahaffey KW, Garg J, et al, The ROCKET AF Steering Committee for the ROCKET AF Investigators. Rivaroxaban versus warfarin in nonvalvular atrial fibrillation. N Engl J Med 2011; 365:883–91.
56. Granger CB, Alexander JH, McMurray JJ, et al. Apixaban versus warfarin in patients with atrial fibrillation. N Engl J Med 2011;365:981–92.
57. Flaker GC, Gruber M, Connolly SJ, et al, SPORTIF Investigators. Risks and benefits of combining aspirin with anticoagulant therapy in patients with atrial fibrillation: an exploratory analysis of stroke prevention using an oral thrombin inhibitor in atrial fibrillation (SPORTIF) trials. Am Heart J 2006;152: 967–73.
58. Alexander JH, Lopes RD, James S, et al, APPRAISE-2 Investigators. Apixaban with antiplatelet therapy after acute coronary syndrome. N Engl J Med 2011;365(8):699–708.
59. Ezekowitz MD, Connolly S, Parekh A, et al. Rationale and design of RE-LY: randomized evaluation of long-term anticoagulant therapy, warfarin, compared with dabigatran. Am Heart J 2009;157: 805–10.
60. ROCKET AF Study Investigators. Rivaroxaban-once daily, oral, direct factor Xa inhibition compared with vitamin K antagonism for prevention of stroke and Embolism Trial in Atrial Fibrillation: rationale and design of the ROCKET AF Study. Am Heart J 2010; 159:340–7.
61. Lopes RD, Alexander JH, Al-Khatib SM, et al, ARISTOTLE Investigators. Apixaban for reduction in stroke and other ThromboLic events in atrial fibrillation (ARISTOTLE) trial: design and rationale. Am Heart J 2010;159:331–9.
62. Ruff CT, Giugliano RP, Antman EM, et al. Evaluation of the novel factor Xa inhibitor edoxaban compared with warfarin in patients with atrial fibrillation: design and rationale for the Effective aNticoaGulation with factor xA next GEneration in Atrial Fibrillation-Thrombolysis in Myocardial Infarction study 48 (ENGAGE AF-TIMI 49). Am Heart J 2010;160:635–41.

Common Questions in Anticoagulation Management in Atrial Fibrillation

Pilar Gallego, MD, PhD[a,b], Vanessa Roldán, MD, PhD[b],
Gregory Y.H. Lip, MD[a],*

KEYWORDS

- Atrial fibrillation • New oral anticoagulants • Chronic anticoagulation management

KEY POINTS

- Until recently, the only oral options for chronic anticoagulation were the vitamin K antagonists (VKAs), but their various limitations promoted the development of novel oral anticoagulants (NOACs), with a specific target.
- To assess the probability of good or poor anticoagulation control while taking VKAs, a new score (the SAMe-TT$_2$R$_2$ score) has been developed to help identify patients who are likely to be in the therapeutic range for a long time.
- Not every patient is suitable for NOACs, including pediatric patients, those who are pregnant, and those with prior (particularly gastrointestinal) bleeding.
- Bleeding remains the main complication of all oral anticoagulants.
- Clinical trials of stroke prevention in AF have shown a significant reduction in hemorrhagic stroke and intracranial bleeding with the NOACs. Prescriptions are increasing; therefore, clinicians need to be prepared to manage bleeding complications should they occur.
- More guidance is needed on how to manage patients who require urgent surgery or systemic thrombolysis for ischemic stroke or ST elevation myocardial infarction.

INTRODUCTION

Nonvalvular atrial fibrillation (AF) confers a fivefold increased risk of stroke and thromboembolism, and oral anticoagulation (OAC) is highly effective in preventing both stroke and mortality, compared with placebo or control.[1] Until recently, the only oral options for chronic anticoagulation were the vitamin K antagonists (VKAs), which act by inducing the synthesis of nonfunctioning coagulation factors. When used as thromboprophylaxis for AF, VKAs result in a 64% stroke risk reduction when compared with placebo or control and

a 37% stroke risk reduction compared with antiplatelet therapy.[1] Moreover, VKAs reduce all-cause mortality by 26% compared with placebo or control in AF.

Nonetheless, the efficacy and safety of VKAs strongly depends on time in the therapeutic range (TTR) with an international normalized ratio (INR) between 2.0 and 3.0. VKAs achieve maximum benefit when the TTR is between 70% and 80%[2,3] and a TTR less than 40% offsets the benefit of VKA therapy[4] because poor control of anticoagulation intensity increases the risks for both thrombotic and hemorrhagic events.[3] However,

The authors have nothing to disclose.
[a] University of Birmingham Centre for Cardiovascular Sciences, City Hospital, Dudley Road, Birmingham, B18 7QH, UK; [b] Department of Hematology and Clinical Oncology, Hospital Universitario Morales Meseguer, Avda. Marqués de los Velez s/n. 30004 Murcia, Spain
* Corresponding author.
E-mail address: g.y.h.lip@bham.ac.uk

cardiacEP.theclinics.com

a TTR greater than 70% is seldom accomplished in everyday clinical practice.[2,3]

The inherent limitations of VKA therapy complicate its management[5] and have promoted the development of novel OACs (NOACs), which may offer convenience, efficacy, and safety (with appropriate patient selection).[6]

In contrast to the VKAs, NOACs directly inhibit specific coagulation factors (eg, thrombin for dabigatran and factor Xa for both rivaroxaban and apixaban) and their predictable pharmacology, with a rapid-action onset and offset, leading to a stable dose-related anticoagulant effect. This allows a fixed dose and makes regular monitoring unnecessary.[7]

WHO SHOULD SWITCH?

Patients with difficulties in achieving a stable anticoagulation will benefit from NOACs. In fact, patients with TTR less than 55% or who are treated with interfering drugs proven to cause INR fluctuations might benefit from switching to NOACs.[8] However, such patients should also be carefully considered before switching. Indeed, drug compliance and treatment adherence needs to be assured by focusing on patients' education so they understand which factors under their control might affect efficacy and safety (eg, diet, alcohol, or other medications) while on VKAs. Switching to NOACs will be the best option if labile INR is not caused by poor compliance; keeping in mind that the short half-life of NOACs will leave patients who have poor compliance or treatment nonadherence more likely to be unprotected to a greater degree than will warfarin (indeed, the first marker of noncompliance will probably be a stroke or other thromboembolic complication).[9] Clinicians should remember that nonadherence in patients older than 65 years with chronic conditions such as AF is estimated to range from 40% to 75%,[8] and that once daily regimens could possibly be related to greater adherence than twice daily regimens, which can have a major impact with NOACs.[10]

To assess the probability of achieving a good TTR, the SAMe-TT$_2$R$_2$ score[11] has recently been developed. This acronym is based on several clinical characteristics. It is scored with one point for female Sex; Age (<60 years); Medical history (at least two of the following: hypertension, diabetes, coronary artery disease or myocardial infarction (MI), peripheral arterial disease, congestive heart failure, previous stroke, pulmonary disease, hepatic or renal disease); Treatment with interacting drugs such as amiodarone for rhythm control; and two points for current Tobacco use; and Race (nonwhite) **(Table 1)**. This simple score can

Table 1 The SAMe-TT$_2$R$_2$ score		
S	Sex (female)	1
A	Age (less than 60 y)	1
Me	Medical history[a]	1
T	Treatment (rhythm control strategy)	1
T	Tobacco use (within 2 y)	2
R	Race (nonwhite)	2

[a] Defined as more than two of the following: hypertension, diabetes, coronary artery disease or MI, peripheral arterial disease, congestive heart failure, previous stroke, pulmonary disease, and hepatic or renal disease.

From Apostolakis S, Sullivan RM, Olshansky B, et al. Factors affecting quality of anticoagulation control among patients with atrial fibrillation on warfarin: The SAMe-TT$_2$R$_2$ score. Chest 2013;144(5):1555-63; with permission.

help predict poor INR control and aid decision-making by identifying those AF patients who would do well on VKA (SAMe-TT$_2$R$_2$ score = 0–1) or, conversely, those who require additional interventions to achieve acceptable anticoagulation control (ie, SAMe-TT$_2$R$_2$ score$\geq$2). In that sense, patients with a poor predicted TTR (ie, SAMe-TT$_2$R$_2$ score$\geq$2) would be more suitable for NOACs.

WHO SHOULD NOT SWITCH?
Previous Gastrointestinal Bleeding

A recent meta-analysis[12,13] comparing main trials on dabigatran, rivaroxaban, and apixaban suggests that new oral anticoagulants lower the risk for intracranial bleeding; the data on overall risk of bleeding were inconclusive. In contrast, it suggests an increased risk for gastrointestinal bleeding associated with the new agents (especially dabigatran and apixaban) probably was related to their local absorption. Therefore, patients with previous gastrointestinal bleeding should perhaps stay under VKAs treatment until results are more conclusive.

Previous Acute Coronary Syndrome

Although published data remain controversial, patients with previous acute coronary syndrome (ACS) might benefit from remaining under VKA treatment. In fact, a protective effect of warfarin against MI rather than an inherent dabigatran-related risk is suspected[14–16]; discrepancies among published data prevent making a strong recommendation. Some meta-analyses have reported no differences between NOACs and VKAs[17,18]; however, other studies have reported lower MI rates with warfarin versus other treatments (relative risk = 0.77; 95% CI 0.63–0.95; P<.01).[14]

Populations Excluded from Clinical Trials

Some specific populations (eg, pediatric or pregnant patients) were originally excluded from clinical trials. Until the emergence of new evidence, caution should prevail; therefore, international guidelines recommend against the use of NOACs among populations not included in clinical trials.[19]

Similarly, NOACs have not already been evaluated in patients with heart valve prosthesis (both mechanical and bioprosthesis). The Randomized, phase II study to evaluate the safety and pharmacokinetics of oral dabigatran etexilate in patients after heart valve replacement (RE-ALIGN) was stopped early due to increased risk of both thromboembolism and bleeding in the dabigatran group. Nine patients (5%) in the dabigatran group and no patients in the warfarin group presented a stroke seven patients (4%) suffered from major bleeding (all pericardial), while only two patients (2%) bled in the warfarin group.[20] Dabigatran-targeted action (which exclusively inhibits thrombin) seems to be less effective in halting the coagulation cascade than the ubiquitous warfarin, which inhibits the synthesis of coagulation factor VII (stopping the activation of tissue factor-induced coagulation) and factor IX (stopping contact pathway-induced coagulation), as well as inhibits the synthesis of factor X and thrombin in the common pathway.[20] Because safety and efficacy profiles in such patients cannot be determined, these patients should remain on warfarin.

HOW TO DEAL WITH SURGERY?
Scheduled Surgery

Some invasive procedures might require the temporary discontinuation of anticoagulation. Both surgery and patient characteristics (eg, age, kidney function, concomitant medication) need to be taken into account when discontinuing and restarting NOACs. Bridging therapy is considered in patients at high risk of thromboembolism. However, NOACs allow a predictable waning of the anticoagulation effect, thus short-term cessation can be accurately timed (**Table 2**).[10,21]

Urgent Surgery

NOACs should be discontinued, and the procedure deferred, if possible, at least 1 to 2 days after the last dose intake.[10] The risk of bleeding must be weighed against the risk of delaying surgery in each specific situation. Evaluation of common coagulation tests might be useful; for example, usually a normal prothrombin time (PT) ratio excludes an anticoagulation effect due to rivaroxaban and a normal activated partial thromboplastin (APTT) time could exclude one due to dabigatran.

HOW TO ASSESS AN ANTI-COAGULATION EFFECT?

Unlike warfarin, knowing the exact time lapse between drug intake and coagulation assessment is mandatory because the impact on a coagulation test varies roughly with the peak level.[10,22] Moreover, the high variability in reagent sensitivity leads to a lack of standard measures to quantify the effect, which depends on the specific coagulometer and reagent used in each laboratory[23]; although assay-specific calibrators and calibration curves should be made at each center.[10]

NOACs prolong some laboratory coagulation tests (**Table 3**). However, only qualitative measures can be made of the PT or the APTT with rivaroxaban, or HEMOCLOT (Hyphen BioMed, France) dilute thrombin time (TT) with dabigatran.[7,24] Thus, the anticoagulant intensity of NOACs should not be monitored with any of these laboratory tests. Indeed, the APTT shows a curvilinear dose response to dabigatran and it may be used to reflect that a patient is taking dabigatran treatment, but it does not provide a quantitative measure.[22] The PT shows better linear dose-response to both dabigatran and rivaroxaban, and it might exclude an anticoagulation effect due to rivaroxaban when normal. However,

Table 2				
Timing of last anticoagulant intake before elective surgery				
	Low Bleeding-Risk Surgery		**High Bleeding-Risk Surgery**	
Creatinine Clearance	**Dabigatran**	**Apixaban or Rivaroxaban**	**Dabigatran**	**Apixaban or Rivaroxaban**
>80 mL/min	24 h	24 h	48 h	36 h
50–80 mL/min	36 h		72 h	
30–50 mL/min	48 h	48 h	96 h	48 h

Table 3
Assessment of anticoagulation effect with the NOACs

	VKA	Dabigatran	Rivaroxaban or Apixaban
APTT	Prolonged	Prolonged (curvilinear dose-response)	Prolonged (curvilinear dose-response)
PT or INR	Prolonged (linear relation)	Insensitive	Prolonged (linear dose-response)
TT	Insensitive	Prolonged (linear relation)	Insensitive

Abbreviation: TT, thrombin time.

standardization among different laboratories is needed before widespread clinical use.[8]

The degree of anticoagulation reached can partly be measured by noncoagulation methods (eg, Ecarin clotting time, or chromogenic methods), which are only available for research purposes,[25,26] as well as the HEMOCLOT test, which measures the effect of dabigatran through a modified thrombin clotting time.[27]

HOW TO DEAL WITH SYSTEMIC THROMBOLYSIS FOR ISCHEMIC STROKE OR ST ELEVATION MI?

AF-complicating ACS (with and without ST elevation) and vice versa is not only relatively frequent, but also associated with significantly higher mortality rates. Moreover, AF patients with ACS receive fewer evidence-based therapies or procedures, and antithrombotic cocktails vary considerably.[10] The anticoagulation state or intensity is difficult to interpret through the usual tests: INR, TT, and APTT. This is especially so if other antithrombotics have been administered (eg, bivalirudin, fondaparinux). Their results also depend on both the timing of the last dose and the patient's renal function. Therefore, decisions on thrombolysis that are based on traditional coagulation assessment cannot be made in patients on NOACs.

In case of an ST elevation MI, primary percutaneous coronary intervention is recommended over fibrinolysis by European guidelines, and a radial approach is preferred to reduce the risk of access site bleeding.[10] Additional, parenteral anticoagulation is also recommended, regardless of the timing of the last dose of NOAC.[10]

In acute ischemic stroke, mechanical removal of the clot is sometimes an alternative. Otherwise, measurement of the APTT or PT for dabigatran or rivaroxaban, respectively, before systemic thrombolysis is advised to determine whether there is a systemic anticoagulation effect from the NOAC. However, reliable biomarkers and more definitive practice guidelines are needed to help decision-making regarding thrombolysis in patients presenting with an acute ischemic strokes or ST elevation MI while on NOACs.

HOW TO DEAL WITH ADHERENCE PROBLEMS?

Nonadherence in patients older than 65 years, with chronic conditions such as AF is estimated to range from 40% to 75%.[8] Once-daily regimens are usually associated with greater adherence than are twice daily regimens.[10] Patients with poor compliance or low treatment adherence may not achieve their underprotection against stroke because the anticoagulant effect of NOACs lasts only for 12 to 24 hours after intake.[9] Therefore, patient education (as well as family member involvement) is extremely important to assure strict adherence, which needs to be checked at every follow-up.

FOLLOW-UP

The follow-up of patients taking NOACs is vital, and should be carefully specified and communicated among all involved healthcare staff. Indeed, all anticoagulants have some drug interactions so new prescriptions should be carefully considered. Moreover, routine follow-up increases patient adherence, which is crucial. Therefore, compliance should be periodically checked. Renal function should be assessed frequently because as patients become older some renal impairment may appear. The European guidelines recommend monitoring renal function every 6 months in elderly patients (>75 years) or patients with mild renal impairment (creatinine clearance rate [CrCl] <60 mL/min), and yearly in all other patients.[10]

FRAIL POPULATIONS
Elderly

OAC underuse is particularly pronounced in elderly patients (>80 years). The elderly progressively own certain particular characteristics that make data extrapolation more difficult; therefore, they are often excluded from clinical trials.

The elderly are more prone to achieve high INR levels with low doses of VKA and have a greater likelihood of labile INRs. Given the lower rates of serious bleeding, some physicians may prescribe NOACs to the elderly.[28] Nonetheless, NOACs should be used as they were studied in their respective clinical trials and deviations from studied indications invite disaster. A recent review highlights adverse data from indiscriminate (and often inappropriate) wide-spread use of NOACs in the elderly.[29]

Renal Impairment

Chronic kidney disease increases the risk of both thrombotic and hemorrhagic events.[10,30] Although OAC reduces thrombotic risk, the bleeding risk will also be increased, thus the net clinical benefit should be carefully assessed in each patient. Patients with mild-to-moderate chronic kidney disease might be suitable for some NOACs after some dose reduction (for specific doses, refer to **Fig. 1**). However, this should be avoided in severe renal impairment (CrCl<15 mL/min) pending more clinical trial data.[10]

HOW TO MANAGE BLEEDING?

Bleeding remains the main complication of OACs and the fear of bleeding among physicians has long led to a lack of prescription and reduced uptake particularly when treating patients who may otherwise benefit greatly from its use.[31–34] Although not conclusive, NOACs might have a generally safer profile, with some reduction in all-bleeding rates. However, as NOACs prescriptions increase clinicians need to be prepared to deal with bleeding complications.

While bleeding events are a known adverse effect of all anticoagulants, some safety concerns have been raised regarding the NOACs because of the lack of any specific antidote for a rapid reversal in case of emergencies. Management of bleeding (**Fig. 2**) while on NOACs depends on the elimination half-life of the agent (ranging from 8 hours for rivaroxaban or apixaban to 17 hours for dabigatran). Therefore, stopping the medication rapidly drops the blood levels; restoration of hemostasis is expected within 12 to 24 hours after the last dose.[10] Withholding the drug is usually enough for most patients with mild bleeding. However, in patients with major, life-threatening bleeding, other measures might be necessary.

Fluid replacement and blood transfusion should be part of supportive management (because most NOACs have a renal excretion, maintaining renal perfusion should be a priority) and, in very severe cases, the nonspecific reversal agents may be used. These include fresh frozen plasma (FFP); prothrombin complex concentrates (PCCs), which provide more prothrombin to increase thrombin generation; recombinant activated factor VII (rFVIIa); activated PCCs; and factor eight inhibitor bypass activity (FEIBA), mainly compounded by activated factor times and prothrombin.[35] However, the safety and usefulness of FFP or PCC is still to be definitively established because the drug present in plasma may also block newly administered coagulation factors and the use of rFVIIa may result in a potential risk for arterial thrombosis.[8] For dabigatran, hemodialysis can help reduce dabigatran blood levels[36]; however,

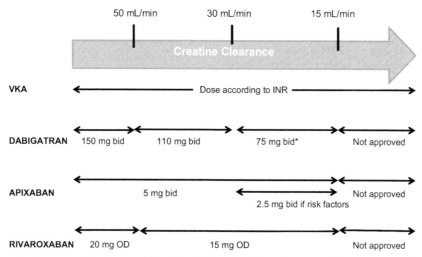

Fig. 1. Dose reduction according to renal function. bid, twice daily; OD, once daily. * Approved in the United States, not in Europe.

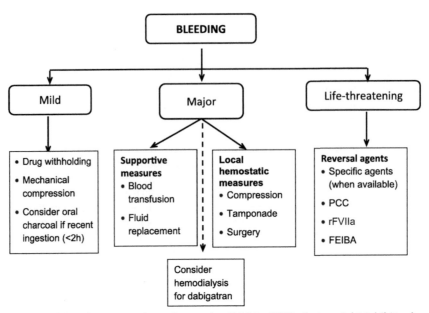

Fig. 2. Management of bleeding events in patients using NOACs. FEIBA, factor eight inhibitor bypass activity; PCC, prothrombin complex concentrates; rFVIIa, recombinant activated factor VII. (*Adapted from* Heidbuchel H, Verhamme P, Alings M, et al. European Heart Rhythm Association Practical Guide on the use of new oral anticoagulants in patients with non-valvular atrial fibrillation. Europace 2013;15:625–51; with permission.)

multiple sessions may be required due to its large distribution volume. The risk of bleeding at venipuncture site should be considered; therefore, it is more suitable for overdose rather than to stop active bleeding. Of note, rivaroxaban and apixaban are not dialyzable due to a high plasma protein binding.[10,27,37]

Specific antidotes, such as PRT064445,[38] or monoclonal antibodies (eg, aDabi-Fab[39]) are currently under development but are not ready for clinical use.

SUMMARY

The widespread use of NOACs has highlighted important management questions. Bleeding remains the main complication of all OACs. Although clinical trials of stroke prevention in AF have shown a significant reduction in hemorrhagic stroke and intracranial bleeding with the NOACs, as prescriptions increase clinicians need to be prepared to manage bleeding complications if they occur. More guidance on how to manage patients who require urgent surgery or systemic thrombolysis for ischemic stroke or ST elevation MI is needed.

REFERENCES

1. Hart RG, Pearce LA, Aguilar MI. Meta-analysis: antithrombotic therapy to prevent stroke in patients who have nonvalvular atrial fibrillation. Ann Intern Med 2007;146(12):857–67.
2. Gallagher AM, Setakis E, Plumb JM, et al. Risks of stroke and mortality associated with suboptimal anticoagulation in atrial fibrillation patients. Thromb Haemost 2011;106(5):968–77.
3. Wan Y, Heneghan C, Perera R, et al. Anticoagulation control and prediction of adverse events in patients with atrial fibrillation: a systematic review. Circ Cardiovasc Qual Outcomes 2008;1(2):84–91.
4. Banerjee A, Marin F, Lip GY. A new landscape for stroke prevention in atrial fibrillation: focus on new anticoagulants, antiarrhythmic drugs, and devices. Stroke 2011;42(11):3316–22.
5. Lip GY, Andreotti F, Fauchier L, et al. Bleeding risk assessment and management in atrial fibrillation patients. Executive Summary of a Position Document from the European Heart Rhythm Association [EHRA], endorsed by the European Society of Cardiology [ESC] Working Group on Thrombosis. Thromb Haemost 2011;106(6):997–1011.
6. Banerjee A, Lane DA, Torp-Pedersen C, et al. Net clinical benefit of new oral anticoagulants (dabigatran, rivaroxaban, apixaban) versus no treatment in a 'real world' atrial fibrillation population: a modelling analysis based on a nationwide cohort study. Thromb Haemost 2012;107(3):584–9.
7. Huisman MV, Lip GY, Diener HC, et al. Dabigatran etexilate for stroke prevention in patients with atrial fibrillation: resolving uncertainties in routine practice. Thromb Haemost 2012;107(5):838–47.

8. Pengo V, Crippa L, Falanga A, et al. Questions and answers on the use of dabigatran and perspectives on the use of other new oral anticoagulants in patients with atrial fibrillation. A consensus document of the Italian Federation of Thrombosis Centers (FCSA). Thromb Haemost 2011;106(5):868–76.

9. Schulman S, Crowther MA. How I treat with anticoagulants in 2012: new and old anticoagulants, and when and how to switch. Blood 2012;119(13): 3016–23.

10. Heidbuchel H, Verhamme P, Alings M, et al. European Heart Rhythm Association Practical Guide on the use of new oral anticoagulants in patients with non-valvular atrial fibrillation. Europace 2013;15: 625–51.

11. Apostolakis S, Sullivan RM, Olshansky B, et al. Factors affecting quality of anticoagulation control among patients with atrial fibrillation on warfarin: The SAMe-TT$_2$R$_2$ score. Chest 2013;144(5): 1555–63.

12. Holster IL, Valkhoff VE, Kuipers EJ, et al. New oral anticoagulants increase risk for gastrointestinal bleeding: a systematic review and meta-analysis. Gastroenterology 2013;145(1):105–12.

13. Miller CS, Grandi SM, Shimony A, et al. Meta-analysis of efficacy and safety of new oral anticoagulants (dabigatran, rivaroxaban, apixaban) versus warfarin in patients with atrial fibrillation. Am J Cardiol 2012; 110(3):453–60.

14. Lip GY, Lane DA. Does warfarin for stroke thromboprophylaxis protect against MI in atrial fibrillation patients? Am J Med 2010;123(9):785–9.

15. Potpara TS, Lip GY, Apostolakis S. New anticoagulant treatments to protect against stroke in atrial fibrillation. Heart 2012;98(18):1341–7.

16. Uchino K, Hernandez AV. Dabigatran association with higher risk of acute coronary events: meta-analysis of noninferiority randomized controlled trials. Arch Intern Med 2012;172(5):397–402.

17. Dentali F, Riva N, Crowther M, et al. Efficacy and safety of the novel oral anticoagulants in atrial fibrillation: a systematic review and meta-analysis of the literature. Circulation 2012;126(20):2381–91.

18. Larsen TB, Rasmussen LH, Skjoth F, et al. Efficacy and safety of dabigatran etexilate and warfarin in 'real world' patients with atrial fibrillation: a prospective nationwide cohort study. J Am Coll Cardiol 2013; 61(22):2264–73.

19. Camm AJ, Lip GY, De CR, et al. 2012 focused update of the ESC Guidelines for the management of atrial fibrillation: an update of the 2010 ESC Guidelines for the management of atrial fibrillation. Developed with the special contribution of the European Heart Rhythm Association. Eur Heart J 2012; 33(21):2719–47.

20. Eikelboom JW, Connolly SJ, Brueckmann M, et al. Dabigatran versus warfarin in patients with mechanical heart valves. N Engl J Med 2013; 369(13):1206–14.

21. Sie P, Samama CM, Godier A, et al. Surgery and invasive procedures in patients on long-term treatment with oral direct thrombin or factor Xa inhibitors. Ann Fr Anesth Reanim 2011;30(9):645–50 [in French].

22. Alikhan R, Rayment R, Keeling D, et al. The acute management of haemorrhage, surgery and overdose in patients receiving dabigatran. Emerg Med J 2013. [Epub ahead of print].

23. Ogata K, Mendell-Harary J, Tachibana M, et al. Clinical safety, tolerability, pharmacokinetics, and pharmacodynamics of the novel factor Xa inhibitor edoxaban in healthy volunteers. J Clin Pharmacol 2010;50(7):743–53.

24. Turpie AG, Kreutz R, Llau J, et al. Management consensus guidance for the use of rivaroxaban–an oral, direct factor Xa inhibitor. Thromb Haemost 2012;108(5):876–86.

25. Baglin T, Keeling D, Kitchen S. Effects on routine coagulation screens and assessment of anticoagulant intensity in patients taking oral dabigatran or rivaroxaban: guidance from the British Committee for Standards in Haematology. Br J Haematol 2012; 159(4):427–9.

26. Montoya RC, Gajra A. Current status of new anticoagulants in the management of venous thromboembolism. Adv Hematol 2012;2012:856341.

27. van RJ, Stangier J, Haertter S, et al. Dabigatran etexilate—a novel, reversible, oral direct thrombin inhibitor: interpretation of coagulation assays and reversal of anticoagulant activity. Thromb Haemost 2010;103(6):1116–27.

28. De CR, Husted S, Wallentin L, et al. New oral anticoagulants in atrial fibrillation and acute coronary syndromes: ESC Working Group on Thrombosis-Task Force on Anticoagulants in Heart Disease position paper. J Am Coll Cardiol 2012;59(16):1413–25.

29. Forman DE, Goyette RE. Oral anticoagulation therapy for elderly patients with atrial fibrillation: utility of bleeding risk covariates to better understand and moderate risks. Clin Appl Thromb Hemost 2013. [Epub ahead of print].

30. Olesen JB, Lip GY, Kamper AL, et al. Stroke and bleeding in atrial fibrillation with chronic kidney disease. N Engl J Med 2012;367(7):625–35.

31. Lip GY, Lane DA. Stroke prevention with oral anticoagulation therapy in patients with atrial fibrillation. Circ J 2013;77(6):1380–8.

32. Ogilvie IM, Welner SA, Cowell W, et al. Characterization of the proportion of untreated and antiplatelet therapy treated patients with atrial fibrillation. Am J Cardiol 2011;108(1):151–61.

33. Waldo AL, Becker RC, Tapson VF, et al. Hospitalized patients with atrial fibrillation and a high risk of stroke are not being provided with adequate anticoagulation. J Am Coll Cardiol 2005;46(9):1729–36.

34. Wilke T, Groth A, Mueller S, et al. Oral anticoagulation use by patients with atrial fibrillation in Germany. Adherence to guidelines, causes of anticoagulation under-use and its clinical outcomes, based on claims-data of 183,448 patients. Thromb Haemost 2012;107(6):1053–65.

35. Marlu R, Hodaj E, Paris A, et al. Effect of non-specific reversal agents on anticoagulant activity of dabigatran and rivaroxaban: a randomised crossover ex vivo study in healthy volunteers. Thromb Haemost 2012;108(2):217–24.

36. Khadzhynov D, Wagner F, Formella S, et al. Effective elimination of dabigatran by haemodialysis. A phase I single-centre study in patients with end-stage renal disease. Thromb Haemost 2013;109(4):596–605.

37. Wong PC, Pinto DJ, Zhang D. Preclinical discovery of apixaban, a direct and orally bioavailable factor Xa inhibitor. J Thromb Thrombolysis 2011;31(4):478–92.

38. Lu G, Deguzman FR, Hollenbach SJ, et al. A specific antidote for reversal of anticoagulation by direct and indirect inhibitors of coagulation factor Xa. Nat Med 2013;19(4):446–51.

39. Schiele F, van RJ, Canada K, et al. A specific antidote for dabigatran: functional and structural characterization. Blood 2013;121(18):3554–62.

Atrial Fibrillation and Stroke
Increasing Stroke Risk with Intervention

Christopher V. DeSimone, MD, PhD[a],
Malini Madhavan, MBBS[a], Elisa Ebrille, MD[b],
Alejandro A. Rabinstein, MD[c], Paul A. Friedman, MD[a],
Samuel J. Asirvatham, MD, FACC, FHRS[a,d],*

KEYWORDS

- Atrial fibrillation - Silent cerebral lesions - Ablation - Embolism - Catheter

KEY POINTS

- Although stroke is a well-recognized but rare complication of atrial fibrillation ablation, recent studies have shown an unexpected and high rate of silent cerebral lesions detected by diffusion-weighted magnetic resonance imaging (MRI).
- MRI-detected silent cerebral lesions that occur during atrial fibrillation ablation pose serious risks and challenges.
- Further prospective trials with longer follow-up periods are required to increase understanding of how best to risk stratify patients who are candidates for atrial fibrillation ablation.
- To achieve improved ablation safety, a multidisciplinary and multi-modal approach is needed in determining the best method to prevent these lesions. This approach will involve innovation in ablation techniques, anticoagulation, and cerebral protection.

Atrial fibrillation (AF) is the most common sustained arrhythmia in adults, with an estimated prevalence of 2.1% in the United States.[1] Catheter ablation for AF is now commonly used in the management of patients with symptomatic drug-refractory arrhythmias.[2] Although increasingly successful approaches for ablation have become available over the last 2 decades, the potential for complications remains a major impediment. However, interventional procedures, including radiofrequency ablation, other ablation strategies, and implanted cardiac devices, particularly in the presence of patent foramen ovale (PFO), may all represent an underappreciated risk for stroke and transient ischemic attack (TIA).[3] Although stroke is a well-recognized but rare complication of AF ablation, recent studies have shown an unexpected and high rate of silent cerebral lesions (SCLs) detected by diffusion-weighted (DW) magnetic resonance imaging (MRI). The cause and consequence of these lesions is currently the subject of intense research. This article discusses the current state of knowledge of the incidence, risk factors, and potential significance of SCL and discusses techniques to prevent them.

SCLS FOLLOWING AF ABLATION: DIAGNOSIS, INCIDENCE, AND RISK FACTORS

Clinically evident stroke or TIA can be a serious complication of AF ablation, but occurs in less than 1% of patients.[2,4] However, the use of

The authors have nothing to disclose.
[a] Division of Cardiovascular Diseases, Mayo Clinic, 200 First Street Southwest, Rochester, MN 55905, USA;
[b] Department of Cardiology, University of Turin, S. Giovanni Battista, Corso Bramante, Turin, Italy;
[c] Department of Neurology, Mayo Clinic, 200 First Street Southwest, Rochester, MN 55905, USA;
[d] Department of Pediatrics and Adolescent Medicine, Mayo Clinic, 200 First Street Southwest, Rochester, MN 55905, USA
* Corresponding author. Division of Cardiovascular Diseases, Mayo Clinic, 200 First Street Southwest, Rochester, MN 55905.
E-mail address: asirvatham.samuel@mayo.edu

postablation MRI of the brain has revealed the frequent occurrence of new lesions in the brain without clinically apparent stroke, labeled as SCLs.[5–9] An SCL is identified as focal, well-demarcated, hyperintense signals on diffusion-weighted MRI with corresponding hypointensity in the apparent diffusion coefficient maps. These MRI findings represent cytotoxic edema caused by ischemia or infarct and are sensitive and specific for acute infarction.[10,11] Ischemic brain injury results in loss of membrane gradient and net movement of water into cells, where movement is more restrained. The hyperintense lesions on diffusion-weighted MRI represent restricted diffusion of water in cells and appear within 30 minutes of the event. SCLs following AF ablation are frequently multiple, occurring in several vascular distributions, again suggesting the embolic nature of these lesions.

The reported incidence of SCL varies from 4.3% to 38.9% depending on several procedural factors.[5–7,12] Although the risk factors for SCL need further study, currently available data suggest that procedural factors are more important than patient-related factors. The type of catheter and energy source has been the subject of several studies. The multielectrode pulmonary vein ablation catheter (PVAC) that delivers phased duty-cycled radiofrequency energy (Medtronic, Minneapolis, MN) has been associated with higher risk of SCL compared with irrigated radiofrequency and cryoablation (38.9%, 8.3%, and 5.6% respectively).[7,12] However, no significant difference has been noted between irrigated radiofrequency catheter versus cryoablation[13] and mesh radiofrequency ablator versus cryoablation.[14] In another study, the number and design of external irrigation ports on the catheter did not affect the incidence of SCL.[15] A comparison between manual and robotic-assisted radiofrequency ablation also did not reveal any differences.[8] Intraprocedural lower activated clotting time (ACT) and electrical cardioversion have been reported to be associated with a higher risk of SCL.[6,15,16] Ablation of complex fractionated atrial electrograms was associated with increased risk in one study, but was not corroborated in another study.[16,17] Patient-related factors such as advanced age, persistent AF, lower left ventricular ejection fraction, and spontaneous echo contrast on transesophageal echocardiography have been associated with SCL in some but not all studies.[13,16,17]

Irrespective of AF ablation, patients with AF are more likely to have silent cerebral ischemic lesions at baseline compared with patients in sinus rhythm.[18] A recent study from Gaita and colleagues[18] showed that patients with paroxysmal and persistent AF had a higher prevalence and number of silent cerebral ischemic lesions per patient than those in sinus rhythm (89%, 92%, and 46% respectively; $P<.01$). Of clinical significance, the silent ischemic lesions in the AF group were associated with worse cognitive performance.[18]

There has been great interest in using different MRI protocols to identify new procedure-related silent ischemic cerebral lesions such as T2-weighted spin echo sequences, fluid-attenuated inversion recovery, and DW echo spin protocols.[19] For example, DW-MRI allows detection of very small as well as acute ischemic lesions.[20] In addition, MRI is able to differentiate between ischemic and embolic origins of brain lesions.[21,22] Small, sharply demarcated lesions, which are often in clusters, with bilateral distribution and located predominantly in the frontal lobe (the so-called spotted pattern) strongly support an embolic mechanism typical of AF origination.[18]

Dynamic Assessment of SCL Using Transcranial Doppler and Intracardiac Echocardiography

Although MRI enables early detection of silent cerebral ischemic events, these lesions are not found until the ablation procedure is completed. A real-time assessment of emboli during ablation, with the potential to guide energy delivery, is paramount to improving overall ablation procedural safety. Two methods have been used for this purpose: (1) monitoring for the formation of microbubbles on intracardiac echocardiography (ICE), and (2) detection of microembolic signals (MESs) in the cerebral arteries by transcranial Doppler (TCD). Kilicaslan and colleagues[23] first reported on MESs detected by TCD during pulmonary vein isolation, finding a close correlation between MESs and the amount of microbubble formation detected by ICE. Future research must focus on the correlation between MESs on TCD and the occurrence of SCLs on MRI as well as long-term neurologic outcome before this technology finds widespread use in AF ablation.

SCLS: SIGNIFICANCE AND LONG-TERM FOLLOW-UP

Although SCLs in patients with AF are associated with cognitive decline,[18] whether SCLs after AF ablation lead to long-term cognitive dysfunction is not well understood. Investigation of mild neurocognitive effects of SCLs have so far focused on short-term outcomes. Medi and colleagues[24] recently reported higher prevalence of cognitive dysfunction based on neuropsychiatric testing, with an incidence of 28% in paroxysmal AF and 27% in the persistent AF ablation groups (compared with the nonablative group in which no patients developed cognitive dysfunction). These findings occurred at 24 to 48 hours after the procedure and remained significant in the ablative compared with the control groups at 90 days (13% paroxysmal, 20% persistent AF, 0 in nonablative group).[24] The data become even more striking when taking into account that most patients included in the study had low CHADS2 (congestive heart failure, hypertension, age >75 years, diabetes mellitus, stroke) scores (0–1). Similarly Schwartz and colleagues[25] showed decline in verbal memory 3 months following AF ablation. In contrast, Haeusler and colleagues[14] did not note any change in cognitive function in the postablation period despite a 40% incidence of new SCLs. However, these studies used different tools for neuropsychiatric assessment, which can influence the findings significantly.

Despite the high incidence of cerebral lesions after ablation, current data suggest that most these resolve in the long term without discernible changes on MRI. In a long-term follow-up study of 9 patients with new silent cerebral infarcts after AF ablation, there was an attenuation of radiological lesions over time with no residual lesions seen on repeat MRI after 21 months.[8] Deneke and colleagues[5] similarly showed that 94% of asymptomatic lesions resolved at about 1 year after ablation, with only large (>10 mm) acute lesions producing chronic glial scars at long-term follow-up. This finding was also confirmed by a study using 3-T MRI, enabling a higher contrast/noise ratio and improving diagnostic reliability of ischemic lesion detection.[14] In light of these findings, more research is needed to fully characterize the long-term neurologic effects of these resolved lesions.

CAUSE OF SCL DURING ABLATION AND TECHNIQUES TO REDUCE INCIDENCE

Several factors can cause silent ischemic lesions and these may coexist during ablation procedures.[26] The proposed mechanisms involved include (1) thromboembolism, (2) air embolism, (3) coagulum formation, and (4) hypoperfusion or hypoxia.[27,28] Several recent studies have focused on the potential cause of SCL and techniques to reduce the risk. In addition to the major factors involved in generation of this embolic phenomenon, this article reviews the relevant considerations that have been studied to date in an attempt to reduce the incidence of these lesions.

Thromboembolism

Thromboembolism is often diagnosed as the cause of stroke in patients with AF including following an ablation procedure. Thromboembolism has similarly been proposed as an important cause of SCL after ablation. Thrombus can form on the catheter, sheath, or ablated endocardial surface during ablation. The risk of thrombus formation is modulated by several procedural factors including anticoagulation, type of catheter, energy source for ablation, and cardioversion during the procedure. These factors each lend an opportunity to reduce the risk of SCL.

Heparinization: robust ACT goal

Heparin use during AF ablation should in theory limit or reduce formation of thrombus while ablating in the left-sided circulation. Ren and colleagues[29] investigated the effects of heparin in trying to reduce left atrial thrombus formation through a robust ACT goal of greater than 300 seconds (301–400 seconds) compared with 250 to 300 seconds during AF ablation. The investigators found a significant difference in the higher intensity ACT (>300 seconds) group with respect to a lower incidence of left atrial thrombus in patients with spontaneous echo contrast (SEC).[29] This finding led them to conclude that patients with SEC may benefit from more aggressive ACT goals during AF ablation procedures.[29] Consistent with these findings, Scaglione and colleagues[15] found that a high intraprocedural mean ACT value was the only independent protective factor against thromboembolic lesion formation in patients undergoing AF ablation. Furthermore, consistent with the positive correlation between a more aggressive heparinization strategy and lower embolic risk, Scaglione and colleagues[15] found that an incremental increase of 1 second in ACT was associated with a decreased risk of 0.4% in developing silent embolic lesions during catheter ablation. The risk of SEC is also an independent predictor of cerebral embolic lesions despite the continued use of oral anticoagulation.[16,30]

Heparinization: importance of timing

In addition to an adequate heparinization strategy, the timing of heparin administration is crucial. Bruce and colleagues[31] found that administration of heparin before a transseptal puncture was critical in reducing left atrial thrombus formation during ablation procedures. Moreover, this early heparinization approach did not increase the risk of bleeding complications.[31]

Current guidelines on catheter ablation of AF recommend an ACT goal of 300 to 400 seconds and administration of heparin before or soon after transseptal puncture.[2] We prefer the administration of heparin before transseptal puncture.

Periprocedural oral anticoagulation

The continuation of therapeutic warfarin anticoagulation during AF ablation has been proposed to reduce the risk of thromboembolism and bleeding complications related to vascular access. Verma and colleagues[32] recently reported a lower incidence of SCL with the use of multielectrode, duty-cycled, phased radiofrequency ablation with the institution of several procedural changes including the continuation of therapeutic oral anticoagulation during the procedure. However, the continuation of warfarin during the procedure did not remove the risk of SCL in another study, with 12% of patients experiencing SCLs during open irrigated catheter ablation on therapeutic anticoagulation.[16] Data on the safety and efficacy of continuation of newer oral anticoagulants during AF ablation are lacking.

Although the timing and intensity of heparin anticoagulation during the procedure and periprocedural anticoagulation can lessen the risk of thromboembolic events during AF ablation, they are not adequate to prevent all events, which highlights the importance of sources of embolism apart from thrombi during the ablation procedure, such as air and coagulum (this is discussed later).

Air Embolism

Air embolism has been proposed as a potential cause for SCL based on observations in animal models and human studies. Potential sources of air embolism include (1) catheter exchange after transseptal puncture, (2) irrigation of sheaths, and (3) microbubble formation during ablation.

Haines and colleagues[33] reported both particulate and air embolism detected in an extracorporeal circulation during ablation in a swine model. Furthermore, in another elegant proof-of-concept study, they showed that injection of air or coagulum into the carotids caused MRI-detected lesions that reflected what was seen on histologic review at autopsy.[34] Studies in humans using ICE imaging and TCD for monitoring of cerebral microembolic signals have shown a correlation between microbubbles during ablation and cerebral emboli during radiofrequency ablation with both irrigated and nonirrigated catheters.[23,35] These studies suggest that most microemboli are gaseous in nature. Furthermore, nonirrigated multielectrode catheters resulted in more microbubbles compared with the open irrigated catheter.[23,35] The exact cause of microbubbles during radiofrequency ablation is not known. Potential causes include tissue heating leading to an endocavitary pop and electrolysis. Wood and colleagues[36] have suggested that, once the presence of microbubbles are seen during radiofrequency ablation application, it may be prudent to cease radiofrequency energy or slowly decrement energy in order to prevent further propagation of microbubbles. Kilicaslan and colleagues[23] further showed that the titration of radiofrequency energy output to minimize microbubbles detected by ICE can reduce the number of microembolic signals and symptomatic neurologic events. This technique warrants further study and validation.

Air embolism can also occur during catheter exchange through the transseptal sheath and with irrigation of sheaths. Air can also be introduced into the sheath during introduction of a catheter. Catheters with a more complex design, such as circular catheters and cryoballoons, are more prone to this than catheters with a smooth bullet-shaped tip. Furthermore, sheaths with a lumen introduced into the left atrium can be more thrombogenic than a solid catheter, increasing the risk of thromboembolism.[37,38] Meticulous attention should be paid to management of the sheath to minimize these complications. The sheath should also be maintained on a continuous flush of normal saline. Cauchemez and colleagues[37] showed that a high-flow continuous flush at 180 mL/h is more effective that a low-flow flush at 3 mL/h in preventing clinical stroke. Rapid withdrawal of the catheter through the sheath can cause aspiration of blood into the tip of the sheath, predisposing to thrombus. All catheter exchanges must be performed slowly during continuous flushing of the sheath. Catheter introduction under submersion should also be considered, especially for catheters with complex geometry. Many operators withdraw the long transseptal sheath into the right atrium during catheter manipulation in the left atrium.[39]

Coagulum Formation

The risk of embolic showering during an AF ablation procedure can result from formation of coagulum.[40] Coagulum forms because of heat-induced denaturation and aggregation of components of the fibrin clot (platelets, red blood cells, and most notably fibrin) at the electrode-tissue interface.[40,41] The use of irrigated-tip catheters has significantly reduced the risk of coagulum formation.[42] The critical part in the pathway to coagulum formation is electrostatic conformational changes in fibrinogen polymers and the subsequent attachments of these aggregates to the catheter surface.[40] Lim and colleagues[40] showed that applying a negative charge to the catheter surface prevents aggregation of these fibrinogen polymers, and thus provides an innovative technique to reduce coagulum formation.

Hypotension, Hypoxia, and Cerebral Hypoperfusion

Although embolism is considered the major cause of SCL, infarction in watershed regions of the brain caused by hypoperfusion cannot be ruled out. Several procedural factors predispose to hypoperfusion and hypoxia, including hypotension from anesthesia and arrhythmia induction and transient right-to-left shunting across the transseptal puncture. Measures should be taken to prevent hypotension during the procedure.

Impact of Energy Source and Catheter Design on SCL

Observational studies have shown significant differences in rate of SCL between various catheter designs and energy sources, as discussed previously. The use of saline irrigation of catheters for active cooling of the catheter tip can reduce the risk of thrombus and coagulum formation on the catheter.[42] Furthermore, open-irrigation catheters have been shown to be more effective in reducing coagulum formation than internally cooled catheters in a swine model.[42]

The nonirrigated, multielectrode, duty-cycled, phased radiofrequency ablation catheter (PVAC) has been particularly associated with a high risk of SCL; as high as 38%.[7,12] Observations from swine and human studies with the PVAC catheter are instructive in understanding the combination of factors that lead to SCL.[33] The PVAC is a decapolar nonirrigated catheter capable of duty-cycled unipolar-bipolar radiofrequency ablation. Although duty cycling and phasing of radiofrequency delivery is expected to allow periodic cooling of the tissue-catheter interface, clinical studies showed a higher incidence of SCL with this catheter. The following mechanisms have been proposed to explain the higher risk of SCL with the PVAC catheters: (1) the multipolar catheter design can result in variable tissue contact on each electrode, predisposing to overheating of some poles and coagulum formation; (2) the lack of external irrigation may result in variable cooling of each electrode by blood flow; (3) the complex catheter geometry can result in air embolism during introduction across the hemostatic valve; and (4) excessive microbubble formation during accidental overlap of electrodes 1 and 10 on the catheter caused by shunting of excess current density and overheating.[7,12,33] Verma and colleagues[32] showed that meticulous attention to preventing these factors can significantly reduce the risk of SCL with PVAC ablation. The investigators systematically introduced 3 procedural changes: (1) either electrode 1 or electrode 10 was deactivated

to prevent accidental bipolar interaction, (2) introduction of the catheter into a introducer under saline to prevent ingress of air, and (3) therapeutic anticoagulation with warfarin and heparin to maintain ACT greater than 350 milliseconds. These measures resulted in a reduction in rate of SCL to 1.7% with use of the PVAC catheter.

The use of cryoablation to limit thermal injury of tissue at the catheter contact interface has been evaluated for its potential to reduce embolic lesions during ablation. Although histopathologic studies have shown a lower risk of endocardial thrombus formation with cryoablation compared with radiofrequency, this has not been borne out in clinical studies, which have shown a similar rate of SCL with the cryoballoon and irrigated radiofrequency catheter.[7,13,27] This finding may be explained by microemboli and air emboli introduced by multiple catheter manipulations and thrombus formation at the catheter sheath interface. Sauren and colleagues[43] reported fewer microembolic signals using TCD during cryoablation compared with radiofrequency ablation. However, most emboli with cryoablation occurred during catheter manipulation and at the end of each cryoablation, in contrast with radiofrequency ablation, which produced microemboli predominantly during energy delivery.

RECENT STUDIES, REMAINING CHALLENGES, AND FUTURE CONSIDERATIONS
Benefits of Catheter Ablation in Patients with AF

Recent findings discussed earlier should prompt a reassessment of the risks associated with AF ablation. However, these findings should also be interpreted in light of the potential benefits of AF ablation. Bunch and colleagues[44] showed that patients who had undergone AF ablation had a lower long-term incidence of stroke compared with patients who had not undergone an ablation procedure. This finding held true even after stratifying for baseline propensity for stroke using CHADS2 scores, as well as comparing for stroke across age groups.[44] In a prior study from the same investigators, findings of reduced stroke, dementia, and mortality were found in patients who underwent AF ablation compared with those with AF who did not undergo ablation.[45]

Need for Future Studies and Innovation

Although several recent studies have provided data on the magnitude of the problem and potential solutions for embolic lesions occurring during catheter ablation of AF, several questions remain unanswered. Future studies should focus on better defining patient-related and procedure-related factors that affect the incidence of SCL and the pathogenesis of these lesions. Longer term follow-up of patients with SCL after ablation and assessment of impact on neurocognitive function are required to better understand the true impact of these lesions. In addition, innovative strategies are needed to significantly reduce the risk of cerebral embolism. These innovations can take the form of better anticoagulation strategies, radically different approaches to AF ablation, or exploration of cerebral protection strategies, including devices.

As the new oral anticoagulants continue to be accepted in clinical practice, future studies evaluating safety are needed to balance potential reduction in embolic lesions associated with ablation with the risk of increased bleeding.[46] A large number of studies[47–53] have been conducted of drugs such as dabigatran and warfarin during procedures to reduce embolic complications from left-sided ablation, and also assessing for hemorrhagic complications. A recent editorial called for a prospective trial including one of the new anticoagulants to assess for SCL during AF ablation.[46]

An epicardial approach to AF ablation can eliminate the risk of cerebrovascular accidents associated with endocardial ablation. Sauren and colleagues[54] reported a reduced incidence of cerebral microembolic signals during thoracoscopic epicardial pulmonary vein isolation compared with percutaneous endocardial ablation. However, currently available strategies for epicardial ablation are significantly invasive, making them undesirable for most patients. Future innovations focused on minimally invasive percutaneous epicardial ablation are required. The use of carotid protection devices in patients with thrombus during ablation has been reported in individual cases.[55] However, currently available devices have problems such as a prothrombotic tendency, prohibiting the widespread use of these devices. Future technical innovations in cerebral protection are needed.

SUMMARY

MRI-detected SCLs that occur during AF ablation pose serious risks and challenges. Further prospective trials with longer follow-up periods are required to increase understanding of how best to risk stratify patients who are candidates for AF ablation. To achieve improved ablation safety, a multidisciplinary and multimodal approach is needed to determine the best method to prevent these lesions. This approach will involve innovation in ablation techniques, anticoagulation, and cerebral protection.

REFERENCES

1. Miyasaka Y, Barnes ME, Gersh BJ, et al. Secular trends in incidence of atrial fibrillation in Olmsted County, Minnesota, 1980 to 2000, and implications on the projections for future prevalence. Circulation 2006;114:119–25.
2. Calkins H, Kuck KH, Cappato R, et al. 2012 HRS/EHRA/ECAS expert consensus statement on catheter and surgical ablation of atrial fibrillation: recommendations for patient selection, procedural techniques, patient management and follow-up, definitions, endpoints, and research trial design: a report of the Heart Rhythm Society (HRS) Task Force on Catheter and Surgical Ablation of Atrial Fibrillation. Developed in partnership with the European Heart Rhythm Association (EHRA), a registered branch of the European Society Of Cardiology (ESC) and the European Cardiac Arrhythmia Society (ECAS); and in collaboration with the American College Of Cardiology (ACC), American Heart Association (AHA), the Asia Pacific Heart Rhythm Society (APHRS), and the Society Of Thoracic Surgeons (STS). Endorsed by the governing bodies of the American College Of Cardiology Foundation, the American Heart Association, the European Cardiac Arrhythmia Society, the European Heart Rhythm Association, the Society of Thoracic Surgeons, the Asia Pacific Heart Rhythm Society, and the Heart Rhythm Society. Heart Rhythm 2012;9:632–96.e21.
3. Desimone CV, Friedman PA, Noheria A, et al. Stroke or transient ischemic attack in patients with transvenous pacemaker or defibrillator and echocardiographically detected patent foramen ovale. Circulation 2013;128:1433–41.
4. Cappato R, Calkins H, Chen SA, et al. Updated worldwide survey on the methods, efficacy, and safety of catheter ablation for human atrial fibrillation. Circ Arrhythm Electrophysiol 2010;3:32–8.
5. Deneke T, Shin DI, Balta O, et al. Postablation asymptomatic cerebral lesions: long-term follow-up using magnetic resonance imaging. Heart Rhythm 2011;8:1705–11.
6. Gaita F, Caponi D, Pianelli M, et al. Radiofrequency catheter ablation of atrial fibrillation: a cause of silent thromboembolism? Magnetic resonance imaging assessment of cerebral thromboembolism in patients undergoing ablation of atrial fibrillation. Circulation 2010;122:1667–73.
7. Gaita F, Leclercq JF, Schumacher B, et al. Incidence of silent cerebral thromboembolic lesions after atrial fibrillation ablation may change according to technology used: comparison of irrigated

radiofrequency, multipolar nonirrigated catheter and cryoballoon. J Cardiovasc Electrophysiol 2011;22:961–8.

8. Rillig A, Meyerfeldt U, Tilz RR, et al. Incidence and long-term follow-up of silent cerebral lesions after pulmonary vein isolation using a remote robotic navigation system as compared to manual ablation. Circ Arrhythm Electrophysiol 2012;5(1):15–21.

9. Schrickel JW, Lickfett L, Lewalter T, et al. Incidence and predictors of silent cerebral embolism during pulmonary vein catheter ablation for atrial fibrillation. Europace 2010;12:52–7.

10. Gonzalez RG, Schaefer PW, Buonanno FS, et al. Diffusion-weighted MR imaging: diagnostic accuracy in patients imaged within 6 hours of stroke symptom onset. Radiology 1999;210:155–62.

11. Lovblad KO, Laubach HJ, Baird AE, et al. Clinical experience with diffusion-weighted MR in patients with acute stroke. AJNR Am J Neuroradiol 1998; 19:1061–6.

12. Herrera Siklody C, Deneke T, Hocini M, et al. Incidence of asymptomatic intracranial embolic events after pulmonary vein isolation: comparison of different atrial fibrillation ablation technologies in a multicenter study. J Am Coll Cardiol 2011;58: 681–8.

13. Neumann T, Kuniss M, Conradi G, et al. Medafi-trial (micro-embolization during ablation of atrial fibrillation): comparison of pulmonary vein isolation using cryoballoon technique vs. radiofrequency energy. Europace 2011;13:37–44.

14. Haeusler KG, Koch L, Herm J, et al. 3 Tesla MRI-detected brain lesions after pulmonary vein isolation for atrial fibrillation: results of the MACPAF study. J Cardiovasc Electrophysiol 2013;24:14–21.

15. Scaglione M, Blandino A, Raimondo C, et al. Impact of ablation catheter irrigation design on silent cerebral embolism after radiofrequency catheter ablation of atrial fibrillation: results from a pilot study. J Cardiovasc Electrophysiol 2012;23: 801–5.

16. Martinek M, Sigmund E, Lemes C, et al. Asymptomatic cerebral lesions during pulmonary vein isolation under uninterrupted oral anticoagulation. Europace 2013;15:325–31.

17. Ichiki H, Oketani N, Ishida S, et al. Incidence of asymptomatic cerebral microthromboembolism after atrial fibrillation ablation guided by complex fractionated atrial electrogram. J Cardiovasc Electrophysiol 2012;23:567–73.

18. Gaita F, Corsinovi L, Anselmino M, et al. Prevalence of silent cerebral ischemia in paroxysmal and persistent atrial fibrillation and correlation with cognitive function. J Am Coll Cardiol 2013;62(21): 1990–7.

19. Sommer T, Vahlhaus C, Lauck G, et al. MR imaging and cardiac pacemakers: in-vitro evaluation and

in-vivo studies in 51 patients at 0.5 t. Radiology 2000;215:869–79.

20. Lickfett L, Hackenbroch M, Lewalter T, et al. Cerebral diffusion-weighted magnetic resonance imaging: a tool to monitor the thrombogenicity of left atrial catheter ablation. J Cardiovasc Electrophysiol 2006;17:1–7.

21. Svensson LG, Robinson MF, Esser J, et al. Influence of anatomic origin on intracranial distribution of micro-emboli in the baboon. Stroke 1986;17: 1198–202.

22. Zhu L, Wintermark M, Saloner D, et al. The distribution and size of ischemic lesions after carotid artery angioplasty and stenting: evidence for microembolization to terminal arteries. J Vasc Surg 2011;53: 971–6.

23. Kilicaslan F, Verma A, Saad E, et al. Transcranial Doppler detection of microembolic signals during pulmonary vein antrum isolation: implications for titration of radiofrequency energy. J Cardiovasc Electrophysiol 2006;17:495–501.

24. Medi C, Evered L, Silbert B, et al. Subtle postprocedural cognitive dysfunction after atrial fibrillation ablation. J Am Coll Cardiol 2013;62:531–9.

25. Schwarz N, Kuniss M, Nedelmann M, et al. Neuropsychological decline after catheter ablation of atrial fibrillation. Heart Rhythm 2010;7:1761–7.

26. Madhavan M, Govil SR, Asirvatham SJ. Signals. Circ Arrhythm Electrophysiol 2012;5:2–4.

27. Khairy P, Chauvet P, Lehmann J, et al. Lower incidence of thrombus formation with cryoenergy versus radiofrequency catheter ablation. Circulation 2003;107:2045–50.

28. Tse HF, Kwong YL, Lau CP. Transvenous cryoablation reduces platelet activation during pulmonary vein ablation compared with radiofrequency energy in patients with atrial fibrillation. J Cardiovasc Electrophysiol 2005;16:1064–70.

29. Ren JF, Marchlinski FE, Callans DJ, et al. Increased intensity of anticoagulation may reduce risk of thrombus during atrial fibrillation ablation procedures in patients with spontaneous echo contrast. J Cardiovasc Electrophysiol 2005;16:474–7.

30. Bernhardt P, Schmidt H, Hammerstingl C, et al. Patients with atrial fibrillation and dense spontaneous echo contrast at high risk a prospective and serial follow-up over 12 months with transesophageal echocardiography and cerebral magnetic resonance imaging. J Am Coll Cardiol 2005;45: 1807–12.

31. Bruce CJ, Friedman PA, Narayan O, et al. Early heparinization decreases the incidence of left atrial thrombi detected by intracardiac echocardiography during radiofrequency ablation for atrial fibrillation. J Interv Card Electrophysiol 2008;22:211–9.

32. Verma A, Debruyne P, Nardi S, et al. Evaluation and reduction of asymptomatic cerebral embolism in

ablation of atrial fibrillation, but high prevalence of chronic silent infarction: results of the evaluation of reduction of asymptomatic cerebral embolism trial. Circ Arrhythm Electrophysiol 2013;6:835–42.

33. Haines DE, Stewart MT, Ahlberg S, et al. Microembolism and catheter ablation I: a comparison of irrigated radiofrequency and multielectrode-phased radiofrequency catheter ablation of pulmonary vein ostia. Circ Arrhythm Electrophysiol 2013;6: 16–22.

34. Haines DE, Stewart MT, Barka ND, et al. Microembolism and catheter ablation II: effects of cerebral microemboli injection in a canine model. Circ Arrhythm Electrophysiol 2013;6:23–30.

35. Nagy-Baló E, Tint D, Clemens M, et al. Transcranial measurement of cerebral microembolic signals during pulmonary vein isolation: a comparison of two ablation techniques. Circ Arrhythm Electrophysiol 2013;6:473–80.

36. Wood MA, Shaffer KM, Ellenbogen AL, et al. Microbubbles during radiofrequency catheter ablation: composition and formation. Heart Rhythm 2005;2: 397–403.

37. Cauchemez B, Extramiana F, Cauchemez S, et al. High-flow perfusion of sheaths for prevention of thromboembolic complications during complex catheter ablation in the left atrium. J Cardiovasc Electrophysiol 2004;15:276–83.

38. Maleki K, Mohammadi R, Hart D, et al. Intracardiac ultrasound detection of thrombus on transseptal sheath: incidence, treatment, and prevention. J Cardiovasc Electrophysiol 2005;16:561–5.

39. Haines DE. ERACEing the risk of cerebral embolism from atrial fibrillation ablation. Circ Arrhythm Electrophysiol 2013;6:827–9.

40. Lim B, Venkatachalam KL, Jahangir A, et al. Concurrent application of charge using a novel circuit prevents heat-related coagulum formation during radiofrequency ablation. J Cardiovasc Electrophysiol 2008;19:843–50.

41. Demolin JM, Eick OJ, Münch K, et al. Soft thrombus formation in radiofrequency catheter ablation. Pacing Clin Electrophysiol 2002;25(8):1219–22.

42. Dorwarth U, Fiek M, Remp T, et al. Radiofrequency catheter ablation: different cooled and noncooled electrode systems induce specific lesion geometries and adverse effects profiles. Pacing Clin Electrophysiol 2003;26:1438–45.

43. Sauren LD, van Belle Y, de Roy L, et al. Transcranial measurement of cerebral microembolic signals during endocardial pulmonary vein isolation: comparison of three different ablation techniques. J Cardiovasc Electrophysiol 2009;20:1102–7.

44. Bunch TJ, May HT, Bair TL, et al. Atrial fibrillation ablation patients have long-term stroke rates similar to patients without atrial fibrillation regardless of CHADS2 score. Heart Rhythm 2013;10: 1272–7.

45. Bunch TJ, Crandall BG, Weiss JP, et al. Patients treated with catheter ablation for atrial fibrillation have long-term rates of death, stroke, and dementia similar to patients without atrial fibrillation. J Cardiovasc Electrophysiol 2011;22:839–45.

46. Noheria A, Asirvatham S. Periprocedural dabigatran anticoagulation for atrial fibrillation ablation: do we have enough information to make a rational decision. J Interv Card Electrophysiol 2013;37: 209–11.

47. Lakkireddy D, Reddy YM, Di Biase L, et al. Feasibility and safety of dabigatran versus warfarin for periprocedural anticoagulation in patients undergoing radiofrequency ablation for atrial fibrillation: results from a multicenter prospective registry. J Am Coll Cardiol 2012;59:1168–74.

48. Santangeli P, Di Biase L, Horton R, et al. Ablation of atrial fibrillation under therapeutic warfarin reduces periprocedural complications: evidence from a meta-analysis. Circ Arrhythm Electrophysiol 2012; 5:302–11.

49. Steinberg B, Hasselblad V, Atwater B, et al. Dabigatran for periprocedural anticoagulation following radiofrequency ablation for atrial fibrillation: a meta-analysis of observational studies. J Interv Card Electrophysiol 2013;37:213–21.

50. Kaiser D, Streur M, Nagarakanti R, et al. Continuous warfarin versus periprocedural dabigatran to reduce stroke and systemic embolism in patients undergoing catheter ablation for atrial fibrillation or left atrial flutter. J Interv Card Electrophysiol 2013;37:241–7.

51. Imamura K, Yoshida A, Takei A, et al. Dabigatran in the peri-procedural period for radiofrequency ablation of atrial fibrillation: efficacy, safety, and impact on duration of hospital stay. J Interv Card Electrophysiol 2013;37:223–31.

52. Maddox W, Kay GN, Yamada T, et al. Dabigatran versus warfarin therapy for uninterrupted oral anticoagulation during atrial fibrillation ablation. J Cardiovasc Electrophysiol 2013;24:861–5.

53. Kim JS, She F, Jongnarangsin K, et al. Dabigatran vs warfarin for radiofrequency catheter ablation of atrial fibrillation. Heart Rhythm 2013;10:483–9.

54. Sauren LD, la Meir M, de Roy L, et al. Increased number of cerebral emboli during percutaneous endocardial pulmonary vein isolation versus a thoracoscopic epicardial approach. Eur J Cardiothorac Surg 2009;36:833–7.

55. Munir A, Safian RD, Haines DE. Use of embolic protection to prevent stroke during catheter ablation of atrial fibrillation. Circulation 2011;124:965–6.

Anticoagulation Issues in Atrial Fibrillation Ablation

Michael P. Riley, MD, PhD

KEYWORDS

- Atrial fibrillation ablation • Anticoagulation • Intracardiac echocardiography • Reversal agents
- Novel oral anticoagulants • Warfarin

KEY POINTS

- Patients undergoing atrial fibrillation ablation should be anticoagulated before, during, and following ablation to reduce the risk of thromboembolic complications.
- The uninterrupted use of warfarin throughout the ablation period seems safe and effective, though benefits are limited by the inherent variability of the international normalized ratio.
- The periprocedural use of the novel oral anticoagulants throughout the ablation period requires additional investigation though their use is increasing. Differences among these novel agents need to be defined.
- The development of safe and effective reversal agents for the novel oral anticoagulants is needed to minimize the bleeding risks associated with their use.
- The long-term use of oral anticoagulants following successful ablation requires ongoing research and investigation.

INTRODUCTION

Patients undergoing atrial fibrillation ablation are anticoagulated before, during, and following their procedure to reduce the serious risk of a thromboembolic complication. Despite this well established recommendation, there remains debate about the optimal nature of anticoagulation and a continuing evolution in practice patterns. This article addresses issues related to anticoagulation in atrial fibrillation ablation focusing on the preprocedural, intraprocedural, and postprocedural periods.

PREPROCEDURAL ANTICOAGULATION

Most patients undergoing atrial fibrillation ablation are maintained on therapeutic oral anticoagulation, with warfarin or one of the novel oral anticoagulants, including dabigatran, rivaroxaban, or apixaban. Selected low-risk patients (with a CHADS2 [congestive heart failure, hypertension, age, diabetes, stroke] score of 0-1) may be maintained without anticoagulation or on aspirin therapy.[1]

The most current guidelines regarding anticoagulation and the performance of transesophageal echocardiography before atrial fibrillation ablation are modeled on the guidelines used to guide anticoagulation before cardioversion.[2] That is, for patients who are persistently in atrial fibrillation or have episodes lasting longer than 48 hours, 3 weeks of therapeutic anticoagulation is recommended. In such patients, the performance of a transesophageal echocardiogram before ablation is not required. In situations in which patients are not anticoagulated, performance of a transesophageal echocardiogram is recommended. Notably, the CHADS2 score (or other scoring system grading thromboembolic risk) is not a part of these recommendations. Uncommonly, these recommendations can lead to some unusual clinical

The author has nothing to disclose.
Department of Medicine, Division of Cardiology, Section of Electrophysiology, Hospital of the University of Pennsylvania, 9 Founders Pavilion, 3400 Spruce Street, Philadelphia, PA 19104, USA
E-mail address: michael.riley@uphs.upenn.edu

Card Electrophysiol Clin 6 (2014) 95–100
http://dx.doi.org/10.1016/j.ccep.2013.10.009

scenarios. For instance, a patient with infrequent paroxysmal atrial fibrillation with a CHADS2 score of 0 who is maintained on aspirin would require a transesophageal echocardiogram, whereas a patient with persistent atrial fibrillation with a CHADS2 score of 3 to 4 who is maintained on warfarin would not require a transesophageal echocardiogram. In scenarios such as these, or when there is any concern for left atrial appendage thrombus, clinical judgment regarding the performance of a transesophageal echocardiogram should take precedence.

Historically, up until a few years ago, warfarin was discontinued before atrial fibrillation ablation and anticoagulation bridging before and after the ablation was performed with heparin (low-molecular-weight or unfractionated). As for many surgical procedures, the rationale for this practice was to attempt to reduce the bleeding risks associated with the procedure. In the case of atrial fibrillation ablation, these risks are often serious and are associated with pericardial tamponade and retroperitoneal bleeding.[3-6] This concern regarding bleeding risks required weighing the relative risks associated with thromboembolic complications during and immediately following the procedure when, in the absence of therapeutic levels of an oral anticoagulant, the patient may have lower levels of systemic anticoagulation.

Recent observational studies have demonstrated that periprocedural continuation of uninterrupted warfarin can be performed safely and it does not seem to increase the rate of bleeding complications.[7-13] One difficulty with the approach of uninterrupted warfarin is the inherent unpredictability of the patient's international normalized ratio (INR) on the day of the procedure. For this reason, the increasingly common practice of performing atrial fibrillation ablations on the day of admission to the hospital (based on insurance company mandate or physician preference) complicates the practice of performing atrial fibrillation ablations on uninterrupted warfarin. Evidence suggests that a supratherapeutic INR can be associated with an increased risk of complications that may minimize the benefit from performing procedures on warfarin.[14] To minimize the elevated risks associated with high INRs, one large center administers fresh frozen plasma to any patient with an INR greater than 3.5 on the day of the procedure.[7] Another approach has been to hold 1 or 2 days of warfarin before the ablation in an attempt to minimize extremely high INRs; however, this approach has not been studied and validated and may negate the benefit in thromboembolism prevention (due to subtherapeutic INRs).

Up until the release of the newer generation novel oral anticoagulants, the choice of anticoagulation was limited to warfarin. The availability of dabigatran, rivaroxaban, and apixaban has led to an increasing number of patients using one of these agents for the prevention of thromboembolism.[15-17] As expected, many of these patients are presenting for atrial fibrillation ablation on one of these novel agents. Periprocedural management of these new agents is less well understood from both evidence-based and experience-based perspectives. Importantly, because of differences in pharmacokinetics as well as mechanism of action, these agents likely will not behave identically to warfarin, or even to each other, in terms of risks and benefits. This emphasizes the need for ongoing investigation regarding the use of these agents periablation for atrial fibrillation. Toward that end, several small observational studies have evaluated the use of periprocedural dabigatran versus uninterrupted warfarin.[18-22] These studies have differed in patient population as well as the number of doses of dabigatran held before the ablation. There are conflicting results between studies related to bleeding complications and thromboembolism complications. They have not yielded clear recommendations and thus there is an ongoing need for large randomized trials of uninterrupted warfarin versus all of the novel oral anticoagulants.

Finally, any interruption of oral anticoagulation raises the issue of whether the performance of a transesophageal echocardiogram is warranted. Strictly speaking, patients presenting for their ablation in atrial fibrillation who have held doses of a novel oral anticoagulant should be considered for transesophageal echocardiography.

INTRAPROCEDURAL ANTICOAGULATION
Heparin Anticoagulation During the Atrial Fibrillation Ablation

As mentioned above, there is ongoing debate regarding the optimal means to manage warfarin and the novel oral anticoagulants immediately before ablation. There is clearly an increasing trend toward uninterrupted (or minimally interrupted) oral anticoagulation throughout the procedure. Despite differences in the management of oral anticoagulants preprocedure, there is nearly universal use of unfractionated heparin during the ablation procedure. Dosing regimens range from 70 mg/kg to 100 mg/kg bolus followed by a continuous infusion.[23] Physician preference dictates the decision about when to administer the heparin bolus. This decision usually revolves around whether to give the heparin bolus before or after transseptal puncture. This timing is largely related to weighing the risks of tamponade during transseptal puncture with the risk of thrombus formation on the sheaths and catheters once they enter the left atrium. In many centers, intracardiac echocardiography is used to minimize the perforation risk associated with transseptal puncture. In the author's laboratory, heparin is administered with the goal of a therapeutic activated clotting time (ACT) before transseptal puncture.

While catheters are in the left atrium performing ablation, the target ACT ranges from 300 to 400 seconds. There is some evidence that higher ACT may reduce the risk of thrombus formation on sheaths in the setting of spontaneous dense smoke.[24,25]

Some published data and much anecdotal experience suggest that bolus heparin dosing requirements may be less when administered in the presence of a therapeutic INR.[14] How heparin dosing is affected by the presence (or acute withdrawal) of the novel oral anticoagulants is not understood.

Currently used transseptal sheaths are coated with polymers to reduce their thrombogenicity. Despite this, thrombus can infrequently form in some patients. The relationship between patient factors such as possible procoagulability and catheter characteristics leading to thrombus formation on the catheter is not understood. The practice of flushing sheaths with heparinized saline at rates ranging from 100 mL per hour to 200 mL per hour may decrease the risk of thrombus formation at the sheath tip by preventing stagnant blood flow near the sheath opening.

Aspirin

The periprocedural use of aspirin as an adjunctive anticoagulant targeting platelet reactivity has not been rigorously studied but is used in some atrial fibrillation centers.[3] Aspirin dosing can range from a single preprocedure dose to weeks of aspirin use before and following the procedure. Obviously, any use of adjunctive anticoagulants raises the risk of bleeding and needs to be weighed against any additive reduction in thromboembolic complications.

INTRACARDIAC ECHOCARDIOGRAPHY

The increased use of intracardiac echocardiography to guide transseptal puncture and for the early recognition of hemorrhagic pericardial effusion has improved the comfort level for the performance of atrial fibrillation ablation with high levels of anticoagulation. The use of intracardiac echo has also demonstrated the low but real issue of

thrombus associated with sheaths and catheters in the left atrium and led to higher target ACT during left atrial ablation.[24–27]

With and without the use of intracardiac echocardiography, vigilance for any type of bleeding complication (pericardial, femoral access) must be maintained given the high levels of anticoagulation during ablation. Given the risks of cardiac perforation and tamponade, physicians performing atrial fibrillation ablations should be well trained and comfortable with epicardial access.

ANTICOAGULATION REVERSAL AGENTS

No currently available reversal agents except Protamine exist for the immediate and specific reversal of anticoagulants. This section describes in general terms the available agents used to reverse anticoagulation during a bleeding complication.[28] The need for prompt reversal of anticoagulation is uncommon due to bleeding complications but potentially life-saving when necessary due to the severity of pericardial effusion/tamponade and retroperitoneal bleeding, the most common bleeding complications.

Reversing Heparin

Protamine administered intravenously can promptly reverse the anticoagulant effect of heparin. There is a dose–response relationship; therefore, the dose of protamine can be titrated to achieve a slow reversal as when reversing heparin in anticipation of groin sheath removal or to achieve a more rapid reversal when dealing with life-threatening bleeding.

Reversing Warfarin

Recently approved for use in the United States, four-factor prothrombin complex concentrate containing factors II, VII, IX, and X targets reversal of high INRs associated with warfarin. Procoagulation is a concern with its use and must be balanced again the bleeding risk. Activated factor VIIa has also been used in some centers. The use of fresh frozen plasma replaces clotting factors more broadly but is limited by the time required to thaw and deliver to the patient. Vitamin K antagonizes warfarin by augmenting the production of new clotting factors but takes substantial time to achieve an effect and is more useful as a longer term means of reversing warfarin anticoagulation.

Reversing Dabigatran

Dabigatran is a direct thrombin (IIa) inhibitor for which no specific reversal agent is currently available. Antibody fragments are undergoing development that should be able to rapidly and specifically reverse the anticoagulant effect of dabigatran. Hemodialysis can reduce the serum concentration of dabigatran in cases of overdose or refractory bleeding. Some evidence suggests that four-factor prothrombin complex concentrate can be used if needed.[28]

Reversing Rivaroxaban or Apixaban

Both rivaroxaban and apixaban are factor Xa inhibitors. There is scarce published evidence for their use during atrial fibrillation ablation and thus the usefulness of reversal agents is less well known. In other cases of bleeding associated with these agents, the use of four-factor prothrombin complex concentrate has been suggested.[28]

POSTPROCEDURAL ANTICOAGULATION
Immediate Postprocedure Time Period

In the hours immediately following atrial fibrillation ablation, the thromboembolic risk remains elevated and anticoagulation must be continued or reinitiated.[6,29] The current guidelines suggest that, unless a therapeutic INR is present, either low-molecular-weight or unfractionated heparin be given.[2] The timing of this varies from 2 to 6 hours after sheath removal and varies by center. Use of the novel oral anticoagulants may be considered as alternatives to heparin and warfarin postablation. The current guidelines and the practice at many centers is to avoid heparin in the presence of a therapeutic INR. This strategy seems to protect against thromboembolic risk while minimizing the risks associated with bleeding due to heparin at the femoral access sites. In selected patients at high risk for a thromboembolic complication, or if it is unknown whether there is a therapeutic INR, the use of heparin immediately following the procedure should be considered.

Short-term Anticoagulation (up to 2 months)

Guidelines regarding anticoagulation following atrial fibrillation ablation recommend therapeutic anticoagulation with either warfarin, a direct thrombin (dabigatran), or factor Xa inhibitor (rivaroxaban or apixaban) for a minimum of 2 months following ablation.[2] This is the practice at most centers.

Two centers have evaluated the usefulness of a less intensive anticoagulation strategy for very low risk patients. One center discharged patients on aspirin therapy only and noted no significant increase in the risk of thromboembolic complications.[30] Another center used an approach of 10 days of low-molecular-weight heparin followed by 2 months of aspirin therapy and also noted no

increase in thromboembolic complications in patients with a CHADS2 score of 0 or 1.[31] Both of these studies raise interesting issues with regard to the usefulness of therapeutic anticoagulation postprocedure in low-risk patients. Before either of these approaches can be broadly recommended, they require validation at other centers and with additional patients.

Despite the paucity of published data regarding the clinical use and usefulness of aspirin and/or clopidogrel following atrial fibrillation ablation, there is some suggestion that this approach is used.[3,4] The world-wide survey by Cappato[3,4] seems to suggest that up to 10% of patients are discharged home on aspirin only and that there is also some use of clopidogrel.

The adjunctive use of aspirin with an oral anticoagulant has also not been studied in a formal way but is used at some centers. The author's practice is to combine an oral anticoagulant with 30 days of aspirin.

Long-term Anticoagulation (beyond 2 months)

Anticoagulation beyond 2 months after atrial fibrillation ablation is an area of active debate and investigation. The issue essentially revolves around whether and how atrial fibrillation ablation influences the long-term risk of thromboembolism. The maintenance of sinus rhythm postablation likely mitigates the thromboembolic risk associated with atrial fibrillation; however, this benefit may be offset by changes in left atrial function following ablation as well as the potential presence of asymptomatic atrial fibrillation following ablation.[32] Addressing this question, the most recent expert consensus document recommends that long-term anticoagulation should be based on a patient's overall risk factors for thromboembolism (CHADS2 or CHA2DS2-VASc [congestive heart failure (1), hypertension (1), age >75 (2), diabetes (1), prior stroke or TIA (2), vascular disease (1), age 65–74 (1), female (1)] score) and not on the presence or absence of atrial fibrillation.[2] Despite this recommendation, many physicians discontinue oral anticoagulation after detailed conversations with selected patients with CHADS2 scores of 2 or higher. This practice is increasingly supported by observational studies that seem to demonstrate lower long-term rates of thromboembolic complications following atrial fibrillation ablation, including in patients selected to discontinue oral anticoagulation.[33–37] These studies are limited by their observational nature. Ongoing randomized studies are needed to better define the role of long-term oral anticoagulation in patients following atrial fibrillation ablation. This is especially true considering the costs and morbidity associated with long-term anticoagulation.

SUMMARY

Anticoagulation management before, during, and following ablation for atrial fibrillation is a complex issue involving the risks of thromboembolism and bleeding. No other widely performed invasive procedure weighs these risks as delicately as that of ablation for atrial fibrillation, largely because neither thromboembolism nor life-threatening bleeding is rare. The complexity of anticoagulation management is compounded by the recent development of the novel oral anticoagulants. Navigating the best course of treatment of each patient can be challenging both periprocedurally and long-term. Ongoing investigation, with randomized trials when possible, should continue to inform our knowledge and decision making.

REFERENCES

1. Fuster V, Ryden L, Cannom D, et al, American College of Cardiology Foundation/American Heart Association Task Force. 2011 ACCF/AHA/HRS focused updates incorporated into the ACC/AHA/ESC 2006 guidelines for the management of patients with atrial fibrillation: a report of the American College of Cardiology Foundation/American Heart Association Task Force on practice guidelines. Circulation 2011;123:e269–367.

2. Calkins H, Kuck KH, Cappato R, et al, Heart Rhythm Society Task Force on Catheter and Surgical Ablation of Atrial Fibrillation. 2012 HRS/EHRA/ECAS expert consensus statement on catheter and surgical ablation of atrial fibrillation: recommendations for patient selection, procedural techniques, patient management and follow-up, definitions, endpoints, and research trial design: a report of the Heart Rhythm Society (HRS) Task Force on Catheter and Surgical Ablation of Atrial Fibrillation. Developed in partnership with the European Heart Rhythm Association (EHRA), a registered branch of the European Society of Cardiology (ESC) and the European Cardiac Arrhythmia Society (ECAS); and in collaboration with the American College of Cardiology (ACC), American Heart Association (AHA), the Asia Pacific Heart Rhythm Society (APHRS), and the Society of Thoracic Surgeons (STS). Endorsed by the governing bodies of the American College of Cardiology Foundation, the American Heart Association, the European Cardiac Arrhythmia Society, the European Heart Rhythm Association, the Society of Thoracic Surgeons, the Asia Pacific Heart Rhythm Society, and the Heart Rhythm Society. Heart Rhythm 2012;9:632–96.e21.

3. Cappato R, Calkins H, Chen SA, et al. Updated worldwide survey on the methods, efficacy, and safety of catheter ablation for human atrial fibrillation. Circ Arrhythm Electrophysiol 2010;3:32–8.

4. Cappato R, Calkins H, Chen SA, et al. Worldwide survey on the methods, efficacy, and safety of catheter ablation for human atrial fibrillation. Circulation 2005;111:1100–5.

5. Bertaglia E, Zoppo F, Tondo C, et al. Early complications of pulmonary vein catheter ablation for atrial fibrillation: a multicenter prospective registry on procedural safety. Heart Rhythm 2007;4:1265–71.

6. Oral H, Chugh A, Ozaydin M, et al. Risk of thromboembolic events after percutaneous left atrial radiofrequency ablation of atrial fibrillation. Circulation 2006;114:759–65.

7. Gopinath D, Lewis WR, Di Biase L, et al. Pulmonary vein antrum isolation for atrial fibrillation on therapeutic coumadin: special considerations. J Cardiovasc Electrophysiol 2011;22:236–9.

8. Hussein AA, Martin DO, Saliba W, et al. Radiofrequency ablation of atrial fibrillation under therapeutic international normalized ratio: a safe and efficacious periprocedural anticoagulation strategy. Heart Rhythm 2009;6:1425–9.

9. Santangeli P, Di Biase L, Horton R, et al. Ablation of atrial fibrillation under therapeutic warfarin reduces periprocedural complications: evidence from a meta-analysis. Circ Arrhythm Electrophysiol 2012;5:302–11.

10. Schmidt M, Segerson NM, Marschang H, et al. Atrial fibrillation ablation in patients with therapeutic international normalized ratios. Pacing Clin Electrophysiol 2009;32:995–9.

11. Wazni OM, Beheiry S, Fahmy T, et al. Atrial fibrillation ablation in patients with therapeutic international normalized ratio: comparison of strategies of anticoagulation management in the periprocedural period. Circulation 2007;116:2531–4.

12. Latchamsetty R, Gautam S, Bhakta D, et al. Management and outcomes of cardiac tamponade during atrial fibrillation ablation in the presence of therapeutic anticoagulation with warfarin. Heart Rhythm 2011;8:805–8.

13. Kuwahara T, Takahashi A, Takahashi Y, et al. Prevention of periprocedural ischemic stroke and management of hemorrhagic complications in atrial fibrillation ablation under continuous warfarin administration. J Cardiovasc Electrophysiol 2013;24:510–5.

14. Kim JS, Jongnarangsin K, Latchamsetty R, et al. The optimal range of international normalized ratio for radiofrequency catheter ablation of atrial fibrillation during therapeutic anticoagulation with warfarin. Circ Arrhythm Electrophysiol 2013;6:302–9.

15. Granger CB, Alexander JH, McMurray JJ, et al, ARISTOTLE Committees and Investigators. Apixaban versus warfarin in patients with atrial fibrillation. N Engl J Med 2011;365:981–92.

16. Patel MR, Mahaffey KW, Garg J, et al, ROCKET AF Investigators. Rivaroxaban versus warfarin in nonvalvular atrial fibrillation. N Engl J Med 2011;365: 883–91.

17. Connolly SJ, Ezekowitz MD, Yusuf S, et al, RE-LY Steering Committee and Investigators. Dabigatran versus warfarin in patients with atrial fibrillation. N Engl J Med 2009;361:1139–51.

18. Lakkireddy D, Reddy YM, Di Biase L, et al. Feasibility and safety of dabigatran versus warfarin for periprocedural anticoagulation in patients undergoing radiofrequency ablation for atrial fibrillation: results from a multicenter prospective registry. J Am Coll Cardiol 2012;59:1168–74.

19. Maddox W, Kay G, Yamada T, et al. Dabigatran versus warfarin therapy for uninterrupted oral anticoagulation during atrial fibrillation ablation. J Cardiovasc Electrophysiol 2013;24:861–5.

20. Pelargonio G, Perna F. Periprocedural dabigatran in atrial fibrillation ablation: a new kid on the block. J Cardiovasc Electrophysiol 2013;24:866–8.

21. Winkle RA, Mead RH, Engel G, et al. Safety of dabigatran versus warfarin for periprocedural anticoagulation in patients undergoing ablation for atrial fibrillation. J Am Coll Cardiol 2012;60:1118–9.

22. Nin T, Sairaku A, Yoshida Y, et al. A randomized controlled trial of dabigatran versus warfarin for peri-ablation anticoagulation in patients undergoing ablation of atrial fibrillation. Pacing Clin Electrophysiol 2013;36:172–9.

23. Vazquez SR, Johnson SA, Rondina MT. Peri-procedural anticoagulation in patients undergoing ablation for atrial fibrillation. Thromb Res 2010;126: e69–77.

24. Ren JF, Marchlinski FE, Callans DJ, et al. Increased intensity of anticoagulation may reduce risk of thrombus during atrial fibrillation ablation procedures in patients with spontaneous echo contrast. J Cardiovasc Electrophysiol 2005;16:474–7.

25. Wazni OM, Rossillo A, Marrouche NF, et al. Embolic events and char formation during pulmonary vein isolation in patients with atrial fibrillation: impact of different anticoagulation regimens and importance of intracardiac echo imaging. J Cardiovasc Electrophysiol 2005;16:576–81.

26. Ren JF, Marchlinski FE, Callans DJ. Left atrial thrombus associated with ablation for atrial fibrillation: identification with intracardiac echocardiography. J Am Coll Cardiol 2004;43:1861–7.

27. Bruce CJ, Friedman PA, Narayan O, et al. Early heparinization decreases the incidence of left atrial thrombi detected by intracardiac echocardiography during radiofrequency ablation for atrial fibrillation. J Interv Card Electrophysiol 2008;22: 211–9.

28. Kalus J. Pharmacologic interventions for reversing the effects of oral anticoagulants. Am J Health Syst Pharm 2013;70:S12–21.

29. Scherr D, Sharma K, Dalal D, et al. Incidence and predictors of periprocedural cerebrovascular accident in patients undergoing catheter ablation of atrial fibrillation. J Cardiovasc Electrophysiol 2009; 20:1357–63.

30. Bunch TJ, Crandall BG, Weiss JP, et al. Warfarin is not needed in low-risk patients following atrial fibrillation ablation procedures. J Cardiovasc Electrophysiol 2009;20:988–93.

31. Duytschaever M, Berte B, Acena M, et al. Catheter ablation of atrial fibrillation in patients at low thrombo-embolic risk: efficacy and safety of a simplified periprocedural anticoagulation strategy. J Cardiovasc Electrophysiol 2013;24:855–60.

32. Hindricks G, Piorkowski C, Tanner H, et al. Perception of atrial fibrillation before and after radiofrequency catheter ablation: relevance of asymptomatic arrhythmia recurrence. Circulation 2005; 112:307–13.

33. Bunch T, May H, Bair T, et al. Atrial fibrillation ablation patients have long-term stroke rates similar to patients without atrial fibrillation regardless of CHADS2 Score. Heart Rhythm 2013;10:1272–7.

34. Bunch TJ, Crandall BG, Weiss JP, et al. Patients treated with catheter ablation for atrial fibrillation have long-term rates of death, stroke, and dementia similar to patients without atrial fibrillation. J Cardiovasc Electrophysiol 2011;22:839–45.

35. Guiot A, Jongnarangsin K, Chugh A, et al. Anticoagulant therapy and risk of cerebrovascular events after catheter ablation of atrial fibrillation in the elderly. J Cardiovasc Electrophysiol 2012;23:36–43.

36. Hunter RJ, McCready J, Diab I, et al. Maintenance of sinus rhythm with an ablation strategy in patients with atrial fibrillation is associated with a lower risk of stroke and death. Heart 2012;98:48–53.

37. Themistoclakis S, Corrado A, Marchlinski FE, et al. The risk of thromboembolism and need for oral anticoagulation after successful atrial fibrillation ablation. J Am Coll Cardiol 2010;55:735–43.

Illustrated Atlas of Post-AF Ablation Cerebral Abnormalities

Fiorenzo Gaita, MD[a,*], Maria Consuelo Valentini, MD[b],
Laura Corsinovi, MD, PhD[a], Martina Pianelli, MD[a],
Davide Castagno, MD[a], Federico Cesarani, MD[c],
Marco Scaglione, MD[d]

KEYWORDS

- Atrial fibrillation • Atrial fibrillation transcatheter ablation • Cardioembolic risk • Cognitive decline
- Silent cerebral ischemia • Magnetic resonance imaging

KEY POINTS

- Atrial fibrillation (AF) is one of the most common cardiac arrhythmias and relates to high morbidity and mortality due to thromboembolic events, especially ischemic stroke.
- Transcatheter AF ablation is a well-established treatment for symptomatic patients refractory to antiarrhythmic drugs, but this procedure implies a relevant risk of cerebral ischemia, especially silent.
- Most AF-ablation-related silent cerebral ischemias were detected by means of magnetic resonance imaging mainly at cortical level with a preferential clustering in the frontal and parietal lobes and in the cerebellum.
- The clinical impact of silent cerebral ischemia is not fully understood, but this cerebral damage seems to affect cognitive performance.

INTRODUCTION

Atrial fibrillation (AF) is one of the most common cardiac arrhythmias, affecting 1% to 2% of the worldwide population, and its burden is expected to increase in the next decades.[1,2] Prevalence of AF increases with age, from less than 0.4% at 40 to 50 years of age up to 15% over the age of 80.[3,4] Independently from the presence of comorbidities, AF relates to enhanced mortality and thromboembolism,[5] particularly to the brain.

The cerebral thromboembolic damage secondary to AF may be clinically overt or appear as a silent phenomenon.[6] If symptomatic brain damage is easily diagnosed and has been thoroughly analyzed, the relationship between AF and silent cerebral ischemia (SCI) needs further evaluation.

SCI has been proven not to be "really silent" from a clinical point of view and to deserve attention by the worldwide medical community, especially as a possible complication of transcatheter ablation.[7]

As a matter of fact, the presence of silent cerebral damage resulted in a higher incidence of stroke, physical disability, death, and with worsening cognitive function.[8–10] In addition, a recent study[11] underlined that the greater SCI burden typical of patients with AF can negatively impact neuropsychological performance as compared with a control group.

Disclosure: The authors have nothing to disclose.
[a] Division of Cardiology, Department of Medical Sciences, Città della Salute e della Scienza, University of Turin, Corso A.M. Dogliotti 14, 10126 Turin, Italy; [b] Division of Neuroradiology, Città della Salute e della Scienza, Via Zuretti, 29, 10126 Turin, Italy; [c] Division of Radiology, Cardinal Guglielmo Massaia Hospital, Corso Dante 202, 14100 Asti, Italy; [d] Division of Cardiology, Cardinal Guglielmo Massaia Hospital, Corso Dante 202, 14100 Asti, Italy
* Corresponding author.
E-mail address: fiorenzo.gaita@unito.it

CEREBRAL ISCHEMIA AND AF ABLATION

During the last 15 years, transcatheter ablation of AF has emerged as an effective therapeutic option to restore sinus rhythm, relieve symptoms, and prevent thromboembolic events in patients refractory or intolerant to antiarrhythmic medications.[12]

As any invasive procedure, AF ablation carries a risk of possible complications; the occurrence of cerebrovascular accidents is one of the most frequent and severe.

If the incidence of clinically relevant brain alterations following AF ablation can reach 0.9%,[13] the occurrence of SCI is much more common and ranges from 7% to 50%. This broad variation can be attributed to the different patient characteristics, anticoagulation protocol, and type of energy used to perform the ablation among different studies.[14–17]

Patients' clinical characteristics, such as age,[18,19] previous episodes of AF,[20] presence of preablation SCI,[21] coronary artery disease, left ventricular hypertrophy or dilatation,[14] as well as procedural aspects (ie, intraprocedural cardioversion, activated clotting time <250 seconds,[7] complex fractionated atrial electrograms ablation[18]) were associated with the occurrence of SCI following transcatheter ablation.

Being that SCI related not only to AF itself but also to AF transcatheter ablation performed to cure this arrhythmia, the authors' group, as other research teams, tested different interventional protocols, ablation tools, and energy sources, to minimize the occurrence of such complication.

The anatomic features and distribution of SCI occurring after transcatheter ablation represent a crucial and unresolved issue. In addition, the effective clinical impact of these lesions and whether they persist or disappear at follow-up[21,22] remain still unclear and represent a matter of debate.[23]

Although computed tomography scans were previously performed to evaluate the possible occurrence of post-AF ablation brain alterations,[24–26] more recently, magnetic resonance (MR) imaging has become the preferred technique used to investigate this problem because of its high sensitivity and accuracy.

Accordingly, fruitful collaborations between cardiologists and neuroradiologists have been started in many centers to achieve thorough cerebral MR scans analyses of patients with AF.

The aim of this article is to discuss the current knowledge about post-AF ablation cerebral abnormalities with particular attention toward their MR features.

RESEARCH PROTOCOL ON CEREBRAL ISCHEMIA FOLLOWING AF ABLATION

The authors examined, by means of cerebral MR imaging, a large population of about 900 AF patients undergoing AF transcatheter ablation, of which a group resulted that was affected by SCI following this intervention.

In general all patients included in studies on cerebral ischemia following AF ablation performed by this group were evaluated by the protocol summarized as follows:

- Medical history (specifically focused on AF subtype and duration, comorbidities, and presence of underlying structural heart disease).
- Thromboembolic risk assessment performed by means of systematic calculation of $CHADS_2$ (congestive heart failure, hypertension, age >75 years, diabetes mellitus, and prior stroke or transient ischemic attack)[27] and CHA_2DS_2-VASc (congestive heart failure/left ventricular dysfunction; hypertension; age; diabetes; stroke/transitory ischemic attack, thromboembolism; vascular disease)[28] scores.
- Pharmacologic history (with particular attention to the anticoagulation regimen used).
- Standardized neurologic examination based on the National Institute of Health Stroke Scale administered by certified neurologists (at the time of admission, after the neuroimaging investigation, and during follow-up) to exclude clinical signs and symptoms suggestive of focal or global deficits.
- Echocardiographic assessment (both transthoracic and transesophageal).
- MR scans were performed 1 day before and the day following the ablation. All MR scans were collected and assessed by 2 certified neuroradiologists blinded to clinical details. Eventually, a subgroup of patients underwent follow-up MR after 3 months.
- Evaluation of cognitive function by means of Repeatable Battery for the Assessment of Neuropsychological Status.[29]
- Different ablation technologies and protocols were evaluated.
- Exclusion criteria have been described elsewhere.[7,11]

CEREBRAL MR IMAGING PROTOCOL AND DEFINITION OF CEREBRAL ISCHEMIC LESIONS FOLLOWING AF TRANSCATHETER ABLATION

The imaging protocol used in the authors' center is summarized in **Fig. 1**.

Brain MR imaging examinations were obtained with an 8-channel head coil on Magnetom Avanto

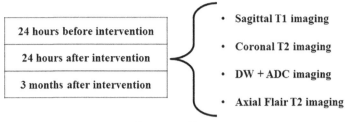

24 hours before intervention		• Sagittal T1 imaging
24 hours after intervention		• Coronal T2 imaging
3 months after intervention		• DW + ADC imaging
		• Axial Flair T2 imaging

Fig. 1. MR research protocol. ADC, apparent diffusion coefficient.

1.5 T (Siemens, Erlangen, Germany) following an imaging protocol including a sagittal T1- and coronal T2-weighted spin-echo sequence (repetition time/echo time 400/13 milliseconds) and an axial T2-fluid attenuated inversion recovery (FLAIR; repetition time/echo time 8500/112 milliseconds; TI, 2500 milliseconds) scan, with a 240-mm field-of-view, 5-mm section thickness, and 154 × 256 matrix. A diffusion-weighted (DW) and an apparent diffusion coefficient mapping sequence with a single-shot spin-echo with echo-planar imaging technique (repetition time/echo time 3200/99 milliseconds, field-of-view 230 mm, matrix 128 × 128, bandwidth 1502 Hz, gradient strength 22 mT, duration of diffusion gradient 31 milliseconds, gradient separation 42 milliseconds in 3 orthogonal directions, acquisition time 43 seconds) was also used.

A standardized definition of AF ablation-related SCI unfortunately is still lacking.

In the authors' studies an acute embolic lesion was defined as a focal hyperintense area on T2-FLAIR sequences or isointense in T1-weighted images, not present at the preprocedural scan, corresponding to a restricted diffusion signal in the DW sequence and confirmed by apparent diffusion coefficient mapping to rule out a shine-through artifact.[7]

Perivascular spaces were differentiated from small (<3 mm) lacunar ischemic lesions because of their location, form, surrounding gliosis, and T2-FLAIR-weighted sequences[30] (the former appearing as hypointense and the latter appearing as hyperintense). Leukoaraiosis was defined as bilateral and either patchy or diffuse areas of hyperintensity on T2-weighted and hypointense on T1-weighted MR sequences confined to the periventricular regions or extending into the centrum semiovale.[31]

Size and localization of the focal lesions were recorded according the classification shown in **Table 1**.

MAIN FINDINGS OF THE STUDIES

The prevalence of SCI reported in the authors' studies ranges from 5% to 38.9%: more details on SCI incidence and different ablation protocols and techniques tested by the group are given in **Table 2**.

SCI showed a cortical and bilateral distribution with a typical preferential localization within the context of the frontal and parietal lobes as well as in the cerebellum.

ATLAS OF CEREBRAL ALTERATIONS FOLLOWING AF ABLATION

The following MR images provide some examples of cerebral alterations occurring in patients with different clinical characteristics after AF transcatether ablation performed with alternative ablation tools.

Patient 1

Cerebral MR imaging of a 64-year-old female patient with persistent AF who underwent irrigated radiofrequency (RF) ablation (**Fig. 2**).

Patient 2

Cerebral MR imaging of 67-year-old female patient with paroxysmal AF (**Fig. 3**).

Table 1 Anatomic classification and brain distribution of SCI	
Dimensions	• Small (<5 mm) • Medium (≥5 and <10 mm) • Large (≥10 mm)
Cerebral hemisphere	• Right hemisphere • Left hemisphere
Brain region	• Frontal lobe • Parietal lobe • Temporal lobe • Occipital lobe • Cerebellum • Basal ganglia • Nucleus caudatus • Internal capsule • Corpus callosum
Brain tissue depth	• Cortical region • Subcortical white matter • Deep white matter

Table 2
SCI incidence following AF transcatheter ablation in the different studies

Patients (n)	Anticoagulation Protocol	Source of Energy Used	SCI Incidence	SCI Predictors
232[7]	UFH, ACT >250 s	Irrigated RF	14.0%	Cardioversion ACT <250 s
95[32]	UFH, ACT >250 s	Irrigated RF	6.0%	Cardioversion
80[33]	UFH, ACT >300 s	Irrigated RF Superirrigated RF	7.5% 5.0%	ACT <320 s
108[15]	UFH, ACT >300 s	Irrigated RF Cryoballoon PVAC	8.3% 5.6% 38.9%	PVAC

Abbreviations: ACT, activated clotting time; PVAC, pulmonary veins ablation catheter associated with duty-cycled radio-frequency generator; UFH, unfractionated heparin.

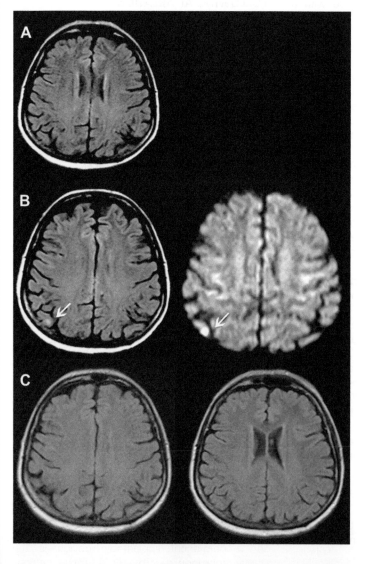

Fig. 2. Cerebral MR imaging of a 64-year-old female patient with persistent AF who underwent irrigated RF ablation. (*A*) Preprocedural scan without brain lesions. (*B*) T2-FLAIR and DW images postprocedural scans showing the appearance of a single bright cortical lesion in the right parietal lobe (maximum dimensions 6 × 4 mm) consistent with an acute embolic cerebral infarction (*white arrows*). (*C*) Three-month follow-up T2-FLAIR scan demonstrates that the small lesion has disappeared. To better visualize the region of interest, 2 adjacent images are provided.

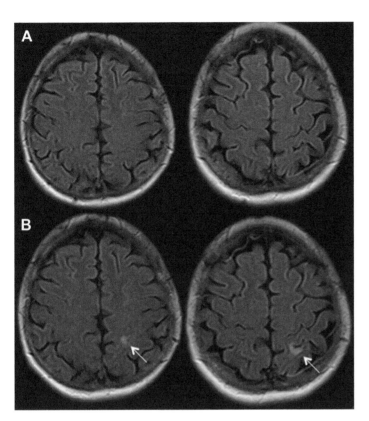

Fig. 3. Cerebral MR imaging of 67-year-old female patient with paroxysmal AF. MR scans pre- (*row A*) and post-RF ablation with pulmonary vein ablation catheter-associated with duty-cycled RF generator (*row B*): a new cortical-subcortical single ischemic lesion is present in the left parietal lobe (maximum dimension 10 × 3 mm) (see *white arrows*).

Patient 3

Cerebral MR imaging of a 63-year-old male patient with persistent AF; an example of SCI occurring after irrigated RF ablation was performed with a mean activated clotting time of 220 seconds. Moreover, an electrical cardioversion was administered at the end of this procedure (**Fig. 4**).

Patient 4

Cerebral MR imaging of 71-year-old female patient, with a CHA_2DS_2Vasc score of 4, who underwent cryoablation for persistent AF (**Fig. 5**).

Patient 5

Multiple new ischemic lesions following irrigated RF ablation are visible in the MR scans of a 54-year-old female patient with paroxysmal AF (**Fig. 6**).

Patient 6

Cerebral MR imaging of a 59-year-old female patient with paroxysmal AF and hypertension (**Fig. 7**).

Patient 7

Cerebral scans of 64-year-old male patient with paroxysmal AF (**Fig. 8**).

CONSIDERATIONS REGARDING SCI AFTER AF TRANSCATHETER ABLATION

In the authors' population experiencing SCI, following AF transcatheter ablation SCI prevalence ranges from 5% to 38.9%: this broad variation depends on the different ablation protocols and tools used (activating clotting time value, electrical cardioversion at the end of procedure, type of energy sources applied). Concerning the pathophysiology of silent embolic lesions, 3 main mechanisms are responsible for the occurrence of SCI during transcatheter ablation: clot formation, char formation, and air/gas embolism. In particular, the following are potential causes of thromboembolism: endothelial disruption, electroporation injury, heating of circulating blood elements,[34,35] and gaseous[36] or solid embolism due to catheter movement within the left atria.

SCI mostly showed a cortical and bilateral distribution with a typical preferential localization in the parietal and frontal lobes as well as in the cerebellum. These findings are in line with results previously reported by other groups, although in smaller study populations. For instance, Schrickel and colleagues[14] outlined a similar distribution of periprocedural cerebral microemboli in the

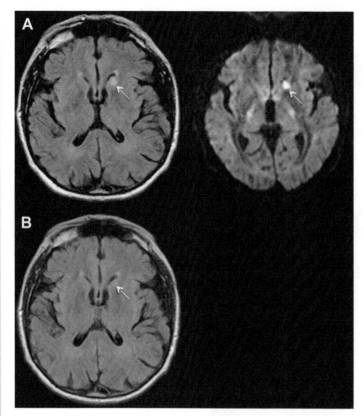

Fig. 4. Cerebral MR imaging of a 63-year-old male patient with persistent AF. An example of SCI occurring after irrigated RF ablation performed with a mean activated clotting time of 220 seconds. Moreover, an electrical cardioversion was administered at the end of this procedure. Postprocedural cerebral MRI (*row A*) T2-FLAIR and DW image indicate a single new ischemic lesion in the left head of the caudate nucleus (*white arrows*) (maximum dimensions 4 × 4 mm). Three-month follow-up T2-FLAIR scan (*row B*) demonstrates the persistence of a lesion of reduced dimensions (see *white arrow*).

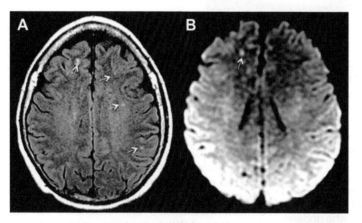

Fig. 5. Cerebral MR imaging of 71-year-old female patient, with a CHA$_2$DS$_2$Vasc score of 4, who underwent cryoablation for persistent AF. The T2-FLAIR scan (*A*) shows multiple cortical-subcortical hyperintense cerebral lesions (*white arrows*). However, only one lesion in the superior frontal gyrus is recent, as demonstrated in the DW image (*B*) (*arrow*). The other lesions are attributable to older ischemic brain damage.

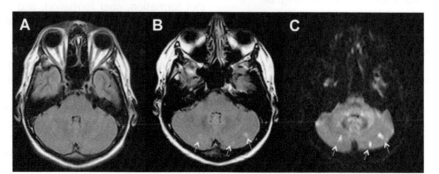

Fig. 6. Multiple new ischemic lesions following irrigated RF ablation are visible in the MR scans of a 54-year-old female patient with paroxysmal AF. Preprocedural (*A*), postprocedural T2-FLAIR (*B*), and postprocedural DW (*C*): (*white arrows*) new multiple lesions in the left cerebellum (maximum dimensions 8 × 6 mm).

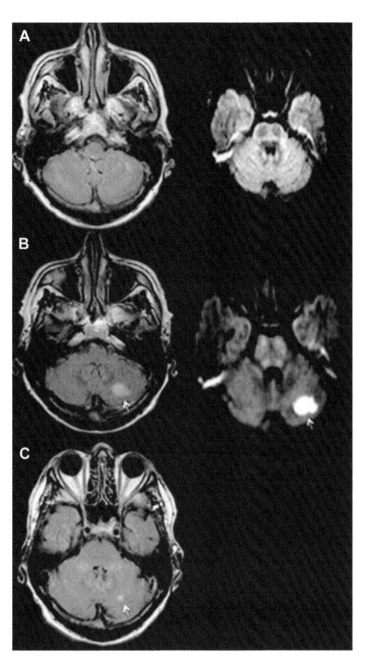

Fig. 7. Cerebral MR imaging of a 59-year-old female patient with paroxysmal AF and hypertension. (*row A*) The basal T2-FLAIR and DW image scans are shown. After irrigated RF ablation (*row B*) a new hyperintense lesion with reduced diffusion (*white arrows*) is visible in the right cerebellum. After 3 months of follow-up, a smaller lesion is still visible in T2-FLAIR image (*row C*) (indicated by the *white arrow*).

frontoparietal regions and in the cerebellum in patients with persistent or paroxysmal AF undergoing transcatheter pulmonary vein isolation. The reasons for this preferential localization might be related to the high blood volume and to the vast distribution of the middle cerebral and vertebrobasilar arteries, easily accessed by periprocedural microemboli.

Despite the cortical localization of SCI, none of the patients with postprocedural cerebral alterations had neurologic symptoms; this may sound surprising considering that most of the lesions were localized in the cortical region and in the parietal, frontal lobes, and cerebellum.

At present, the neurocognitive implications of periprocedural SCI still remain uncertain and many doubts concerning the persistence or the disappearing of these cerebral lesions at follow-up need to be clarified.[19–21]

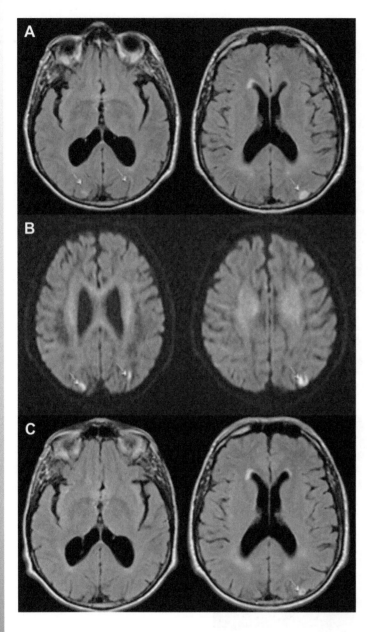

Fig. 8. Cerebral scans of a 64-year-old male patient with paroxysmal AF, another example of SCI detected after irrigated RF ablation followed by electrical cardioversion at the end of the procedure. The mean activated clotting time was 250 seconds. Post-procedural T2-FLAIR (*row A*) and DW images (*row B*) indicate 2 new bilateral lesions (maximum dimensions 20 × 10 mm), the first located in the right occipital-parietal lobe and the second in the left parietal lobe. Three-month follow-up T2-FLAIR scans (*row C*) demonstrate the disappearance of the first lesion and a reduction of the second one (*white arrow*).

In particular, even if a large study showed a lower incidence of cerebrovascular events and dementia among AF patients undergoing RF ablation compared with AF patients not treated with ablation,[37] other experiences[22,38] highlighted the presence of some cognitive alterations after this type of interventional procedure.

Although some information has been acquired concerning the neuropsychological significance of SCI due to AF,[11] further research must be performed to fully understand the impact of ablating new cerebral embolic lesions in regard to cognitive function at long-term follow-up.

SUMMARY

SCI following transcatheter AF ablation is generally localized in the cortex of the frontal, in the parietal lobes, and in the cerebellum.

It seems to be crucial to continue testing and optimizing AF ablation techniques and protocols to reduce their possible embolic complications. In this regard, cerebral MR scans of AF patients have emerged as a fundamental evaluation tool.

Also, it is relevant to create a cardiologic and radiologic shared knowledge base about cerebral damage secondary to AF, because the frequency of these problems is already very high and expected to increase in the future.

Eventually much attention should be paid to the long-term neurologic impact of AF-related silent cerebral damage. In the near future, more studies specifically investigating its influence on cognitive function are warranted.

REFERENCES

1. Feinberg WM, Blackshear JL, Laupacis A, et al. Prevalence, age distribution and gender of patients with atrial fibrillation. Analysis and implications. Arch Intern Med 1995;155:469–73.

2. Go AS, Hylek EM, Phillips KA, et al. Prevalence of diagnosed atrial fibrillation in adults: national implications for rhythm management and stroke prevention: the anticoagulation and risk factors in atrial Fibrillation (ATRIA) study. JAMA 2001;285:2370–5.

3. Miyasaka Y, Barnes ME, Gersh BJ, et al. Secular trends in incidence of atrial fibrillation in Olmsted County, Minnesota, 1980 to 2000, and implications on the projections for future prevalence. Circulation 2006;114:119–25.

4. Naccarelli GV, Varker H, Lin J, et al. Increasing prevalence of atrial fibrillation and flutter in the United States. Am J Cardiol 2009;104:1534–9.

5. Benjamin EJ, Wolf PA, D'Agostino RB, et al. Impact of atrial fibrillation on the risk of death: the Framingham Heart Study. Circulation 1998;98:946–52.

6. Vermeer SE, Longstreth WT Jr, Koudstaal PJ. Silent brain infarcts: a systematic review. Lancet Neurol 2007;6:611–9.

7. Gaita F, Caponi D, Pianelli M, et al. Radiofrequency catheter ablation of atrial fibrillation: a cause of silent thromboembolism? Magnetic resonance imaging assessment of cerebral thromboembolism in patients undergoing ablation of atrial fibrillation. Circulation 2010;122:1667–73.

8. Vermeer SE, Prins ND, den Heijer T, et al. Silent brain infarcts and the risk of dementia and cognitive decline. N Engl J Med 2003;348:1215.

9. Santangeli P, Di Biase L, Bai R, et al. Atrial fibrillation and the risk of incident dementia: a meta-analysis. Heart Rhythm 2012;9(11):1761–8. http://dx.doi.org/10.1016/j.hrthm.2012.07.026.

10. Asirvatham SJ, Friedman PA. Silent cerebral thromboembolism with left atrial ablation: a lurking danger. J Cardiovasc Electrophysiol 2006;17:8–10.

11. Gaita F, Corsinovi L, Anselmino M, et al. Prevalence of silent cerebral ischemia in paroxysmal and persistent atrial fibrillation and correlation with cognitive function. J Am Coll Cardiol 2013;62:1990–7.

12. Calkins H, Kuck KH, Cappato R, et al. 2012 HRS/EHRA/ECAS expert consensus statement on catheter and surgical ablation of atrial fibrillation: recommendations for patient selection, procedural techniques, patient management and follow-up, definitions, endpoints, and research trial design. Europace 2012;14(4):528–606.

13. Cappato R, Calkins H, Chen SA, et al. Updated worldwide survey on the methods, efficacy, and safety of catheter ablation for human atrial fibrillation. Circ Arrhythm Electrophysiol 2010;3(1):32.

14. Schrickel JW, Lickfett L, Lewalter T, et al. Incidence and predictors of silent cerebral embolism during pulmonary vein catheter ablation for atrial fibrillation. Europace 2010;12:52–7.

15. Gaita F, Leclercq JF, Schumacher B, et al. Incidence of silent cerebral thromboembolic lesions after atrial fibrillation ablation may change according to technology used: comparison of irrigated radiofrequency, multipolar nonirrigated catheter and cryoballoon. J Cardiovasc Electrophysiol 2011;22:961–8.

16. Herrera Siklódy C, Deneke T, Hocini M, et al. Incidence of asymptomatic intracranial embolic events after pulmonary vein isolation: comparison of different atrial fibrillation ablation technologies in a multicenter study. J Am Coll Cardiol 2011;58:681–8.

17. Anselmino M, Matta M, Toso E, et al. Silent cerebral embolism during atrial fibrillation ablation: pathophysiology, prevention and management. J Atr Fibrillation, in press.

18. Martinek M, Sigmund E, Lemes C, et al. Asymptomatic cerebral lesions during pulmonary vein isolation under uninterrupted oral anticoagulation. Europace 2013;15(3):325–31.

19. Neumann T, Kuniss M, Conradi G, et al. MEDAFI-Trial (Micro-embolization during ablation of atrial fibrillation): comparison of pulmonary vein isolation using cryoballoon technique vs. radiofrequency energy. Europace 2011;13(1):37–44.

20. Haeusler KG, Koch L, Herm J, et al. 3 Tesla MRI-detected brain lesions after pulmonary vein isolation for atrial fibrillation: results of the MACPAF study. J Cardiovasc Electrophysiol 2013;24(1):14–21.

21. Deneke T, Shin DI, Balta O, et al. Postablation asymptomatic cerebral lesions: long-term follow-up using magnetic resonance imaging. Heart Rhythm 2011;8:1705–11.

22. Schwarz N, Kuniss M, Nedelmann M, et al. Neuropsychological decline after catheter ablation of atrial fibrillation. Heart Rhythm 2010;7(12):1761–7.

23. Ringer TM, Neumann-Haefelin T, Sobel RA, et al. Reversal of early diffusion-weighted magnetic resonance imaging abnormalities does not necessarily reflect tissue salvage in experimental cerebral ischemia. Stroke 2001;32:2362–9.

24. Feinberg WM, Seeger JF, Carmody RF, et al. Epidemiologic features of asymptomatic cerebral infarction in patients with nonvalvular atrial fibrillation. Arch Intern Med 1990;150:2340–4.

25. Ezekowitz MD, James KE, Nazarian SM, et al. Silent cerebral infarction in patients with nonrheumatic atrial fibrillation. The Veterans Affairs Stroke Prevention in Nonrheumatic Atrial Fibrillation Investigators. Circulation 1995;92:2178–82.

26. EAFT Study Group. European atrial fibrillation trial. Silent brain infarction in nonrheumatic atrial fibrillation. Neurology 1996;46:159–65.

27. Gage BF, Waterman AD, Shannon W, et al. Validation of clinical classification schemes for predicting stroke: results from the National Registry of Atrial Fibrillation. JAMA 2001;285:2864–70.

28. Lip GY, Nieuwlaat R, Pisters R, et al. Refining clinical risk stratification for predicting stroke and thromboembolism in atrial fibrillation using a novel risk factor-based approach: the euro heart survey on atrial fibrillation. Chest 2010;137(2):263–72.

29. Randolph C, Tierney MC, Mohr E, et al. The repeatable battery for the assessment of neuropsychological status (RBANS): preliminary clinical validity. J Clin Exp Neuropsychol 1998;20(3):310–9.

30. Kwee RM, Kwee TC. Virchow-Robin spaces at MR imaging. Radiographics 2007;27:1071–86.

31. Pantoni L, Garcia JH. Pathogenesis of leukoaraiosis. A review. Stroke 1997;28:652–9.

32. Pianelli M, Scaglione M, Anselmino M, et al. Delaying cardioversion following 4-week anticoagulation in case of persistent atrial fibrillation after a transcatheter ablation procedure to reduce silent cerebral thromboembolism: a single-center pilot study. J Cardiovasc Med (Hagerstown) 2011; 12(11):785–9.

33. Scaglione M, Blandino A, Raimondo C, et al. Impact of ablation catheter irrigation design on silent cerebral embolism after radiofrequency catheter ablation of atrial fibrillation: results from a pilot study. J Cardiovasc Electrophysiol 2012;23(8):801–5.

34. Anfinsen OG, Gjesdal K, Brosstad F, et al. The activation of platelet function, coagulation, and fibrinolysis during catheter radiofrequency ablation in heparinized patients. J Cardiovasc Electrophysiol 1999;10:503–12.

35. Lee DS, Dorian P, Downar E, et al. Thrombogenicity of radiofrequency ablation procedures: what factors influence thrombin generation? Europace 2001;3: 195–200.

36. Wood MA, Shaffer KM, Ellenbogen AL, et al. Microbubbles during radiofrequency catheter ablation: composition and formation. Heart Rhythm 2005;2: 397–403.

37. Bunch TJ, Crandall BG, Weiss JP, et al. Patients treated with catheter ablation for atrial fibrillation have long-term rates of death, stroke, and dementia similar to patients without atrial fibrillation. J Cardiovasc Electrophysiol 2011;22:839–45.

38. Medi C, Evered L, Silbert B, et al. Subtle postprocedural cognitive dysfunction after atrial fibrillation ablation. J Am Coll Cardiol 2013;62:531–9.

Cerebrovascular Complications Related to Atrial Fibrillation Ablation and Strategies for Periprocedural Stroke Prevention

Zoltan Csanadi, MD, PhD[a],*, Edina Nagy-Baló, MD[a],
Stephan Danik, MD[d], Conor Barrett, MD[d],
J. David Burkhardt, MD[e], Javier Sanchez, MD[e],
Pasquale Santangeli, MD[f,g], Francesco Santoro, MD[g],
Luigi Di Biase, MD, PhD[e,g,h,i],
Andrea Natale, MD, FACC, FHRS[b,c,e,i]

KEYWORDS

- Atrial fibrillation • Stroke • Silent cerebral ischemia
- Diffusion-weighted cerebral magnetic resonance imaging • Transcranial Doppler

KEY POINTS

- Manifest, clinical stroke related to ablation of atrial fibrillation occurs in about 1% of patients.
- Silent cerebral ischemia can be detected by diffusion-weighted magnetic resonance imaging (MRI) in as many as 50% of patients postablation.
- The long-term significance of these silent lesions is not yet known.
- Postablation diffusion-weighted MRI and intraprocedural transcranial Doppler recordings of cerebral microemboli can be used to compare the thrombogenic potential of different ablation techniques.
- A safe periprocedural strategy using novel oral anticoagulants needs to be determined.
- Prospective randomized trials are needed to establish the optimal postablation care of patients regarding long-term anticoagulation.

INTRODUCTION

Transcatheter treatment of atrial fibrillation (AF) is a complex intervention requiring the introduction of hardware into the left atrium (LA), energy applications over a large area of the LA endocardium, and prolonged instrumentation in the systemic circulation.[1] Furthermore, these procedures are

---

The authors have nothing to disclose.
[a] Department of Cardiology, University of Debrecen, 22 Móricz Zs, Debrecen H4032, Hungary; [b] Case Western Reserve University, Cleveland, OH, USA; [c] Interventional Electrophysiology, Scripps Clinic, San Diego, CA, USA; [d] Al-Sabah Arrhythmia Institute (AI), St. Luke's Hospital, NY, USA; [e] Texas Cardiac Arrhythmia Institute, St. David's Medical Center, Austin, TX, USA; [f] Clinical Cardiac Electrophysiology, University of Pennsylvania, Philadelphia, PA, USA; [g] Department of Cardiology, University of Foggia, Foggia, Italy; [h] Albert Einstein College of Medicine, Montefiore Hospital, Bronx, NY, USA; [i] Department of Biomedical Engineering, University of Texas, Austin, TX, USA
* Corresponding author.
E-mail address: drcsanadi@hotmail.com

Card Electrophysiol Clin 6 (2014) 111–123
http://dx.doi.org/10.1016/j.ccep.2013.10.003

performed in patients who are at inherently increased risk of a thromboembolic complication, including stroke. It is therefore not surprising that cerebrovascular accidents have been among the most feared complications since the inception of AF ablation, evoking significant concern.

INCIDENCE OF CEREBROVASCULAR COMPLICATIONS RELATED TO AF ABLATION
Stroke and Transient Ischemic Attack

The first worldwide survey on catheter ablation for AF concluded that clinical stroke occurred in 0.28% and transient ischemic attack (TIA) in 0.66% of patients. The update of that survey, relating to AF ablations performed between 2003 and 2006, indicated similar rates of cerebrovascular complications (0.23% for stroke, 0.71% for TIA) despite an apparently more challenging patient population with a more enlarged LA and more persistent AF.[2] A meta-analysis based on the data of 6936 patients who underwent AF ablation by the end of 2006 found that stroke and TIA occurred in 0.3% and 0.2%, respectively.[3] Stroke incidences as high as 5%[4] and as low as 0%[5] have also been reported as single-center findings. Although the complication rates associated with any procedure, including AF ablation, generally decrease with increasing experience, this was not demonstrated in a high-volume center: while the overall complication rate decreased over a 10-year period from 11.1% to 1.6%, the incidence of stroke and TIA remained unchanged.[6] Thromboembolic events typically occur within 24 hours of the ablation procedure, with the high-risk period extending for 2 weeks thereafter.[7] Stroke is a significant cause of periprocedural death during AF ablation. An international survey on AF ablation in 162 centers reported details of 32 deaths in 32,569 patients. The fatal outcome was attributed to stroke in 5 (16%) of these 32 cases.[8] On the other hand, patients who survive a stroke associated with AF ablation often have a favorable long-term prognosis. During a mean 38-month follow-up of 26 patients who suffered AF ablation–related stroke in a high-volume center (2 patients died), complete long-term functional and neurocognitive recovery was documented in most patients, irrespective of the severity of the periprocedural stroke.[9]

Silent Cerebral Ischemia

It has recently been recognized that silent cerebral ischemia (SCI) can be demonstrated by diffusion-weighted cerebral magnetic resonance imaging (DW-MRI) in a much higher proportion of patients undergoing LA ablation than in those with manifest stroke.[10–17] Lickfett and colleagues[10] performed DW-MRI before and after a Lasso-guided pulmonary vein (PV) ostium isolation (PVI), and demonstrated new cerebral lesions in 2 (10%) of 20 patients without overt clinical symptoms. Similarly, an 11% incidence of SCI was reported from the same center in a larger population of 53 patients.[11] In a large-scale study[12] of 232 patients undergoing PVI with or without linear lesions and targeting of complex fractionated electrograms (CFE) with irrigated radiofrequency (RF) ablation, new silent brain lesions were found on DW-MRI in 33 patients (14%). These initial results were followed by several single-center studies[13–18] that reported widely variable results, including an incidence as high as 50% for a new SCI depending on the ablation and the MRI technology used (**Table 1**). A recent study examined the ability of a 3-T MRI scan to detect cerebral injury. Of 22 patients who had undergone PVI using cryoenergy, the incidence of SCI was 50% as opposed to 27% of 15 patients who had undergone PVI using RF energy.[17]

Clinical Relevance of SCI

The clinical significance of SCI after AF ablation is at present uncertain. Deneke and colleagues[18] repeated DW-MRI 2 to 56 weeks (median 12 weeks) after ablation in 14 patients in whom a total of 50 new-onset, clinically silent white matter lesions were identified within 48 hours after ablation. No lesion with a diameter smaller than 10 mm could be identified on the repeated MRI even as early as 2 weeks after the ablation, whereas 3 larger lesions (>10 mm) were still detected. Of note, all of these follow-up lesions demonstrated a reduction in size with no hemorrhagic component in any of them, despite the patients being on oral anticoagulation (OAC). The disappearance or shrinkage of these lesions, although reassuring to some extent, does not imply the full recovery of pathologic alterations in the brain. In an elegant canine model, typical lesions were demonstrated on DW-MRI and fluid-attenuated inversion recovery images after the injection of gaseous and particulate microemboli.[19] Clear evidence of ischemic injury, including severe endothelial proliferation, moderate glia cell activation, and mild perivascular lymphocytic infiltrate, was present on histopathologic examination of brain specimens, despite the resolution of most lesions on MRI by day 4 postembolism.

In the general population of patients with AF, a high prevalence of SCI has consistently been detected on DW-MRI. These subclinical lesions were linked to an unfavorable long-term clinical

Table 1
Silent cerebral ischemia detected by DW-MRI in various studies

Authors,[Ref.] Year	ACT	N	Ablation Technique	Positive DW-MRI
Lickfett et al,[10] 2006	>250	10	Irrigated RF ablation	1 (10%)
Schwarz et al,[13] 2010	>300	13	Irrigated RF ablation	3 (14.3%)
		9	Cryoballoon	
Neumann et al,[14] 2011	>300	44	Irrigated RF	3 (6.8%)
		45	Cryoballoon	4 (8.9%)
Gaita et al,[12] 2010	250–300	232	Irrigated RF ablation	33 (14%)
Schrickel et al,[11] 2010	>250	53	Irrigated RF ablation	6 (11%)
Herrera Siklódy et al,[15] 2011	>300	27	RF	2 (7.4%)
		23	Cryoballoon	1 (4.3%)
		24	Phased RF	8 (33%)
Gaita et al,[16] 2011	>300	36	Irrigated RF ablation	3 (8.3%)
		36	Phased RF	14 (38.9%)
		36	Cryoballoon	2 (5.6%)

Abbreviations: ACT, activated clotting time; DW-MRI, diffusion-weighted cerebral magnetic resonance imaging; RF, radiofrequency.

outcome, including an impaired cognitive function, an increased risk of dementia, and a worse prognosis of AF-related strokes in comparison with those of non-AF etiology.[20,21] A recent cross-sectional study of 180 patients with variable forms of AF demonstrated an 82% (paroxysmal) and a 92% (persistent AF) prevalence of SCI on MRI; the number of lesions per person was significantly higher in the patients with persistent AF than in those with paroxysmal AF.[22] Furthermore, the performance in cognitive function tests was significantly poorer in AF patients compared with matched controls.

However, these observations indicating the clinical significance of spontaneous ischemic lesions in AF patients may not be extrapolated to SCI induced by AF ablation. Whereas postablation SCIs are attributed to microembolization during or shortly after the procedure, the mechanism in patients with AF of variable duration is likely to be multifactorial, with the potential importance of both progressive atherosclerosis and showers of microemboli from the LA. Limited data are available on the cognitive function after AF ablation. Schwarz and colleagues[13] compared the results of neurophysiologic tests before and 3 months after PVI in 21 patients and found a poorer neurophysiologic outcome in verbal memory, but no difference in the other 4 cognitive domains evaluated (attention, verbal fluency, executive functioning, and visual memory). A battery of 8 neuropsychological tests was performed in a recent study on 150 patients, including 90 undergoing wide encircling antrum ablation for paroxysmal (60 patients) or persistent (25 patients) AF, 30 patients

undergoing ablation for supraventricular tachycardia (SVT), and 30 patients scheduled for ablation of AF as a matched nonoperative control group.[23] The results at 90 days after ablation indicated postoperative cognitive dysfunction in 13% of the paroxysmal AF patents, 20% of the persistent AF patients, 3% of the SVT patients, and none in the control group. The only predictor of negative changes was the LA access time. The clinical significance of the subtle changes suggested by these data warrants further exploration.

Although direct evidence is still lacking, it is reasonable to assume that SCI lesions detected by DW-MRI are indicators of the thromboembolic consequences related to AF ablation; a preventive measure that successfully limits the subclinical event rate will also reduce the risk of manifest stroke. Its relatively high incidence therefore makes SCI a logical and practical surrogate of clinically overt cerebrovascular events in future clinical studies.

MECHANISM OF PERIPROCEDURAL THROMBOEMBOLIZATION

The postulated mechanisms of AF ablation–related cerebral embolization include embolism of particulate debris, thrombus, char, or gas bubbles at the site of the ablation in the LA.

Particulate Debris

Transseptal puncture may produce particulate debris in 2 different ways:

1. While advancing, the transseptal needle scrapes plastic particles off the inner wall of

the transseptal dilator, thereby creating embolic material.[24]

2. The coring of cardiac tissue into the tip of the open-ended needle creates a small plug of cardiac tissue regardless of the puncture site and the type of the needle, including RF.[25]

Thrombus

The generation of thrombi relies on Virchow's triad: endothelial injury, hemodynamic changes (stasis and turbulence), and a hypercoagulable state.

Energy application during ablation injures endothelial cells. When the continuity of the endothelium is interrupted, its natural anticoagulation properties are lost and blood components come into direct contact with subendothelial procoagulant proteins, such as collagen, tissue factor, and von Willebrand factor. Consequently, thrombus formation is initiated through platelet adhesion and activation, and thrombin production.[26] Thrombi adherent to the endothelium may dislodge spontaneously or as a result of catheter manipulation, mechanical trauma resulting from electric cardioversion, and restoration of atrial contractility in sinus rhythm.[12] Of importance is that the thrombogenic potential is related to the energy applied: cryoablation has been shown to be less thrombogenic than RF.[27] The difference is explained by the histologic characteristics of RF lesions and cryolesions. Whereas those produced by the latter are well circumscribed with sharp borders, with sparing of most of the endothelial lining, RF lesions are characterized by intralesional hemorrhage and ragged edges, with a marked endothelial injury. Similarly to RF, all energy sources that ablate through heating, such as the microwave and the laser, carry an increased risk of thrombus formation.[26]

Energy delivery can also lead to embolization through the direct embolization of small myocardial fragments generated by steam-pops. This event is more likely to occur when the tissue is overheated because of the high contact forces and/or the high energy delivered during the ablation.[28] Char formation at the tip of the catheter in these situations is not uncommon, and may also be a potential source of embolization.[29]

Hemodynamic changes, including stasis and turbulence, may also contribute to thrombus formation during LA ablation. Stasis can occur in the transseptal sheath and in the trapped blood column in the PV behind an occluding cryoballoon, providing the proper milieu for thrombus formation, which may enter the systemic circulation during catheter exchange or deflation of the balloon.[12,30] The turbulent blood flow created by the catheter manipulation or the rapid injection of contrast material may induce a response that results in platelet activation, which in turn may begin the process ultimately leading to embolization.[31]

A hypercoagulable state develops during PVI through 2 main mechanisms. Heating of the circulating blood elements during RF energy delivery has been demonstrated to activate platelets and the clotting system.[32] However, the introduction of the catheters and sheaths themselves activates the coagulation cascade and induces a prothrombotic state.[33] This concept was demonstrated by Ren and colleagues,[34] who detected fresh thrombi attached to a sheath or mapping catheter by intracardiac echocardiography (ICE) in as many as 10% of the cases.

Gas Bubbles

As transseptal sheaths may potentially connect the LA with the room air, flushing through these sheaths, or introducing or exchanging catheters and guide wires, pose the risk of air embolization, even with the protection of hemostatic valves. The risk of air embolization is higher when catheters with a complex configuration are used.[35] Furthermore, gas embolization can occur during other phases of these procedures, including the energy delivery period, PV angiography, and catheter manipulation.[36] Microcavitation visualized as bubbles by ICE occurs during RF delivery, especially when the tissue temperature exceeds 60°C.[37] The phenomenon of cavitation, well known in stainless-steel turbines, dam outlets, and ship propellers, and first described in a cardiovascular context in connection with mechanical heart valves, involves the rapid formation of vaporous microbubbles in a fluid owing to a local reduction of pressure to below the vapor pressure.[38]

INTRAPROCEDURAL ASSESSMENT OF THROMBOEMBOLIC RISK DURING LA ABLATION

DW-MRI has become the gold standard for assessment of cerebral ischemia, either symptomatic or asymptomatic, after ablation. A real-time assessment of the thromboembolic risk during the ablation may improve the safety of the procedure. Two methods have been used for this purpose: the monitoring of microbubbles on ICE, and the detection of microembolic signals (MES) in the cerebral arteries by transcranial Doppler (TCD).

Monitoring of Bubble Formation by ICE During Ablation; Power Titration Strategy

ICE was originally introduced to interventional electrophysiology as a simple and reliable tool to display different cardiac structures and the positions of catheters in the heart,[39] to ensure safe transseptal puncture and the early recognition of complications during the procedure. ICE-detectable bubble formation during RF delivery was first described in an experimental model by Kalman and colleagues,[37] who noticed that showers of microbubbles often preceded an increase in impedance, indicating overheating of tissue during ablation. The concept was first tested in humans by Marrouche and colleagues,[40] who developed an energy titration strategy based on the microbubble density detected by ICE. Two types of bubble-generation patterns were defined: scattered microbubbles (type 1), indicating early tissue overheating, and a brisk shower of dense microbubbles (type 2) (**Fig. 1**). The energy was increased in stepwise fashion until the appearance of the type 1 pattern, and the power was then reduced. Energy delivery was immediately terminated in the event of the type 2 pattern. This strategy prevented any thromboembolic complication in 152 patients undergoing circular mapping–guided PVI, whereas stroke/TIA occurred in 3% of patients without ICE-guided power titration. Ablation of complex substrates including AF under ICE guidance with power titration has become a routine practice in many centers, although the assessment of bubble density is compromised by echogenic microbubble formation caused by the irrigation flow when open irrigated catheters are used. A semiquantitative scale describing the

bubble density of 3 different patterns as few, moderate, or shower has also been used.

Microembolic Signal Detection by Transcranial Doppler

Circulating cerebral emboli can be detected by TCD when imaging the middle cerebral arteries (**Fig. 2**). MES are characterized by short-term, high-intensity ultrasonic signals with characteristic audible chirps.[41,42] With older devices, the differentiation between true embolic signals and artifacts (probe dislocation or noise from external devices) requires an experienced observer. MES may be due to solid particles, or gaseous in nature. As there is a difference in their acoustic impedance, solid and gaseous emboli can be differentiated. The latter reflect the ultrasonic beam with a higher intensity than do denser particles. The use of novel multifrequency TCDs with imaging at 2 different frequencies (2 and 2.5 MHz) can automatically differentiate true signals from noise, and gaseous from solid emboli, thereby improving the practicality of the technique for routine clinical use.[43] Results of several studies have been reported with MES detection during cardiopulmonary bypass surgery and carotid interventions.[44] The clinical significance of these microemboli with regard to the postoperative neurologic state or the cognitive function of the patients is less well established.

Limited data are available on the number of MES during LA ablation for AF. Kilicaslan and colleagues[45] compared MES counts recorded during PV antrum isolation with ICE-guided power titration (as described earlier) versus that with conventional power-limited RF delivery in 202 patients. A good correlation was found between the intensity of bubble formation and the MES count. The power titration strategy resulted in half the total number of MES (mean = 1015) in comparison with the conventional approach (mean = 2250), and acute neurologic complications occurred in 0.9% and 3.1% of patients, respectively. Sauren and colleagues[46] reported a virtually negligible number of MES (mean = 5) during epicardial AF ablation in comparison with endocardial ablation (mean = 3908). In another study from the same group,[30] the MES counts detected during AF ablation demonstrated significant differences between 3 different techniques (cryoballoon, irrigated RF, and nonirrigated RF), in line with previous MRI results. Nagy-Baló and colleagues[36] recently reported on the results of intraoperative TCD and ICE recording in 34 patients undergoing PVI with either cryoballoon or phased-RF ablation. It is noteworthy that multifrequency TCD capable of

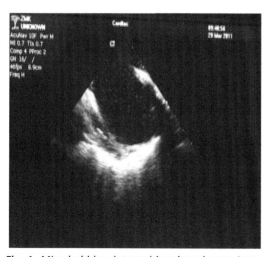

Fig. 1. Microbubbles detected by phased-array intracardiac echocardiography.

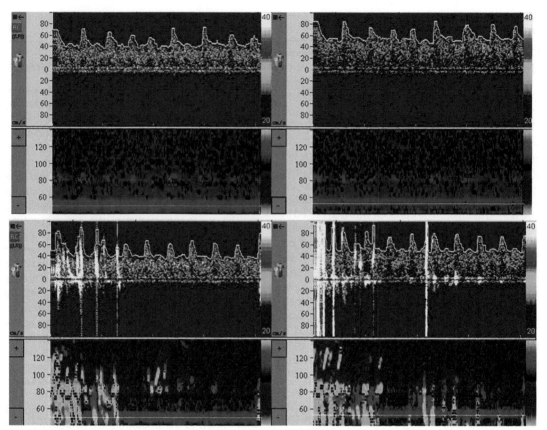

Fig. 2. Bilateral transcranial Doppler recording of microembolic signals (MES) during radiofrequency ablation in the left atrium. MES can be observed on the lower but not on the upper panels.

automatic differentiation of gaseous and solid emboli was used to study the nature of the MES. A very significant correlation was demonstrated between the microbubble density and the MES count, confirming previous observations.[45] In line with published DW-MRI results, significantly lower total numbers of MES were detected during cryo-balloon ablation in comparison with phased-RF ablation. This study was the first to investigate the nature of the MES, and demonstrated that 80% of them were of gaseous origin regardless of the ablation technique. The significance of the composition of the microemboli at this time is unclear. In theory, gaseous bubbles are expected to be less durable and less harmful than particles. With no data available on the relationship between the MES count recorded during ablation and post-procedural DW-MRI findings or manifest cerebral ischemia, it is not possible even to estimate the microembolic load that would indicate a significant risk of a symptomatic or an MRI-detectable lesion. However, MES detection promises to be a valuable tool to compare the thromboembolic potentials of different ablation techniques and

strategies, and to gain further insight into the mechanisms of embolus formation relating to different stages of AF ablation.

CLINICAL AND ABLATION TECHNOLOGY–RELATED PREDICTORS OF CEREBRAL VASCULAR EVENTS

The risk of a periprocedural cerebral ischemic event, either symptomatic or subclinical, is influenced by multiple factors, including the baseline characteristics of patients and the technical aspects of the ablation procedure.

Patients' Characteristics

In a prospective multicenter study[47] on 6454 patients undergoing RF ablation for AF in 9 centers, stroke/TIA occurred in 27 patients (1.1%). Among the characteristics of the cohort, diabetes mellitus, congestive heart failure, and the type of AF (paroxysmal or nonparoxysmal) proved to be independent predictors of a periprocedural cerebrovascular event on multivariate analysis. In a single-center study,[48] 10 (1.4%) of 721 patients suffered a stroke/TIA during or within 30 days after AF ablation, and a CHADS2 score of 2 or higher and a history of previous stroke/TIA remained independent predictors of cerebral ischemia in 2 multivariate models.

Inconsistent DW-MRI results have been published regarding clinical predictors of SCI. In the largest population studied so far,[12] none of the clinical characteristics were predictive of SCI. Schrickel and colleagues[11] reported 6 new cases of SCI in 53 patients after focal RF ablation. Coronary artery disease; the number of failed antiarrhythmic drugs, an enlarged left ventricular volume, and septal-wall thickness were predictors of a positive DW-MRI finding. A Japanese study[49] found only left ventricular ejection fraction to be a positive predictor. In the MEDAFI trial,[14] which compared cryoablation and irrigated RF ablation (nonrandomized) in 89 patients, age was the only predictor of SCI.

Technical Aspects of the Ablation Procedure

Besides the ablation technology, consideration must also be given to the manipulation of the sheaths placed in the LA, and the types of energy and catheter used for the ablation.

Long sheaths, including those used to establish LA access during transseptal puncture and steerable sheaths designed to facilitate maneuvering in the LA, pose well-known hazards of air embolism during injections or flushing through these devices, and also during catheter exchange, as removal of the catheter can create a vacuum inside the lumen. These devices, mostly at their distal segment, are a source of thrombus formation, especially in the absence of appropriate and timely anticoagulation (**Fig. 3**). Continuous flushing

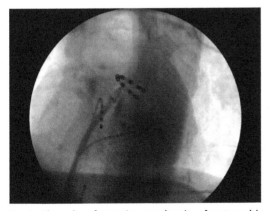

Fig. 3. Thrombus formation on the tip of a steerable sheath in the left atrium. Thrombus attached to the tip of the sheath is visible on fluoroscopy after contrast injection.

of these sheaths and meticulous care to eliminate air bubbles are essential for procedure safety.[50] Furthermore, any catheter removal should be performed slowly with continuous suction on the side arm of the sheaths, followed by careful flushing. It is a common practice in many centers to keep the sheaths in the right atrium once the diagnostic and ablation catheters have been placed in the LA, thereby mitigating the risk and consequences of thrombus formation on the tip of the sheath. Besides other advantages, the routine use of ICE offers an opportunity for the continuous monitoring of all catheters placed in the heart, with the recognition of thrombus formation on them.[34]

The ablation technology, including the type of energy and the catheter used for AF ablation, can lead to different risks. Since the early days of AF ablation, when RF energy was used exclusively with conventional 4-mm and then 8-mm tip ablation catheters, alternative energy sources including cryoenergy and laser have been introduced. In the present era, irrigation RF catheters have become the standard, and balloon-based and multipolar ablation technologies are popular in many centers. It is reasonable to assume that significant differences in thromboembolic risk may be associated with these different technologies. However, conclusive evidence as to the advantage of one technology over another, measured as a difference in the rates of manifest stroke/TIA, is not yet available, largely because of the relatively low occurrence of clinically overt events.

The much higher incidence of SCI events offers a better opportunity for the comparison of these ablation methods. In fact, significant differences have been demonstrated in the rate of SCI. Gaita and colleagues[16] reported a striking ablation technology-dependent difference in the incidence of SCI detected by MRI. In a randomized comparison of 108 patients, phased-RF ablation with a pulmonary vein ablation catheter (PVAC) was associated with a significantly higher (38.9%) incidence of acute lesions than was observed with irrigated focal ablation (8.3%) or cryoablation (5.6%). In 74 patients, Herrera Siklódy and colleagues[15] found new ischemia on DW-MRI in 37.5% after PVAC ablation, compared with 7.4% and 4.3% after irrigated RF and cryoablation, respectively. In a recent report,[51] the use of phased-RF ablation with a new generator and modified software to control power handling during RF applications decreased the incidence of positive findings on DW-MRI to 27%. Another publication by the same group[52] indicated that simultaneous RF delivery to no more than 2 electrode pairs and exclusion of the first and the last poles from the simultaneous energy application further reduced the incidence of SCI to 11.7%, at the price of a prolonged procedure time.

Although it seems reasonable to assume that the procedure (and/or the LA) time and the amount of ablation with the addition of lines or atrial defragmentation may also influence the thromboembolic risk, this has not been confirmed.[12,49] However, coronary angiography performed together with AF ablation[49] and cardioversion (either pharmacologic or electrical) during ablation[12] have been found to be positive predictors.

The available data on the number of MES detected by TCD during AF ablation also demonstrate marked technology-dependent differences (Table 2). Sauren and colleagues[30] observed significantly more MES during ablation with nonirrigated RF (mean = 3908) compared with irrigated RF (1404) and cryoablation (935). In a recent study, Nagy-Baló and coleagues[36] compared the number of MES during cryoablation and PVAC ablation using lower (≥250) and higher (≥320) minimum intraprocedural activated clotting time (ACT) target levels for PVAC. Irrespective of the level of anticoagulation, ablation with the PVAC (means = 3143 and 2205) resulted in significantly higher MES counts in comparison with cryoablation (mean = 834).

PERIPROCEDURAL THROMBOEMBOLISM PROPHYLAXIS AND LONG-TERM ANTICOAGULATION AFTER AF ABLATION
Thromboembolism Prophylaxis Before Ablation

Many patients undergoing AF ablation are at an elevated risk of a thromboembolic complication, and therefore require oral anticoagulation with a vitamin K antagonist (VKA) or a novel oral anticoagulant (NOAC) according to recent guidelines.[53,54] The 2012 expert consensus statement specified that all patients who have been in AF for 48 hours or longer or for an unknown duration need effective anticoagulation for at least 3 weeks before the procedure, or should undergo transesophageal echocardiography (TEE) to exclude LA thrombus.[50] The common practice in the past was bridging. The VKA was discontinued and changed to low molecular weight heparin (LMWH) a few days before the procedure, then switched back afterward. Performing AF ablation on a therapeutic level of anticoagulation (international normalized ratio [INR] 2–3.5) has recently evolved as the preferred approach in many centers, after several studies demonstrated its safety.[55,56] In fact, the risk of both thromboembolism and bleeding was reduced. With the recent introduction and rapid adoption of NOACs for thromboembolism prophylaxis in AF patients, a new strategy for the perioperative management of these patients is urgently needed. Comparison of uninterrupted warfarin and the direct thrombin inhibitor dabigatran, based on data from a multicenter prospective registry,[57] indicated significantly higher rates of major bleeding and the composite of bleeding and thromboembolic complications (6% and 16%) with dabigatran in comparison with warfarin (1% and 6%). All patients with thromboembolic complications who were on dabigatran had nonparoxysmal AF and more extensive LA ablation. It should be noted that dabigatran was suspended at least 12 hours (mean 16 hours) before the procedure, and was restarted within 3 hours after hemostasis. In another study,[58] dabigatran was used in 123 patients with paroxysmal AF with no bleeding or

Table 2				
Microembolic signals detected by transcranial Doppler in different studies				
Authors,[Ref.] Year	**ACT**	**N**	**Ablation Technique**	**MES**
Kilicaslan et al,[45] 2006	350–400	202	RF	1793 ± 547
Sauren et al,[30] 2009	>350	10	RF	3908 ± 2816
	200–250	10	Irrigated RF	1404 ± 981
	>350	10	Cryoballoon	935 ± 463
				P<.05
Sauren et al,[46] 2009	—	10	Epicardial RF ablation	5 ± 6
	>350	10	Endocardial RF	3908 ± 2816
				P<.0001
Nagy-Baló et al,[36] 2013	>250	10	Cryoballoon	834 ± 727
	>250	12	PVAC	3142 ± 1736
	>320	13	PVAC	2204 ± 1078

Abbreviations: MES, microembolic signal; PVAC, pulmonary vein ablation catheter.

thromboembolic complications. However, in this study dabigatran was discontinued 5 days before ablation, a lower intraprocedural ACT target was set, and LMWH was started immediately after the procedure, with dabigatran being resumed 22 hours later. Dabigatran is known to intensify the effect of unfractionated heparin (UFH) on the activated partial thromboplastin time in vitro. As UFH is administered during ablation, this drug-drug interaction may increase the bleeding risk unless dabigatran is withdrawn at least 1 to 2 days in advance. Therefore, starting dabigatran 3 hours after the procedure, with another 2 to 3 hours required for it to reach its full anticoagulation effect, results in an unprotected time window of 5 to 6 hours during the early postablation period unless LMWH is used for bridging.

One study[59] examined the use of interrupted rivaroxaban (n = 321) in comparison with warfarin (n = 321) for patients undergoing PVI. Fifty-one percent of patients in both groups had paroxysmal AF. The respective rates of major bleeding (1.6% vs 1.9%) and embolic events (0.3% vs 0.3%) were not significantly different between those on rivaroxaban and those on warfarin. Further studies using rivaroxaban, as well as other NOACs (apixaban), will be needed to determine whether these agents offer a safer alternative for periprocedural anticoagulation without the need for bridging.

Preablation Exclusion of LA Thrombus

The presence of a thrombus in the LA should be excluded before ablation in all patients unless adequate anticoagulation is documented for at least 3 weeks before the procedure. However, it is the routine in many centers for all patients to undergo an evaluation shortly before the ablation, regardless of the presenting rhythm and previous anticoagulation. The gold-standard method is TEE. Multidetector computed cardiac tomography (CCT) has also been proposed to assess the LA appendage for thrombus, but good sensitivity was associated with poor specificity in several reports.[60] In recent publications,[61,62] further assessment with delayed CCT at 1 or 3 minutes improved the specificity and positive predictive value to 100%. In many centers, CCT is part of the routine preprocedure; because the CCT data are used for image integration with the electroanatomic mapping system, patient discomfort and the additional costs related to the TEE could be avoided by extending its use to exclude a preexisting thrombus. ICE has also been advocated as a supplementary tool to assess LA thrombus in the event of an equivocal TEE finding.[63]

Intraprocedural Heparin Administration

Intraprocedural anticoagulation involves UFH administered as an intravenous bolus followed by continuous infusion to maintain a target ACT. As thrombus can build up on the transseptal sheath within a very short time, after or even before crossing the septum, it has become a common practice to give the bolus before or immediately after the transseptal puncture.[64] The recommended ACT target is 300 to 400 seconds; some centers aim at a level of more than 350 seconds. The target ACT should be reached before the first energy delivery, and then checked regularly (every 20–30 minutes) throughout the procedure. Extra boluses of UFH should be given if the ACT level drops below the target value. UFH administration is discontinued once all catheters and sheaths have been withdrawn from the LA; sheaths from the groin can be removed at an ACT level lower than 200 seconds. Heparin is reversed with protamine in some centers at the end of the procedure.

Postablation Anticoagulation

Both theoretical considerations and clinical observations recommend oral anticoagulation for at least 2 months for all patients after AF ablation. A variable degree of atrial stunning, similar to that occurring with direct-current cardioversion, is present after AF ablation. Moreover, the fresh endothelial damage resulting from energy application in the LA itself is thrombogenic. It has been demonstrated that most post–AF ablation strokes occur within 2 weeks after the procedure.[7] In patients undergoing the ablation with therapeutic INR, VKA should be continued for at least 2 months according to current recommendations.[50] In those managed with the bridging strategy, LMWH should be restarted after sheath removal and continued until the therapeutic INR is reached. Alternatively, oral anticoagulation can be followed by an NOAC.

With no evidence from large-scale randomized trials regarding the long-term thromboembolic risk in these patients, the same therapeutic principles as in patients without ablation are to be applied. The decision should therefore be based on the CHADS2 or CHADS2-VASC score,[53,54,65] and not on the presence or type of AF after ablation. The prognostic value of these scores after ablation has recently been demonstrated.[66] The available, but as yet insufficient, data suggest that successful AF ablation does reduce the stroke risk, and that long-term antithrombotic prophylaxis may not be required in all patients. In a nonrandomized study 755 patients were followed for a mean of 25 months postablation. Late thromboembolic events were noted in 2 of 755 patients

(0.3%), both of whom were on OAC.[7] No cerebral complication occurred in 180 patients who had at least 1 risk factor for stroke, remained in sinus rhythm, and in whom anticoagulant therapy was stopped a median of 5 months postablation. In a recent observational study[67] on 3344 patients who underwent AF ablation in 5 centers, OAC was discontinued and aspirin was prescribed, regardless of the CHADS2 score, in those who had no recurrence of an atrial tachyarrhythmia or a severe LA mechanical dysfunction. In those with a CHADS2 score of 1 or more, anticoagulation was restarted in the event of recurrence of atrial arrhythmia. In 347 patients with a CHADS2 score of greater than 2, no thromboembolic events were observed during a mean follow-up of 28 months. Bleeding complications were significantly more frequent among those on chronic anticoagulant therapy.

SUMMARY

While improvements have been made to limit the incidence of thromboembolic events, especially stroke, during catheter ablation of AF, the optimal strategy to minimize such complications has yet to be determined. Although operator experience certainly plays a role in limiting the incidence of stroke, periprocedural anticoagulation strategies that minimize both bleeding and stroke in a standardized fashion have yet to be universally agreed upon. It is hoped that larger trials can be undertaken to definitively address these important concerns.

REFERENCES

1. Cappato R, Calkins H, Chen SA, et al. Worldwide survey on the methods, efficacy, and safety of catheter ablation for human atrial fibrillation. Circulation 2005;111:1100.
2. Cappato R, Calkins H, Chen SA, et al. Updated worldwide survey on the methods, efficacy, and safety of catheter ablation for human atrial fibrillation. Circ Arrhythm Electrophysiol 2010;3:32–8.
3. Calkins H, Reynolds MR, Spector P, et al. Treatment of atrial fibrillation with antiarrhythmic drugs or radiofrequency ablation: two systematic literature reviews and meta-analyses. Circ Arrhythm Electrophysiol 2009;2:349–61.
4. Kok LC, Mangrum JM, Haines DE, et al. Cerebrovascular complication associated with pulmonary vein ablation. J Cardiovasc Electrophysiol 2002; 13:764–7.
5. Lee G, Sparks PB, Morton JB, et al. Low risk of major complications associated with pulmonary vein antral isolation for atrial fibrillation: results of 500 consecutive ablation procedures in patients with low prevalence of structural heart disease from a single center. J Cardiovasc Electrophysiol 2011; 22:163–8.
6. Hoyt H, Bhonsale A, Chilukuri K, et al. Complications arising from catheter ablation of atrial fibrillation: temporal trends and predictors. Heart Rhythm 2011;8(12):1869–74.
7. Oral H, Chugh A, Özaydin M, et al. Risk of thromboembolic events after percutaneous left atrial radiofrequency ablation of atrial fibrillation. Circulation 2006;114:759–65.
8. Cappato R, Calkins H, Chen SA, et al. Prevalence and causes of fatal outcome in catheter ablation of atrial fibrillation. J Am Coll Cardiol 2009;53: 1798–803.
9. Patel D, Bailey SM, Furlan AJ, et al. Long-term functional and neurocognitive recovery in patients who had an acute cerebrovascular event secondary to catheter ablation for atrial fibrillation. J Cardiovasc Electrophysiol 2010;21:412–7.
10. Lickfett L, Hackenbroch M, Lewalter T, et al. Cerebral diffusion-weighted magnetic resonance imaging: a tool to monitor the thrombogenicity of left atrial catheter ablation. J Cardiovasc Electrophysiol 2006;17:1–7.
11. Schrickel JW, Lickfett L, Lewalter T, et al. Incidence and predictors of silent cerebral embolism during pulmonary vein catheter ablation for atrial fibrillation. Europace 2010;12:52–7.
12. Gaita F, Caponi D, Pianelli M, et al. Radiofrequency catheter ablation of atrial fibrillation: a cause of silent thromboembolism? Magnetic resonance imaging assessment of cerebral thromboembolism in patients undergoing ablation of atrial fibrillation. Circulation 2010;122:1667–73.
13. Schwarz N, Kuniss M, Nedelmann M, et al. Neuropsychological decline after catheter ablation of atrial fibrillation. Heart Rhythm 2010; 7(12):1761–7.
14. Neumann T, Kuniss M, Conradi G, et al. MEDAFI-trial (micro-embolization during ablation of atrial fibrillation): comparison of pulmonary vein isolation using cryoballoon technique vs. radiofrequency energy. Europace 2011;13:37–44.
15. Herrera Siklódy C, Deneke T, Hocini M, et al. Incidence of asymptomatic embolic events following pulmonary vein isolation procedures: comparison between different ablation devices. J Am Coll Cardiol 2011;58:681–8.
16. Gaita F, Leclercq JF, Schumacher B, et al. Incidence of silent cerebral thromboembolic lesions after atrial fibrillation ablation may change according to technology used: comparison of irrigated radiofrequency, multipolar nonirrigated catheter and cryoballoon. J Cardiovasc Electrophysiol 2011;22: 961–8.

17. Haeusler KG, Koch L, Herm J, et al. 3 Tesla MRI-detected brain lesions after pulmonary vein isolation for atrial fibrillation: results of the MACPAF study. J Cardiovasc Electrophysiol 2013;24(1):14–21.

18. Deneke T, Shin DI, Balta O, et al. Post-ablation asymptomatic cerebral lesions—long-term follow-up using magnetic resonance imaging. Heart Rhythm 2011;8:1705–11.

19. Haines DE, Stewart MT, Barka ND, et al. Microembolism and catheter ablation II: effects of cerebral microemboli injections in a canine model. Circ Arrhythm Electrophysiol 2013;6:23–30.

20. Kalantarian S, Stern TA, Mansour M, et al. Cognitive impairment associated with atrial fibrillation: a meta-analysis. Ann Intern Med 2013;158(5 Pt 1): 338–46.

21. Vermeer SE, Prins ND, den Heier T, et al. Silent brain infarcts and the risk of dementia and cognitive decline. N Engl J Med 2013;348:1215–22.

22. Gaita F, Corsinovi L, Anselmino M, et al. Prevalence of silent cerebral ischemia in paroxysmal and persistent atrial fibrillation and correlation with cognitive function. J Am Coll Cardiol 2013. http://dx.doi.org/10.1016/jacc2013.05.074.

23. Medi C, Evered L, Silbert B, et al. Subtle postprocedural cognitive dysfunction after atrial fibrillation ablation. J Am Coll Cardiol 2013;62:531–9.

24. Feld GK, Tiongson J, Oshodi G. Particle formation and risk of embolization during transseptal catheterization: comparison of standard transseptal needles and a new radiofrequency transseptal needle. J Interv Card Electrophysiol 2011;30:31–6.

25. Greenstein E, Passman R, Lin AC, et al. Knight incidence of tissue coring during transseptal catheterization when using electrocautery and a standard transseptal needle. Circ Arrhythm Electrophysiol 2012;5(2):341–4.

26. Zhou L, Keane D, Reed G, et al. Thromboembolic complications of cardiac radiofrequency catheter ablation: a review of the reported incidence, pathogenesis and current research directions. J Cardiovasc Electrophysiol 1999;10(4):611–20.

27. Khairy P, Chauvet P, Lehmann J, et al. Lower incidence of thrombus formation with cryoenergy versus radiofrequency catheter ablation. Circulation 2003;107(15):2045–50.

28. Di Biase L, Natale A, Barrett C, et al. Relationship between catheter forces, lesion characteristics, "popping," and char formation: experience with robotic navigation system. J Cardiovasc Electrophysiol 2009;20(4):436–40.

29. Nath S, DiMarco JP, Haines DE. Basic aspects of radiofrequency catheter ablation. J Cardiovasc Electrophysiol 1994;5(10):863–76.

30. Sauren LD, Van Belle Y, De Roy L, et al. Transcranial measurement of cerebral microembolic signals during endocardial pulmonary vein isolation: comparison of 3 different ablation techniques. J Cardiovasc Electrophysiol 2009;20(10):1102–7.

31. Nesbitt WS, Mangin P, Salem HH, et al. The impact of blood rheology on the molecular and cellular events underlying arterial thrombosis. J Mol Med 2006;84:989–95.

32. Van Oeveren W, Crijns HJ, Korteling BJ, et al. Blood damage, platelet and clotting activation during application of radiofrequency or cryoablation catheters: a comparative in vitro study. J Med Eng Technol 1999;23(1):20–5.

33. Dorbala S, Cohen AJ, Hutchinson LA, et al. Does radiofrequency ablation induce a prethrombotic state? Analysis of coagulation system activation and comparison to electrophysiologic study. J Cardiovasc Electrophysiol 1998;9(11): 1152–60.

34. Ren JF, Marchlinski FE, Callans DJ. Left atrial thrombus associated with ablation for atrial fibrillation: identification with intracardiac echocardiography. J Am Coll Cardiol 2004;43:1861–7.

35. Haines DE, Stewart MT, Ahlberg S, et al. Microembolism and catheter ablation I: a comparison of irrigated radiofrequency and multielectrode-phased radiofrequency catheter ablation of pulmonary vein ostia. Circ Arrhythm Electrophysiol 2013;6: 16–22.

36. Nagy-Baló E, Tint D, Clemens M, et al. Transcranial measurement of cerebral microembolic signals during pulmonary vein isolation: a comparison of two ablation techniques. Circ Arrhythm Electrophysiol 2013;6:473–80.

37. Kalman JM, Fitzpatrick AP, Olgin JE, et al. Biophysical characteristics of radiofrequency lesion formation in vivo: dynamics of catheter tip-tissue contact evaluated by intracardiac echocardiography. Am Heart J 1997;133(1):8–18.

38. Johansen P. Mechanical heart valve cavitation. Expert Rev Med Devices 2004;1(1):95–104.

39. Szili-Torok T, Kimman GP, Theuns D, et al. Visualisation of intracardiac structures and radiofrequency lesions using intracardiac echocardiography. Eur J Echocardiogr 2003;4: 17–22.

40. Marrouche NS, Martin DO, Wazni O, et al. Phased-array intracardiac echocardiography monitoring during pulmonary vein isolation in patients with atrial fibrillation: impact on outcome and complications. Circulation 2006;107:2710–6.

41. Ringelstein EB, Droste DW, Babikian WL, et al. Consensus on microembolus detection by TCD. International consensus group on microembolus detection. Stroke 1998;29:725–9.

42. Grosset DG, Georgiadis G, Kelman AW, et al. Detection of microemboli by transcranial Doppler ultrasound. Tex Heart Inst J 1996;23:289–92.

43. Russell D, Brucher R. Online automatic discrimination between solid and gaseous cerebral microemboli with the first multifrequency transcranial Doppler. Stroke 1998;29:725–9.

44. Borger MA, Peniston CM, Weisel RD, et al. Neurophysiologic impairment after coronary bypass surgery: effect of gaseous microemboli during perfusionist interventions. J Thorac Cardiovasc Surg 2001;121:743–9.

45. Kilicaslan F, Verma A, Saad E, et al. Transcranial Doppler detection of microembolic signals during pulmonary vein antrum isolation: implications for titration of radiofrequency energy. J Cardiovasc Electrophysiol 2006;17:495–501.

46. Sauren LD, La Meir M, de Roy L, et al. Increased number of cerebral emboli during percutaneous endocardial pulmonary vein isolation versus a thoracoscopic epicardial approach. Eur J Cardiothorac Surg 2009;36:833–7.

47. Di Biase L, Burkhardt JD, Mohanty P, et al. Periprocedural stroke and management of major bleeding complications in patients undergoing catheter ablation of atrial fibrillation: the impact of periprocedural therapeutic international normalized ratio. Circulation 2010;121:2550–6.

48. Scherr D, Sharma K, Dalal D, et al. Incidence and predictors of periprocedural cerebrovascular accident in patients undergoing catheter ablation of atrial fibrillation. J Cardiovasc Electrophysiol 2009;20(12):1357–63.

49. Ichiki H, Oketani N, Ishida S, et al. Incidence of asymptomatic cerebral microthromboembolism after atrial fibrillation ablation guided by complex fractionated atrial electrogram. J Cardiovasc Electrophysiol 2012;23(6):567–73.

50. Calkins H, Kuck KH, Cappato R, et al. 2012 HRS/EHRA/ECAS expert consensus statement on catheter and surgical ablation of atrial fibrillation: recommendations for patient selection, procedural techniques, patient management and follow-up, definitions, endpoints, and research trial design. Heart Rhythm 2012;9(4):632–89.

51. Wieczorek M, Lukat M, Hoeltgen R, et al. Investigation into causes of abnormal cerebral MRI findings following PVAC duty cycled phased RF ablation of atrial fibrillation. J Cardiovasc Electrophysiol 2013; 24(2):121–8.

52. Wieczorek M, Hoeltgen R, Brueck M. Does the number of simultaneously activated electrodes during phased RF multielectrode ablation of atrial fibrillation influence the incidence of silent cerebral microembolism? Heart Rhythm 2013;10(10):953–9.

53. American College of Cardiology Foundation, American Heart Association, European Society of Cardiology, Heart Rhythm Society, Wann LS, Curtis AB, Ellenbogen KA, et al. Management of patients with atrial fibrillation (Compilation of 2006 ACCF/AHA/ESC and 2011 ACCF/AHA/HRS Recommendations): a report of the American College of Cardiology/American Heart Association Task Force on Practice Guidelines. Circulation 2013;127:1916–26.

54. European Heart Rhythm Association, European Association for Cardio-Thoracic Surgery, Camm AJ, Kirchhof P, Lip GY, et al. Guidelines for the management of atrial fibrillation. The Task Force for the Management of Atrial Fibrillation of the European Society of Cardiology. Eur Heart J 2010;31: 2369–429.

55. Wazni OM, Beheiry S, Fahmy T, et al. Atrial fibrillation ablation in patients with therapeutic international normalized ratio: comparison of strategies of anticoagulation management in the periprocedural period. Circulation 2007;116:2531–4.

56. Hussein AA, Martin DO, Patel D, et al. Radiofrequency ablation of atrial fibrillation under therapeutic international normalized ratio: a safe and efficacious periprocedural anticoagulation strategy. Heart Rhythm 2009;6:1425–9.

57. Lakkireddy D, Reddy YM, Di Biase L, et al. Feasibility and safety of dabigatran versus warfarin for periprocedural anticoagulation in patients undergoing radiofrequency ablation for atrial fibrillation. results from a multicenter prospective registry. J Am Coll Cardiol 2012;59:1168–74.

58. Winkle RA, Mead RH, Engel G, et al. The use of dabigatran immediately after atrial fibrillation ablation. J Cardiovasc Electrophysiol 2011;23:264–8.

59. Lakkireddy D, Reddy YM, Vallakati A, et al. Feasibility and safety of uninterrupted rivaroxaban for periprocedural anticoagulation in patients undergoing radiofrequency ablation for atrial fibrillation: results from a multicenter prospective registry. J Am Coll Cardiol 2012;13:1168–74.

60. Romero J, Husain SA, Kelesidis I, et al. Detection of left atrial appendage thrombus by cardiac computed tomography in patients with atrial fibrillation: a meta-analysis. Circ Cardiovasc Imaging 2013;6(2):185–94.

61. Sawit ST, Garcia-Alvarez A, Suri B, et al. Usefulness of cardiac computed tomographic delayed contrast enhancement of the left atrial appendage before pulmonary vein ablation. Am J Cardiol 2012;109:677–84.

62. Hur J, Pak HN, Kim YJ, et al. Dual-enhancement cardiac computed tomography for assessing left atrial thrombus and pulmonary veins before radiofrequency catheter ablation for atrial fibrillation. Am J Cardiol 2013;112:238–44.

63. Ren JF, Marchlinski FE, Supple GE, et al. Intracardiac echocardiographic diagnosis of thrombus formation in the left atrial appendage: a complementary role to transesophageal echocardiography. Echocardiography 2013;30:72–80.

64. Bruce CJ, Friedman PA, Narayan O, et al. Early heparinization decreases the incidence of left atrial thrombi detected by intracardiac echocardiography during radiofrequency ablation for atrial fibrillation. J Interv Card Electrophysiol 2008;22:211–9.

65. Camm AJ, Lip GY, De Caterina R, et al. 2012 focused update of the ESC guidelines for the management of atrial fibrillation. Eur Heart J 2012;33: 2719–47.

66. Chao TF, Lin YJ, Tsao HM, et al. CHADS2 and CHA2DS2-VASc scores in the prediction of clinical outcomes in patients with atrial fibrillation after catheter ablation. J Am Coll Cardiol 2011;58: 2380–5.

67. Themistoclakis S, Corrado A, Marchlinski FE, et al. The risk of thromboembolism and need for oral anticoagulation after successful atrial fibrillation ablation. J Am Coll Cardiol 2010;55:735–43.

The Impact of Early Detection of Atrial Fibrillation on Stroke Outcomes

Todd T. Tomson, MD[a], Philip Greenland, MD[b],
Rod Passman, MD, MSCE[a],*

KEYWORDS

- Atrial fibrillation • Stroke • Cardiac monitoring

KEY POINTS

- Early detection of atrial fibrillation (AF) before an AF-related stroke occurs could potentially allow for the initiation of preventive therapy.
- The often asymptomatic and paroxysmal nature of AF makes early detection of this disease complex.
- Despite the difficulties surrounding the detection of AF, early detection of AF has been shown to be possible in the general population, in patients with implantable cardiac monitoring devices, and in patients after cryptogenic stroke.
- However, data showing that early detection of AF leads to improved stroke outcomes are still being gathered.

INTRODUCTION

Early detection of any disease before a related adverse event is an intuitively appealing goal of medical care. However, early detection is only useful when the disease itself is serious, when treatment before event onset is more effective than treatment rendered after an adverse event occurs, and when the prevalence of the disease during the detectable preclinical phase is high. In view of the growing prevalence of atrial fibrillation (AF), the increased risk of stroke associated with the disease,[1] the proven efficacy of anticoagulation in preventing thromboembolic events,[2–5] and the significant morbidity and mortality of AF-related strokes,[6–8] AF seems to be an ideal target for screening strategies. Additionally, because stroke is the first manifestation of the arrhythmia in a quarter of all AF-related strokes,[9] early detection has major public health implications.

Although logical in theory, defining what early AF detection entails is quite complex. In regard to stroke, early detection implies finding and treating AF in patients who would otherwise not be diagnosed with the arrhythmia before stroke occurrence. Thus, early detection involves screening of patients who are at risk for both AF and AF-related thromboembolic events but who have not yet had the arrhythmia detected. The issues surrounding the screening process itself are particularly complicated. An ideal screening test should be inexpensive, easy to administer,

Disclosures: No disclosures (T.T. Tomson and P. Greenland). Medtronic, consultant, research support, speakers bureau; Boehringer Ingelheim, speakers bureau; Janssen Pharmaceuticals, speakers bureau; Pfizer/BMS, speakers bureau; UpToDate, author royalties; NIH, research support (R. Passman).
[a] Department of Preventive Medicine, Bluhm Cardiovascular Institute, Northwestern University Feinberg School of Medicine, 676 North Street Claire, Suite 600, Chicago, IL 60611, USA; [b] Department of Preventive Medicine, Bluhm Cardiovascular Institute, Northwestern University Feinberg School of Medicine, 680 North Lake Shore Drive, Suite 680, Chicago, IL 60611, USA
* Corresponding author.
E-mail address: r-passman@northwestern.edu

cardiacEP.theclinics.com

reliable, and valid. However, given the often paroxysmal nature of AF and the uncertainties surrounding the burden of AF worthy of detection, long periods of monitoring could potentially be required to detect brief and infrequent paroxysmal AF.

This article discusses whether early detection of AF is possible and whether such detection can improve outcomes. Although AF is associated with early mortality, congestive heart failure, and dementia, this article focuses solely on the outcome of stroke. Methods of detecting AF and the early detection of AF by population screening are discussed first. Early detection in the subset of patients with implantable cardiac rhythm management devices is discussed next. The evidence that early detection leads to improved stroke outcomes is then evaluated, followed by a discussion of AF detection in patients with cryptogenic stroke. Finally, areas of uncertainty and future directions for research are presented.

HOW TO SCREEN FOR AF

The diagnosis of AF requires documentation of the arrhythmia by ECG or reliable surrogate. Though physical examination and self-assessment of pulse, either through palpation or smart phone-based technologies, are expected to detect some AF, paroxysmal AF may be most reliably found with cardiac monitoring. With the duration of monitoring needed to detect AF inversely proportional to the AF burden, long periods of monitoring or frequent short monitoring periods may be necessary to detect infrequent paroxysmal AF. In patient with infrequent paroxysmal AF, the sensitivity of a single ECG is likely low, although true sensitivity cannot be determined without continuously monitoring the population of interest. Short-term external monitors, such as 24-hour Holter or 30-day monitors, are expected to have a better sensitivity for detecting paroxysmal AF than a single ECG. Unfortunately, the sensitivity of these approaches for detecting paroxysmal AF seems modest. This fact was demonstrated in a study of 574 permanent pacemaker (PPM) patients with a known history of atrial arrhythmia.[10] A statistical simulation was performed and showed that the sensitivities of a single annual 24-hour Holter for paroxysmal AF was only 31.3%, quarterly 24-hour Holter monitoring was 54.2%, and monthly 24-hour Holter monitoring was 71.0%. Seven-day and 30-day monitoring had sensitivities of only 48.9% and 64.6%, respectively. The negative predictive value of each of these methods of monitoring was 21.5%, 29.2%, 39.4%, 26.9%, and 34.7%, respectively.

In contrast to short-term external monitors, implantable cardiac rhythm management devices, including PPMs and implantable cardioverter-defibrillators (ICDs) with transvenous atrial leads, have the capability to monitor the cardiac rhythm continuously, and they have been shown to be highly accurate for detecting AF.[11,12] Although these patients clearly have different comorbidities than the general population, they are a source of important information concerning the relationship between AF burden and stroke, and they provide a unique opportunity to evaluate the feasibility and impact of early AF detection and treatment. Several studies have demonstrated that a substantial proportion of patients with these devices have a high burden of AF, even if they have no clinical history of the arrhythmia before implant. Between 10% and more than 50% of patients with PPMs or ICDs and no known history of AF before device implantation have device-detected asymptomatic AF.[13–19] Furthermore, these device-detected AF episodes of durations spanning minutes to hours are associated with a two to three times increased risk of stroke, regardless of the presence or absence of symptoms.[15–17,19,20]

Although PPMs and ICDs are only indicated in a minority of the population at risk for AF, leadless subcutaneous implantable cardiac monitors (ICMs) can provide long-term, continuous rhythm monitoring in patients without other device indications. These devices are highly accurate for detecting AF with an overall accuracy reported at 98.5% for total AF duration compared with external monitoring.[21,22] Currently, these devices are indicated for patients with clinical syndromes or situations that increase the risk of cardiac arrhythmias or in patients who experience transient symptoms such as dizziness, palpitations, syncope, or chest pain that may suggest a cardiac arrhythmia. In the future, they could prove useful in detecting AF in a wider range of patients.

POPULATION SCREENING FOR AF

Although short-duration ECGs and short-term external monitors have limited sensitivity for detecting asymptomatic paroxysmal AF, using these noninvasive devices to screen for AF makes intuitive sense given that strokes, which could have been prevented by anticoagulation, may occur in patients with AF even in the absence of prior symptoms.[17] However, a fundamental question surrounding early detection of AF is who in the general population should be screened. Ideally, screening should be performed in patients who are at risk for AF and who would benefit from intervention if AF were detected. Epidemiologic studies of AF have provided a foundation for which patients may benefit most from screening. Given the strong association between AF and age, it makes sense to limit screening to older individuals. It is estimated that the prevalence of AF in the general population is less than 1%.[23] However, the prevalence of AF increases exponentially after age 65 with an estimated prevalence of 6% in patients age 65 years or older and 10% in patients age 80 or older.[24] Additionally, more than 70% of people with AF are between the ages of 65 and 85.[24] Although no definitive threshold can be defended, age 65 years or older in the absence of other stroke risk-factors seems reasonable because these patients are at increased risk of AF and because detection of AF in this population would change management based on the CHA_2DS_2-VASc (Congestive heart failure, Hypertension, Age $\geq$75 [double], Diabetes, Stroke [double]; Vascular disease, Age 65 to 74, and Sex [female]) score.[25,26] Studies performed based on this approach do, in fact, show some effectiveness in identifying patients with AF.

In the Screening for AF in the Elderly (SAFE) study of subjects in the United Kingdom, 14,802 subjects age 65 years or older were randomized in a primary care setting to detection of AF by routine care, by opportunistic screening, or by systematic screening.[27,28] Opportunistic screening involved palpation of the pulse by trained personnel during primary care office visits. In subjects with an irregular pulse, an ECG was obtained. In the systematic screening arm, subjects were asked to attend a screening clinic where an office ECG was performed to assess for AF. Both opportunistic screening and systematic screening effectively increased the diagnosis of AF by about 60%, from 1.04% per year in the routine care arm to 1.64% per year in the opportunistic screening arm and 1.62% per year in the systematic screening arm. However, the systematic screening arm cost more per case of AF detected than did the opportunistic screening arm (£1787 vs £363, or roughly $3217 vs $653 in 2005 dollars). Based on these results, current American and European guidelines recommend active opportunistic screening for AF in patients age 65 years and older in the primary care setting by palpation of the pulse followed by an ECG if the pulse is irregular.[29,30]

Focusing on an older population, a Scandinavian study screened all subjects ages 75 to 76 years living in the Swedish municipality of Halmstad.[31] Subjects were first asked to record a 12-lead ECG and report their relevant medical history. Subjects with sinus rhythm on ECG, no history of AF, and greater than or equal to 2 $CHADS_2$ (Congestive heart failure, Hypertension,

Age $\geq$75, Diabetes, Stroke [double]) risk factors were then asked to use a hand-held device to record an ECG twice daily for 2 weeks or if palpitations occurred. The hand-held monitor recorded lead I of the ECG by application of the users' thumbs to the device (Zenicor Medical Systems AB, Stokholm, Sweden). The initial screening ECG uncovered undiagnosed AF in 1% of the study population. Of those in sinus rhythm but with greater than or equal to 2 $CHADS_2$ risk factors, hand-held ECG monitoring diagnosed 7.4% with paroxysmal AF.

Both studies showed that screening for AF in high-risk patients can effectively increase early detection of AF. However, neither can provide insights into the true sensitivity of either approach for detecting asymptomatic paroxysmal AF. Additionally, neither trial was designed to show a reduction in stroke rates or an improvement in stroke outcomes associated with early detection of AF by population screening.

EARLY DETECTION OF AF IN PATIENTS WITH IMPLANTED CARDIAC RHYTHM MANAGEMENT DEVICES

Although population screening efforts have some usefulness in detecting AF in the population at large, the subset of patients with implantable cardiac rhythm management devices are at particularly high risk of AF and are in a unique position to have their rhythm monitored continuously and over long periods of time. These devices have traditionally required periodic manual device interrogations every 3, 6, or 12 months in an outpatient clinic. However, the advent of remote monitoring has the potential to allow for continuous monitoring, which could lead to early detection and treatment of AF. Several studies have already demonstrated this fact.[32–36]

In a retrospective study of 11,624 subjects with PPMs, ICDs, or cardiac resynchronization therapy (CRT) devices with remote data transmission capabilities, Lazarus estimated that using continuous remote monitoring would advance the time to diagnosis of a clinical event by 64 or 154 days when compared with standard 3 or 6 month follow-up, respectively.[33] In a study by Ricci and colleagues, 166 subjects with dual-chambered devices were followed for a mean of 488 days to determine the impact of daily remote monitoring on detection and treatment of AF.[35] An AF alert was transmitted for either new onset AF, AF lasting greater than 10% of the time for more than 5 consecutive days, or AF lasting 100% of the time for 2 consecutive days. During a mean follow-up of 488 plus or minus 203 days, 26% of subjects had alerts for AF. The median time to the first intervention for AF was 50 days, which was 148 days sooner than AF would have been detected if the subjects had waited until their next regularly scheduled device interrogation. Similarly, in the Lumos-T Safely Reduces Routine Office Device Follow-up (TRUST) trial, 1339 subjects with ICDs were randomized to either automatic daily surveillance or conventional follow-up at 3, 6, 9, 12, and 15 months.[36] The primary endpoint was the time from device detection of an event, defined as mode switching for AF of greater than 10% per 24 hours, to physician evaluation of the event. Overall, the median time from any ICD detection to physician evaluation was significantly reduced from 36 days in the conventional group to less than 2 days in the remote monitoring group.

The largest prospective trial of early detection of AF by remote monitoring to date is the Clinical Evaluation of Remote Notification to Reduce Time to Clinical Decision (CONNECT) trial, which randomized 1997 subjects with ICDs or CRT-defibrillator devices to either remote monitoring with wireless clinician alerts or in-office care with follow-up visits at 1, 3, 6, 9, 12, and 15 months.[32] The primary outcome was the time from device detection of an event, including AF more than 12 hours per day, to the clinical decision in response to the event. During the 15 months of follow-up, 11% of subjects had AF. The time to diagnosis of AF was reduced from a mean of 24 days in the in-office arm to 3 days in the remote monitoring arm.

When taken together, these studies show that daily remote monitoring for arrhythmias in patients with PPMs, ICDs, or CRT devices is feasible, can significantly reduce the time to detection of AF, and can reduce the time to a clinical decision being made about AF treatment. However, none of these studies was designed to address the most important issue of whether early detection of AF leads to a clinically significant improvement in stroke outcomes.

PRIMARY PREVENTION OF STROKE VIA EARLY AF DETECTION

Although the ability to detect asymptomatic AF has been demonstrated in both population screening studies and in subjects with implantable cardiac rhythm management devices, whether early detection of AF and early initiation of anticoagulation actually leads to a reduction in stroke rates has not been clearly demonstrated. Robust data on this topic are still awaited, but studies are in progress.

Based on the results of the Scandinavian population screening study,[31] the Population Screening of 75- and 76-year-old Men and Women for Silent Atrial Fibrillation (STROKESTOP) trial was recently initiated and is ongoing.[37] This trial is a prospective, randomized controlled trial of population screening for AF using the methods described earlier to investigate whether screening for silent AF can reduce stroke rates in the screened population and whether this screening is cost-effective. Overall, 25,000 Swedes ages 75 and 76 years will be randomized to either a control arm or a screening arm and followed for 5 years for a reduction in stroke rates.

Regarding the subset of patients with implantable cardiac rhythm management devices, Ricci and colleagues used data from 136 subjects with pacemakers or defibrillators with remote monitoring capabilities to estimate the potential benefits of remote continuous monitoring on stroke outcomes.[38] Monte Carlo modeling was used to simulate stroke rates in subjects monitored via continuous remote monitoring and via standard follow-up. Results suggest that continuous remote monitoring provides a 2-year stroke reduction of between 9% and 18% when compared with standard in-person follow-up with office visits every 6 to 12 months.

In the COMPArative follow-up Schedule with home monitoring (COMPAS) trial, subjects with PPMs showed a trend toward a lower stroke rate when followed by continuous remote monitoring compared with standard in-office follow-up.[34] However, the study was designed primarily to determine the safety of remote monitoring and was neither powered to show a difference in stroke rates between groups nor designed to specify an intervention protocol once AF was discovered. Similarly, the TRUST study of subjects with ICDs showed a nonsignificant trend toward a lower stroke rate in the group of subjects with continuous remote monitoring compared with those monitored with standard in-office follow-up, though the study was not powered for this endpoint.[36] One large-scale study that addresses the issue of early AF detection and management has completed enrollment. The Impact of Biotronik Home Monitoring Guided Anticoagulation on Stroke Risk in Patients With ICD and CRT-D Devices (IMPACT) trial randomized more than two thousand subjects with CRT devices with remote continuous monitoring capabilities (http://clinicaltrials.gov/show/NCT00559988).[39] The goals of the trial are to evaluate the efficacy of remote monitoring in the early detection of AF and to determine if the initiation and withdrawal of oral anticoagulation therapy guided by continuous remote monitoring improves clinical outcomes by reducing the combined rate of stroke, systemic embolism, and major bleeding compared with conventional in-office management. Results of this trial are not yet available.

Although these studies focused on subjects with implanted cardiac rhythm management devices, a novel study is using leadless subcutaneous ICMs to provide further insights into early AF detection. The Reveal XT Implantable Cardiac Monitor (REVEAL AF) study (http://clinicaltrials.gov/ct2/show/NCT01727297) is a prospective, nonrandomized, multicenter study that aims to enroll 450 subjects at high risk for both AF and stroke. The primary outcome of the trial is the incidence of AF lasting longer than 6 minutes detected by the ICM. Secondary aims include changes in management should AF be detected.

SECONDARY PREVENTION OF STROKE VIA AF DETECTION AFTER CRYPTOGENIC STROKE

Extensive evaluation fails to find a cause of stroke in 20% to 40% of ischemic strokes.[40–44] The detection of AF in a patient with so-called cryptogenic stroke mandates a change from antiplatelet therapy to anticoagulation to prevent recurrent events. As a result, early detection of AF in this group of patients carries great clinical importance.

Multiple studies have assessed the yield of various monitoring techniques for asymptomatic paroxysmal AF in the cryptogenic stroke population. External monitors worn for 24 to 72 hours find newly detected AF in 2.4% to 6.0% of these patients.[45–47] One study that looked at 21-day mobile outpatient telemetry showed that 23% of cryptogenic stroke subjects had AF, but most reported episodes lasted only seconds in duration.[48] Unfortunately, external monitors can be anticipated to have a limited sensitivity in this population. In a subgroup analysis of the Clinical Significance of Atrial Arrhythmias Detected by Implanted Device Diagnostics (TRENDS) study, Ziegler and colleagues evaluated 163 subjects with previous ischemic stroke or transient ischemic attack and no known history of AF who had pacemakers or ICDs implanted for approved indications.[49] Newly detected AF, defined as AF lasting greater than or equal to 5 minutes, occurred in 28% of the subjects during the mean follow-up of 1.1 plus or minus 0.7 years. Due to the temporal clustering of paroxysmal AF episodes, nearly three-quarters of subjects had newly detected atrial arrhythmias on less than 10% of the monitoring days. Furthermore, 60% of subjects had their first episode of AF detected beyond 30 days of monitoring, suggesting that a single, short attempt at AF detection may be insufficient in these patients.

The use of ICMs in this population has also been studied. Noncontrolled studies enrolling small numbers of subjects have reported AF detection rates between 17% and 27%.[50–52] Importantly, the time to AF detection ranged from 48 to 161 days, supporting the contention that short-term external monitors may be insufficient in this high-risk population of patients. Recently, the CRYSTAL AF (CRYptogenic STroke And underLying AF) trial completed enrollment and will provide further insights into the early detection of AF after cryptogenic stroke.[53] This international trial randomizes cryptogenic stroke subjects to receive either an ICM or standard clinical follow-up. The primary endpoint of the study is time to first detected AF event, defined as AF lasting more than 30 seconds within the first 6 months of enrollment.

SUMMARY AND FUTURE DIRECTION

Though theoretically desirable and feasible, early detection and treatment of AF is fraught with challenges and many unanswered questions. Screening methods in the general population can correctly identify some AF patients, but those with infrequent and short-lived episodes may go undetected by anything but continuous monitoring. Whether the burden of AF in this latter group is sufficient to warrant intervention is currently unknown but of great importance given the cost associated with continuous monitoring. Timely identification of AF in the subset of patients with PPMs, ICDs, and CRT devices, who seem to be at particular risk for AF, has also been shown to be possible. Although it might be expected that early detection of AF in the general population or in patients with implantable cardiac devices would lead to a reduction in stroke rates by prompt initiation of anticoagulation, studies addressing this assumption are ongoing.

Future studies are needed to refine detection methods for asymptomatic AF. In the area of population screening, the best means of identifying high-risk patients with asymptomatic AF is not known, and identifying the optimal method of screening will be important. In particular, it will be critical to determine which method of screening provides the best combination of sensitivity and cost-effectiveness, as well as to refine which patient variables should prompt screening. With regard to detection of asymptomatic AF in patients with implantable cardiac rhythm management devices, data from randomized controlled trials showing that early anticoagulation of patients with device-detected AF leads to a significant reduction in stroke rates are still being collected but are an important next step in defining monitoring and treatment strategies in this subset of patients.

Given the growing prevalence of AF and the impact of AF-related strokes on both the individual and societal levels, finding and treating AF before a thromboembolic event seems worthy of attention and resources.

REFERENCES

1. Wolf PA, Abbott RD, Kannel WB. Atrial fibrillation as an independent risk factor for stroke: the Framingham Study. Stroke 1991;22(8):983–8.
2. Connolly SJ, Ezekowitz MD, Yusuf S, et al. Dabigatran versus warfarin in patients with atrial fibrillation. N Engl J Med 2009;361(12):1139–51.
3. Granger CB, Alexander JH, McMurray JJ, et al. Apixaban versus warfarin in patients with atrial fibrillation. N Engl J Med 2011;365(11):981–92.
4. Hart RG, Pearce LA, Aguilar MI. Meta-analysis: antithrombotic therapy to prevent stroke in patients who have nonvalvular atrial fibrillation. Ann Intern Med 2007;146(12):857–67.
5. Patel MR, Mahaffey KW, Garg J, et al. Rivaroxaban versus warfarin in nonvalvular atrial fibrillation. N Engl J Med 2011;365(10):883–91.
6. Indredavik B, Rohweder G, Lydersen S. Frequency and effect of optimal anticoagulation before onset of ischaemic stroke in patients with known atrial fibrillation. J Intern Med 2005;258(2):133–44.
7. Kimura K, Minematsu K, Yamaguchi T, et al. Atrial fibrillation as a predictive factor for severe stroke and early death in 15,831 patients with acute ischaemic stroke. J Neurol Neurosurg Psychiatry 2005;76(5):679–83.
8. Saxena R, Lewis S, Berge E, et al. Risk of early death and recurrent stroke and effect of heparin in 3169 patients with acute ischemic stroke and atrial fibrillation in the International Stroke Trial. Stroke 2001;32(10):2333–7.
9. Lin HJ, Wolf PA, Benjamin EJ, et al. Newly diagnosed atrial fibrillation and acute stroke. The Framingham Study. Stroke 1995;26(9):1527–30.
10. Ziegler PD, Koehler JL, Mehra R. Comparison of continuous versus intermittent monitoring of atrial arrhythmias. Heart Rhythm 2006;3(12):1445–52.
11. Passman RS, Weinberg KM, Freher M, et al. Accuracy of mode switch algorithms for detection of atrial tachyarrhythmias. J Cardiovasc Electrophysiol 2004;15(7):773–7.
12. Purerfellner H, Gillis AM, Holbrook R, et al. Accuracy of atrial tachyarrhythmia detection in implantable devices with arrhythmia therapies. Pacing Clin Electrophysiol 2004;27(7):983–92.
13. Cheung JW, Keating RJ, Stein KM, et al. Newly detected atrial fibrillation following dual chamber pacemaker implantation. J Cardiovasc Electrophysiol 2006;17(12):1323–8.
14. Defaye P, Dournaux F, Mouton E. Prevalence of supraventricular arrhythmias from the automated analysis of data stored in the DDD pacemakers of 617 patients: the AIDA study. The AIDA Multicenter Study Group. Automatic Interpretation for Diagnosis Assistance. Pacing Clin Electrophysiol 1998;21(1 Pt 2):250–5.
15. Glotzer TV, Daoud EG, Wyse DG, et al. The relationship between daily atrial tachyarrhythmia burden from implantable device diagnostics and stroke risk: the TRENDS study. Circ Arrhythm Electrophysiol 2009;2(5):474–80.
16. Glotzer TV, Hellkamp AS, Zimmerman J, et al. Atrial high rate episodes detected by pacemaker diagnostics predict death and stroke: report of the Atrial Diagnostics Ancillary Study of the MOde Selection Trial (MOST). Circulation 2003;107(12):1614–9.
17. Healey JS, Connolly SJ, Gold MR, et al. Subclinical atrial fibrillation and the risk of stroke. N Engl J Med 2012;366(2):120–9.
18. Orlov MV, Ghali JK, Araghi-Niknam M, et al. Asymptomatic atrial fibrillation in pacemaker recipients: incidence, progression, and determinants based on the atrial high rate trial. Pacing Clin Electrophysiol 2007;30(3):404–11.
19. Shanmugam N, Boerdlein A, Proff J, et al. Detection of atrial high-rate events by continuous home monitoring: clinical significance in the heart failure-cardiac resynchronization therapy population. Europace 2012;14(2):230–7.
20. Capucci A, Santini M, Padeletti L, et al. Monitored atrial fibrillation duration predicts arterial embolic events in patients suffering from bradycardia and atrial fibrillation implanted with antitachycardia pacemakers. J Am Coll Cardiol 2005;46(10):1913–20.
21. Sarkar S, Ritscher D, Mehra R. A detector for a chronic implantable atrial tachyarrhythmia monitor. IEEE Trans Biomed Eng 2008;55(3):1219–24.
22. Hindricks G, Pokushalov E, Urban L, et al. Performance of a new leadless implantable cardiac monitor in detecting and quantifying atrial fibrillation: results of the XPECT trial. Circ Arrhythm Electrophysiol 2010;3(2):141–7.
23. Fuster V, Ryden LE, Cannom DS, et al. 2011 ACCF/AHA/HRS focused updates incorporated into the ACC/AHA/ESC 2006 guidelines for the management of patients with atrial fibrillation: a report of the American College of Cardiology Foundation/American Heart Association Task Force on practice guidelines. Circulation 2011;123(10):e269–367.
24. Feinberg WM, Blackshear JL, Laupacis A, et al. Prevalence, age distribution, and gender of patients with atrial fibrillation. Analysis and implications. Arch Intern Med 1995;155(5):469–73.

25. Lip GY, Nieuwlaat R, Pisters R, et al. Refining clinical risk stratification for predicting stroke and thromboembolism in atrial fibrillation using a novel risk factor-based approach: the euro heart survey on atrial fibrillation. Chest 2010;137(2):263–72.

26. European Heart Rhythm Association, European Association for Cardio-Thoracic Surgery, Camm AJ, et al. Guidelines for the management of atrial fibrillation: the Task Force for the Management of Atrial Fibrillation of the European Society of Cardiology (ESC). Eur Heart J 2010;31(19): 2369–429.

27. Hobbs FD, Fitzmaurice DA, Mant J, et al. A randomised controlled trial and cost-effectiveness study of systematic screening (targeted and total population screening) versus routine practice for the detection of atrial fibrillation in people aged 65 and over. The SAFE study. Health Technol Assess 2005;9(40):iii–iiv, ix–x, 1–74.

28. Fitzmaurice DA, Hobbs FD, Jowett S, et al. Screening versus routine practice in detection of atrial fibrillation in patients aged 65 or over: cluster randomised controlled trial. BMJ 2007; 335(7616):383.

29. Goldstein LB, Bushnell CD, Adams RJ, et al. Guidelines for the primary prevention of stroke: a guideline for healthcare professionals from the American Heart Association/American Stroke Association. Stroke 2011;42(2):517–84.

30. Camm AJ, Lip GY, De Caterina R, et al. 2012 focused update of the ESC Guidelines for the management of atrial fibrillation: an update of the 2010 ESC Guidelines for the management of atrial fibrillation. Developed with the special contribution of the European Heart Rhythm Association. Eur Heart J 2012;33(21):2719–47.

31. Engdahl J, Andersson L, Mirskaya M, et al. Stepwise screening of atrial fibrillation in a 75-year-old population: implications for stroke prevention. Circulation 2013;127(8):930–7.

32. Crossley GH, Boyle A, Vitense H, et al. The CONNECT (Clinical Evaluation of Remote Notification to Reduce Time to Clinical Decision) trial: the value of wireless remote monitoring with automatic clinician alerts. J Am Coll Cardiol 2011; 57(10):1181–9.

33. Lazarus A. Remote, wireless, ambulatory monitoring of implantable pacemakers, cardioverter defibrillators, and cardiac resynchronization therapy systems: analysis of a worldwide database. Pacing Clin Electrophysiol 2007;30(Suppl 1):S2–12.

34. Mabo P, Victor F, Bazin P, et al. A randomized trial of long-term remote monitoring of pacemaker recipients (the COMPAS trial). Eur Heart J 2012; 33(9):1105–11.

35. Ricci RP, Morichelli L, Santini M. Remote control of implanted devices through home monitoring technology improves detection and clinical management of atrial fibrillation. Europace 2009;11(1): 54–61.

36. Varma N, Epstein AE, Irimpen A, et al. Efficacy and safety of automatic remote monitoring for implantable cardioverter-defibrillator follow-up: the Lumos-T Safely Reduces Routine Office Device Follow-up (TRUST) trial. Circulation 2010;122(4): 325–32.

37. Friberg L, Engdahl J, Frykman V, et al. Population screening of 75- and 76-year-old men and women for silent atrial fibrillation (STROKESTOP). Europace 2013;15(1):135–40.

38. Ricci RP, Morichelli L, Gargaro A, et al. Home monitoring in patients with implantable cardiac devices: is there a potential reduction of stroke risk? Results from a computer model tested through monte carlo simulations. J Cardiovasc Electrophysiol 2009; 20(11):1244–51.

39. Ip J, Waldo AL, Lip GY, et al. Multicenter randomized study of anticoagulation guided by remote rhythm monitoring in patients with implantable cardioverter-defibrillator and CRT-D devices: rationale, design, and clinical characteristics of the initially enrolled cohort the IMPACT study. Am Heart J 2009;158(3):364–70.e1.

40. Adams HP Jr, Bendixen BH, Kappelle LJ, et al. Classification of subtype of acute ischemic stroke. Definitions for use in a multicenter clinical trial. TOAST. Trial of Org 10172 in Acute Stroke Treatment. Stroke 1993;24(1):35–41.

41. Amarenco P, Bogousslavsky J, Caplan LR, et al. New approach to stroke subtyping: the A-S-C-O (phenotypic) classification of stroke. Cerebrovasc Dis 2009;27(5):502–8.

42. Grau AJ, Weimar C, Buggle F, et al. Risk factors, outcome, and treatment in subtypes of ischemic stroke: the German stroke data bank. Stroke 2001;32(11):2559–66.

43. Kolominsky-Rabas PL, Weber M, Gefeller O, et al. Epidemiology of ischemic stroke subtypes according to TOAST criteria: incidence, recurrence, and long-term survival in ischemic stroke subtypes: a population-based study. Stroke 2001;32(12): 2735–40.

44. Schulz UG, Rothwell PM. Differences in vascular risk factors between etiological subtypes of ischemic stroke: importance of population-based studies. Stroke 2003;34(8):2050–9.

45. Jabaudon D, Sztajzel J, Sievert K, et al. Usefulness of ambulatory 7-day ECG monitoring for the detection of atrial fibrillation and flutter after acute stroke and transient ischemic attack. Stroke 2004;35(7): 1647–51.

46. Schuchert A, Behrens G, Meinertz T. Impact of long-term ECG recording on the detection of paroxysmal atrial fibrillation in patients after an

acute ischemic stroke. Pacing Clin Electrophysiol 1999;22(7):1082–4.

47. Shafqat S, Kelly PJ, Furie KL. Holter monitoring in the diagnosis of stroke mechanism. Intern Med J 2004;34(6):305–9.

48. Tayal AH, Tian M, Kelly KM, et al. Atrial fibrillation detected by mobile cardiac outpatient telemetry in cryptogenic TIA or stroke. Neurology 2008; 71(21):1696–701.

49. Ziegler PD, Glotzer TV, Daoud EG, et al. Incidence of newly detected atrial arrhythmias via implantable devices in patients with a history of thromboembolic events. Stroke 2010;41(2):256–60.

50. Ritter MA, Kochhauser S, Duning T, et al. Occult atrial fibrillation in cryptogenic stroke: detection by 7-day electrocardiogram versus implantable cardiac monitors. Stroke 2013; 44(5):1449–52.

51. Etgen T, Hochreiter M, Mundel M, et al. Insertable cardiac event recorder in detection of atrial fibrillation after cryptogenic stroke: an audit report. Stroke 2013;44(7):2007–9.

52. Cotter PE, Martin PJ, Ring L, et al. Incidence of atrial fibrillation detected by implantable loop recorders in unexplained stroke. Neurology 2013; 80(17):1546–50.

53. Sinha AM, Diener HC, Morillo CA, et al. Cryptogenic stroke and underlying atrial fibrillation (CRYSTAL AF): design and rationale. Am Heart J 2010;160(1):36–41.e1.

Stroke Risk in Patients with Implanted Cardiac Devices

Mahmoud Houmsse, MD, FHRS, Emile G. Daoud, MD, FHRS*

KEYWORDS

- Atrial fibrillation • Stroke • Atrial high rate events • Defibrillator • Pacemaker • Thromboembolism

KEY POINTS

- Current technology of cardiac implanted electronic devices (CIED) allows continuous monitoring of atrial tachyarrhythmias and digitally stores the electrograms associated with atrial high rate events (AHRE).
- AHRE of greater than 5 minutes' duration have a 97% accuracy of being atrial fibrillation (AF).
- Newly diagnosed AF, as detected by stored electrograms of CIEDs during routine device interrogation, is often unassociated with symptoms ("silent AF") and occurs with high frequency (≈25% of patients).
- Compared with patients without device-detected AHRE, patients with device-detected AHRE have a significantly greater risk for stroke.
- Data from CIEDs suggest that AF duration is a risk factor for thromboembolic events.
- Currently, there is no consensus on initiation or withdrawal of anticoagulation therapy in response to device-detected AF; however, AHREs detected by device interrogation should prompt the consideration to begin anticoagulation/antiplatelet therapy.

INTRODUCTION

The presence of atrial fibrillation (AF) increases the risk of ischemic stroke by 5-fold.[1] In the Framingham study, it is estimated that AF causes 14% of all stroke, and the mechanism is thromboembolism (TE).[2–4] Primary prevention anticoagulation therapy using warfarin with a target international normalized ratio (2.0–3.0) or the newer oral anticoagulants (direct thrombin inhibitors and factor X antagonists) have demonstrated a significant reduction of stroke as well as all-cause mortality.[5–10] The initiation of anticoagulation for patients with AF and high risk for thromboemboli is thus of critical importance. However, many patients with AF are unaware of their AF episodes (ie, asymptomatic or "silent" AF), which has been reported to occur in 24% of AF patients.[11] For these patients, the first manifestation of AF may be a TE event.

The diagnosis of asymptomatic (silent) AF is increasingly encountered in clinical practice in patients with cardiac implantable electronic devices (CIED) in 2 different clinical presentations. The first is when a CIED is implanted in a patient who has no prior diagnosis of AF; then, during routine follow-up, device-stored electrograms confirm the diagnosis of AF that may have occurred several months earlier and could be of

The authors have nothing to disclose.

Division of Cardiovascular Medicine, Department of Internal Medicine, Electrophysiology Section, Ross Heart Hospital, The Wexner Medical Center at the Ohio State University Medical Center, Columbus, OH, USA; Davis Heart and Lung Research Institute, Suite 200, 473 West 12th Avenue, Columbus, OH 43210, USA

* Corresponding author.

E-mail address: emile.daoud@osumc.edu

Card Electrophysiol Clin 6 (2014) 133–139

http://dx.doi.org/10.1016/j.ccep.2013.10.002

cardiacEP.theclinics.com

long duration. These episodes of newly diagnosed AF (NDAF) may not be associated with any symptoms. The second scenario is device detection of NDAF in patients who have had an embolic cryptogenic stroke before device implantation. The CIED then confirms the diagnosis of asymptomatic AF, which may be the cause of the stroke.

The purpose of this article is to review the data regarding these 2 scenarios and to address clinical management.

ATRIAL HIGH RATE EVENTS DETECTED BY CIED

CIED routinely monitor for atrial high rate events (AHRE). With the current technology of CIEDs, when an AHRE duration exceeds 5 minutes, the accuracy of a diagnosis of AF is 97%. Unlike clinical AF, most device-detected AF is brief in duration, infrequent, and usually asymptomatic.

Clinical data of AHRE detected by CIEDs have been derived from observational studies with no consensus on the definition or management of AHRE. In pooled data from 9 observational studies including a total of 8853 patients who had CIED, NDAF developed in 2040 patients (23%) during an average follow-up of 17 months (**Table 1**).[12–20] The detection rate of NDAF increased during continued follow-up, reaching 35% to 40% at 30 to 40 months (**Fig. 1**).

These same studies also demonstrated that there is poor correlation between device-detected AHRE and symptoms. Orlov and colleagues[14] reported AHRE in 46% of 331 patients with a pacemaker. Nevertheless, when patients

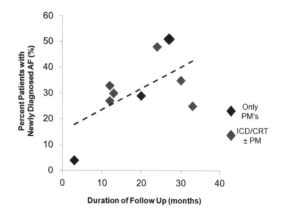

Fig. 1. Relationship between duration of CIED follow-up and NDAF. Data generated from studies presented in **Table 1**. CRT-D, defibrillator with cardiac resynchronization pacing; ICD, implantable cardiac defibrillator; PM, pacemaker.

complained of symptoms, there was no AHRE on 92% of symptomatic days. Another study by Quirino and colleagues[21] confirmed the same observation that 81% of symptomatic days had no AHRE. The correlation between symptoms and AHRE was higher when the duration of AHRE was greater than 24 hours.

Even though the patient is often asymptomatic, AHREs significantly increase the risk of developing clinical AF and has been illustrated in 2 important observational studies. In the Mode Selection Trial (MOST) pacemaker substudy, 312 patients, who did not have a prior diagnosis of AF, were followed for 27 months. AHREs were recorded in 51% of patients and clinical AF subsequently developed

Table 1
Summary of clinical trials of NDAF from CIEDs

Study	Number of Patients	Device	AHRE (bpm)	Duration	Patients with NDAF	F/U (mo)
MOST[12]	312	PM	≥220	≥10 beats	160 (51%)	27
Cheung[13]	262	PM	≥177	≥5 min	77 (29%)	20
Orlov[14]	331	PM	>180	≥1 min	159 (48%)	24
Bunch[15]	1170	ICD	—	≥12 beats	45 (4%)	3
Borleffs[16]	223	CRT-D	>180	≥10 min/d	55 (25%)	33
Caldwell[17]	101	PM/ICD/CRT-D	≥200	>30 s	27 (27%)	12
TRENDS[18]	1428	PM/ICD	≥175	≥5 min	432 (30%)	13
Shanmugam[19]	382	CRT-D	>180	≥14 min/d	127 (33%)	12
ASSERT[20]	2580	PM/ICD	≥190	≥6 min	633 (25%)	30

TOTAL: 6789 patients; NDAF in 1715 (25%) patients during an average follow-up ≈ 17 months.

Abbreviations: CRT-D, defibrillator with cardiac resynchronization pacing; Dx, diagnosis; F/U, follow-up; ICD, implantable cardiac defibrillator; PM, pacemaker.

in 39%. Therefore, the AHRE group had a 5.93 times risk of developing clinical AF compared with the control group that had no AHRE.[12] The second study is the Asymptomatic Atrial Fibrillation and Stroke Evaluation in Pacemaker Patients and the Atrial Fibrillation Reduction Atrial Pacing Trial (ASSERT).[20] Healey and colleagues[20] followed 2580 patients for 2.5 years. Patients were older than 65 years of age and hypertensive and had no history of clinical AF. AHRE of more than 6 minutes was recorded in 35% and clinical AF developed in 16%. Therefore, patients with AHRE had a 5.56 times greater risk of developing clinical AF compared with the control group that had no AHRE. This finding of a significant increase risk of clinical AF associated with AHRE in ASSERT is remarkably similar to that of the MOST study, completed many years earlier.

These studies confirm that asymptomatic AF recorded from CIEDs is part of the clinical spectrum of AF and thus raises the consideration that asymptomatic AF, diagnosed via stored electrograms from a CIED, should be managed in a similar manner as clinical AF.

CORRELATION OF STROKE EVENTS TO DEVICE-DETECTED AF AND TO AF BURDEN

Stroke risk assessment tools and treatment guidelines for initiation of anticoagulation do not differentiate based on detection of asymptomatic AF or AF burden; however, device-detected asymptomatic AF has not been incorporated into stroke risk models.

Multiple observational studies were designed to address the relationship between AHREs and asymptomatic AF burden and TE stroke. These studies have a similar design: enrolled patients who underwent CIED implantation for class I or II clinical indication and, during follow-up, AHREs and TE stroke were tracked. Management of asymptomatic AF and anticoagulation/antiplatelet therapy was at the discretion of the physician.

The ASSERT trial was designed to assess the risk of ischemic stroke in patients with asymptomatic AHRE during their routine pacemaker or defibrillator follow-up. Included in this study were 2580 patients.[20] At 3 months after implantation, AHRE of ≥6 minutes was noted in 261 patients (10.1%). During subsequent follow-up, stroke events were significantly greater in patients with AHRE, and AHREs were independently associated with an increased risk of stroke and TE by 2.50 times compared with patients without AHRE (**Fig. 2**). It was also noticed that the longer the AHRE (>17-hour duration), the higher the risk for ischemic stroke (**Fig. 3**).

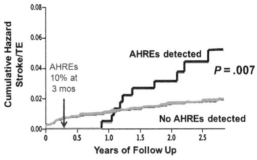

Fig. 2. Detection of the first asymptomatic AHRE and the first clinical stroke/TE in the ASSERT study. AHRE hazard ratio for stroke/TE is 2.50. Also note the time delay between AHREs (10% detection at 3 months after device implantation) and the first stoke, at about 10 months after implantation. (*Data from* Healey JS, Connolly SJ, Gold MR, et al. Subclinical atrial fibrillation and the risk of stroke. N Engl J Med 2012;366:120–9.)

The MOST study, which was designed to assess whether dual-chamber pacing in patients with sick sinus syndrome is superior to single-chamber pacing with respect to subsequent stroke, quality of life, and cost-effectiveness, completed a substudy that included 312 of 2010 patients.[12] All patients had no AF, TE, or stroke. Patients in this observational study were followed for up to 27 months. The investigators of the study concluded that AHRE greater than 5 minutes occurred in 160 of 312 patients (51%) and the mean time to diagnosis of AHRE is 3.5 months. AHRE was an independent predictor of future nonfatal stroke, sustained AF, and death by 2.8 times compared to patients without AHREs.

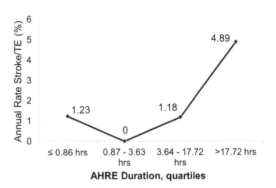

Fig. 3. Data from the ASSERT study demonstrating that longer duration of AHREs may be associated with increased risk of stroke/TE. (*Data from* Healey JS, Connolly SJ, Gold MR, et al. Subclinical atrial fibrillation and the risk of stroke. N Engl J Med 2012;366: 120–9.)

The relationship between AHREs and the duration of AHRE to TE events was assessed in the TRENDS study.[22] This prospective observational study enrolled 2486 patients who had at least one risk factor for stroke (heart failure, hypertension, age 65 or older, diabetes, or previous TE) (mean $CHADS_2$ score of 2.2 ± 1.2) and who required implantation of a CIED. A history of AF was not an exclusion criterion and 20% of patients had paroxysmal AF. During a mean follow-up of 1.4 years, there were 40 of 2486 (1.6%) TE events. The occurrence of TE events was correlated to the occurrence of AHRE and to the AF burden, which was defined as the longest total duration of AF on any given day during the prior 30 days, using the stored device information recorded from CIED. AF burden was stratified into 3 groups based on the study population median AF burden of 5.5 hours: zero burden, low burden with less than 5.5 hours, and high burden with greater than 5.5 hours. Compared with zero and low AF burden groups, the high AF burden group had a 2.2 times greater risk of TE ($P = .06$). This study suggests that stroke risk is a quantitative function of paroxysmal AF burden.

The impact of recurrent clinical AF on development of TE has been evaluated by the Italian AT500 Registry Investigators. Capucci and colleagues[23] enrolled 725 patients with a history of AF and bradycardia requiring a dual-chamber rate-responsive pacemaker, with specific algorithms designated for rhythm discrimination, prevention, and therapy for atrial arrhythmias with antitachycardia pacing. One other purpose of this observational study was to identify specific features that lead to future TE events. Arterial embolic events were independently associated with ischemic heart disease, diabetes mellitus, prior TE, hypertension, and clinical AF. To investigate if there is a correlation between AF duration and TE/stroke, AF that was more than 1 day had a hazard ratio for TE of 3.1 compared with AF of less than 1 day ($P = .04$).

The results of the Italian AT500 Registry highlight that clinical AF and $CHADS_2$ score correlate with TE events. The findings of Italian AT500 Registry are not new; however, this study and an observational study by Botto and colleagues[24] suggest that the risk of AF stroke may not be based merely on the presence of AF and the $CHADS_2$ score, but rather there is a spectrum of risk based on AF duration and $CHADS_2$ score. Botto and colleagues enrolled 568 patients who required a pacemaker and who had a history of AF. During a follow-up of 1 year, stroke events were categorized by a combination of $CHADS_2$ score (4 categories: 0, 1, 2, ≥3) and AF duration

(3 categories: "AF Free" for AF duration <5 minutes on 1 day, "AF-5 minutes" if the duration was 5 minutes to 24 hours on 1 day, and "AF-24 hours" if the duration was >24 hours on 1 day). The study found that there was a progressive increased risk of stroke with increasing $CHADS_2$ score or increasing AF duration or combination of $CHADS_2$ score + AF duration (**Fig. 4**). For example, a high-risk group consisted of $CHADS_2$ score ≥3 + AF-free and $CHADS_2$ score of 1 + AF-24 hours.

There is one other important concept regarding device detection of NDAF and clinical TE stroke. There seems to be a time delay between the first detection of AHRE and clinical stroke. In the ASSERT study, this delay was about 7 months (see **Fig. 2**), and for the MOST study, it was about 10 months (**Fig. 5**). This window of time suggests that if anticoagulation therapy is initiated with detection of AHREs, TE events may be reduced; however, this strategy has not been investigated.

The clinical management of device-detected NDAF has not been defined. With regard to initiation of anticoagulation, of course, the decision to start anticoagulants for asymptomatic AF is based on an assessment of risk for bleeding versus risk for TE. In general, one approach is to initiate anticoagulation therapy for patients with $CHADS_2$ score ≥1 with AF duration of at least 5.5 hours, as demonstrated in the TRENDS study. For patients with low AF burden and $CHADS_2$ score = 0, aspirin seems reasonable.

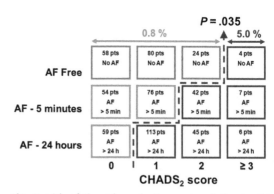

Fig. 4. Risk of thromboembolic events relative to AF duration and $CHADS_2$ score. For those patients with AF duration and/or $CHADS_2$ score that placed them in the red-colored zone (5.0%), the risk of TE/stroke was significantly greater compared with the green-colored zone (0.8%, $P = .035$). (*From* Botto GL, Padeletti L, Santini M, et al. Presence and duration of atrial fibrillation detected by continuous monitoring: crucial implications for the risk of thromboembolic events. J Cardiovasc Electrophysiol 2009;20(3):241–8; with permission.)

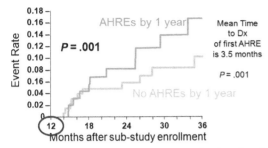

Fig. 5. Kaplan-Meier plot of death or nonfatal stroke after 1 year of ancillary study follow-up in the MOST substudy. There is a time delay from mean diagnosis of AHRE (3.5 months) to first event (≈ 15 months). (*Adapted from* Glotzer TV, Hellkamp AS, Zimmerman J, et al. Atrial high rate episodes detected by pacemaker diagnostics predict death and stroke: report of the atrial diagnostics ancillary study of the Mode Selection Trial (MOST). Circulation 2003;107:1614–9; with permission.)

In summary, these studies elucidate important and new concepts regarding NDAF and AF burden as detected by CIED:

1. Currently, guidelines for initiation of anticoagulation do not differ relative to AF frequency, duration, or symptoms (or absence of symptoms)
2. Asymptomatic AHRE is associated with future clinical episodes of AF
3. Asymptomatic AHRE greater than 5 minutes seem to be associated with increased risk for stroke
   a. MOST study, 5-minute threshold: 2.8× risk for death/nonfatal stroke
   b. ASSERT study, 6-minute threshold: 2.5× risk for stroke
4. Device-measured AF burden is associated with increased risk for stroke
   a. ASSERT study, AF duration of greater than 17-hour duration associated with ≈5× risk
   b. TRENDS study, 5.5-hour threshold associated with 2.2× risk for stroke
   c. Cappucci and colleagues, greater than 1 day AF associated with 3.1× risk (but no increased risk with AF of >5 minutes and <1 day)
   d. Botto and colleagues: AF 5 minutes to 24 hours + CHADS$_2$ ≥2; *or* AF >24 hours + CHADS$_2$ = 1 are associated with increased stroke risk
5. An assessment of AF duration *and* CHADS$_2$ score may improve risk stratification for TE events.

DEVICE DETECTION OF ASYMPTOMATIC AF IN PATIENTS WITH PRIOR STROKE

The TRENDS study completed a retrospective analysis of patients with a prior TE event and who then subsequently underwent implantation of a CIED for a class I or II clinical indication.[18] The purpose of this subgroup analysis was to quantify the incidence of NDAF (>5 minutes) through the use of continuous monitoring by CIEDs in patients without a history of AF, but who had experienced a prior TE event. After excluding patients with a history of warfarin use, or antiarrhythmic drug use (because this may indicate therapy for AF), NDAF was identified via the device in 45 of 116 patients (28%) over a mean follow-up of 1.1 years. The median time from implantation of the CIED until first detection of AF was 1.7 months. This retrospective study was the first to assess the use of stored electrograms from CIED interrogation data to confirm a new diagnosis of AF in patients with stroke.

IS DEVICE-DETECTED AF THE CAUSE OF STROKE?

The information from continuous monitoring provided by CIEDs has led to important observations that challenge the understanding of the mechanism of stroke in patients with AF.

Although AHREs detected by CIEDs are associated with increased risk of TE compared with patients without AHREs, this risk does not seem to be as high as that associated with clinical episodes of AF (**Fig. 6**). For all CHADS$_2$ score, the annual risk of stroke is higher with clinical AF compared with device-detected AF, which implies that in patients with device-detected AF the mechanism of stroke may be attributable to factors other than the AF.

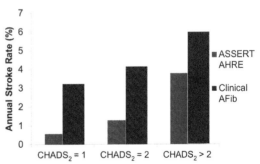

Fig. 6. Annual risk of stroke and TE based on CHADS$_2$ score for asymptomatic atrial tachyarrhythmias detected in ASSERT study (*red bars*) versus clinical AF (*blue bars*). AFib, atrial fibrillation. (*Data from* Healey JS, Connolly SJ, Gold MR, et al. Subclinical atrial fibrillation and the risk of stroke. N Engl J Med 2012;366:120–9; and Gage BF, Waterman AD, Shannon W. Validation of clinical classification schemes for predicting stroke: results from the National Registry of Atrial Fibrillation. JAMA 2001;285:2864–70.)

A second observation was reported by Daoud and colleagues,[25] who evaluated the temporal relationship between AHRE and TE event in the TRENDS study. This retrospective analysis found that most TE did *not* seem to be temporally related to episodes of AF. Of the 40 patients with TE events in the TRENDS study, 20 patients did not have any detection of AF before the stroke, and of the other 20 patients who had AF detected before the stroke, 9 patients (45%) did not have any AF 30 days before the stroke. Therefore, 29 of 40 (73%) patients had zero AF 30 days before their clinical stroke. These data imply that, in most of the study population, a proximate temporal relationship does not exist between device-detected AF episodes and TE. In the 9 patients with AF occurring more than 30 days before the TE event, the mechanism of stroke may be more related to the presence of vascular disease risk factors, which are reflected by the $CHADS_2$ and CHA_2DS_2-VASc risk assessment tools, rather than to episodes of AF.

SUMMARY

Current stroke risk assessment tools for patients with AF and current guideline recommendations for anticoagulation do not consider device-detected asymptomatic AF nor device-measured AF burden. However, the studies presented in this review provide compelling evidence that device-detected AF (the occurrence of AHRE >5 minutes in duration) and AF burden are associated with an increased risk for TE, and, that this data, even though it is detected in asymptomatic patients during a routine device interrogation, should prompt the consideration of initiating anticoagulation therapy. Our approach to managing device-detected AF/AHRE is summarized in **Box 1**. Whether this therapy will have a net benefit in reducing TE events remains to be determined.

REFERENCES

1. Fang MC, Singer DE. Anticoagulation for atrial fibrillation. Cardiol Clin 2004;22:47–62.
2. Wolf PA, Abbott RD, Kannel WB. Atrial fibrillation: a major contributor to stroke in the elderly. The Framingham Study. Arch Intern Med 1987;147:1561–4.
3. Wolf PA, Abbott RD, Kannel WB. Atrial fibrillation as an independent risk factor for stroke: the Framingham Study. Stroke 1991;22:983–8.
4. Camm AJ, Obel OA. Epidemiology and mechanism of atrial fibrillation and atrial flutter. Am J Cardiol 1996;78:3–11.
5. Petersen P, Boysen G, Godtfredsen J, et al. Placebo-controlled, randomized trial of warfarin and aspirin for prevention of thromboembolic complications in chronic atrial fibrillation: The Copenhagen AFASAK Study. Lancet 1989;1:175–8.
6. The Boston Area Anticoagulation Trial for Atrial Fibrillation Investigators. The effect of low-dose warfarin on the risk of stroke in patients with nonrheumatic atrial fibrillation. N Engl J Med 1990;323:1505–11.
7. Stroke Prevention in Atrial Fibrillation Investigators. Stroke Prevention in Atrial Fibrillation study: final results. Circulation 1991;84:527–39.
8. Connolly S, Laupacis A, Gent M, et al. Canadian atrial fibrillation anticoagulation (CAFA) study. J Am Coll Cardiol 1991;18:349–55.
9. Ezekowitz M, Bridgers S, James K, et al. Warfarin in the prevention of stroke associated with

nonrheumatic atrial fibrillation. N Engl J Med 1992; 327:1406–12.

10. Fang MC. Antithrombotic therapy for the treatment of atrial fibrillation in the elderly. J Interv Card Electrophysiol 2009;25:19–23.

11. Ciaroni S, Bloch A. Mid-term clinical and prognostic evaluation of idiopathic atrial fibrillation. Arch Mal Coeur Vaiss 1993;86:1025–30.

12. Glotzer TV, Hellkamp AS, Zimmerman J, et al. Atrial high rate episodes detected by pacemaker diagnostics predict death and stroke: report of the atrial diagnostics ancillary study of the MOde Selection Trial (MOST). Circulation 2003;107:1614–9.

13. Cheung JW, Keating RJ, Stein KM, et al. Newly detected atrial fibrillation following dual chamber pacemaker implantation. J Cardiovasc Electrophysiol 2006;12:1323–8.

14. Orlov MV, Ghali JK, Araghi-Niknam M, et al, Atrial High Rate Trial Investigators. Asymptomatic atrial fibrillation in pacemaker recipients: incidence, progression, and determinants based on the atrial high rate trial. Pacing Clin Electrophysiol 2007;30:404–11.

15. Bunch TJ, Day JD, Olshansky B, et al, INTRINSIC RV Study Investigators. Newly detected atrial fibrillation in patients with an implantable cardioverter-defibrillator is a strong risk marker of increased mortality. Heart Rhythm 2009;6:2–8.

16. Borleffs CJW, Ypenburg C, van Bommel RJ, et al. Clinical importance of new-onset atrial fibrillation after cardiac resynchronization therapy. Heart Rhythm 2009;6:305–10.

17. Caldwell JC, Contractor H, Petkar S, et al. Atrial fibrillation is under-recognized in chronic heart failure: insights from a heart failure cohort treated with cardiac resynchronization therapy. Europace 2009; 11:1295–300.

18. Ziegler PD, Glotzer TV, Daoud EG, et al. Incidence of newly detected atrial arrhythmias via implantable devices in patients with a history of thromboembolic events. Stroke 2010;41:256–60.

19. Shanmugam N, Boerdlein A, Proff J, et al. Detection of atrial high-rate events by continuous home monitoring: clinical significance in the heart failure-cardiac resynchronization therapy population. Europace 2012;14:230–7.

20. Healey JS, Connolly SJ, Gold MR, et al, for the ASSERT Investigators. Subclinical atrial fibrillation and the risk of stroke. N Engl J Med 2012;366: 120–9.

21. Quirino G, Giammaria M, Corbucci G, et al. Diagnosis of paroxysmal atrial fibrillation in patients with implanted pacemakers: relationship to symptoms and other variables. Pacing Clin Electrophysiol 2009;32:91–8.

22. Glotzer TV, Daoud EG, Wyse G, et al. The relationship between daily atrial tachyarrhythmia burden from implantable device diagnostics and stroke risk: The TRENDS Study. Circ Arrhythm Electrophysiol 2009;2:474–80.

23. Capucci A, Santini M, Padeletti L, et al, on behalf of the Italian AT500 Registry Investigators. Monitored atrial fibrillation duration predicts arterial embolic events in patients suffering from bradycardia and atrial fibrillation implanted with antitachycardia pacemakers. J Am Coll Cardiol 2005;46:1913–20.

24. Botto GL, Padeletti L, Santini M, et al. Presence and duration of atrial fibrillation detected by continuous monitoring: crucial implications for the risk of thromboembolic events. J Cardiovasc Electrophysiol 2009;20(3):241–8.

25. Daoud EG, Glotzer TV, Wyse DG, et al, for the TRENDS Investigators. Temporal relationship of atrial tachyarrhythmias, cerebrovascular events, and systemic emboli based on stored device data: a subgroup analysis of TRENDS. Heart Rhythm 2011;8:1416–23.

Left Atrial Appendage Closure for Stroke Prevention
Emerging Technologies

Faisal F. Syed, MBChB, MRCP, Paul A. Friedman, MD, FHRS*

KEYWORDS

- Atrial fibrillation • Left atrial appendage closure • Stroke • Cardioembolic risk

KEY POINTS

- Left atrial appendage closure is a recognized strategy for reducing risk of stroke in atrial fibrillation without utilizing anticoagulation.
- In addition to surgical closure, a number of novel percutaneous approaches have been developed in recent years, each with distinct advantages and limitations.
- The availability of multiple approaches will allow the physician to select the optimal approach for a given patient based on physiologic, anatomic, and clinical considerations.

INTRODUCTION

Atrial fibrillation (AF) affects approximately 2.2 million people in America.[1] The most feared complication of AF is stroke. One in every 6 strokes occurs in patients with AF, with the frequency increasing with age such that 1 of every 3 patients aged 80 to 89 years with stroke has AF.[1] Most strokes in persons with AF are associated with left atrial thrombi, found in 15% to 20% of patients with nonvalvular AF, of which 80% to 90% are located in the left atrial appendage (LAA).[2,3]

To date, antiarrhythmic therapy has not been associated with a reduction in stroke risk, and until recently options were limited to vitamin K antagonism with warfarin. Warfarin reduces the risk of stroke by 60% to 70% compared with no antithrombotic therapy and 30% to 40% compared with aspirin.[1] However, the major limitation of warfarin is its narrow therapeutic window, with both supratherapeutic (15%–30%) and subtherapeutic (up to 45%) international normalized ratios

being common, which are associated with increased bleeding and thromboembolic complications, respectively.[4,5] Other limitations of chronic warfarin therapy include multiple interactions with diet and medications, and management challenges surrounding invasive procedures and the use of adjunctive antiplatelet therapies. The oral direct thrombin inhibitors dabigatran and ximelagatran, and the direct factor Xa inhibitor rivaroxaban, have been demonstrated to be equivalent therapeutically to warfarin and offer a more predictable response,[6–8] while apixiban has been demonstrated to reduce mortality, stroke risk, and bleeding in comparison with warfarin.[9] However, long-term outcome data are lacking and the cost of these agents can be prohibitive. Moreover, these drugs do not eliminate bleeding risk and, like warfarin, subject an increasingly aged patient group to systemic anticoagulation, with significant bleeding complications leading to contraindications for anticoagulation in approximately 40% of subjects at risk.[10,11]

The authors have nothing to disclose.
Division of Cardiovascular Diseases, College of Medicine, Mayo Clinic, 200 1st Street Southwest, Rochester, MN 55905, USA
* Corresponding author.
E-mail address: friedman.paul@mayo.edu

Card Electrophysiol Clin 6 (2014) 141–160
http://dx.doi.org/10.1016/j.ccep.2013.12.002
1877-9182/14/$ – see front matter © 2014 Elsevier Inc. All rights reserved.

These limitations in antithrombotic therapies have led to the development of various ways of obliterating the LAA as a strategy to reduce both stroke risk and the need for anticoagulation. This review summarizes published studies on surgical and transcutaneous approaches to LAA closure, with a focus on emerging technologies. In doing so, the impact of our current understanding of mechanisms of stroke in AF, structure and function of the LAA, and intrinsic variation in procedural techniques on the relative success and limitations of each approach are discussed.

RISK OF STROKE IN AF

Because of its anatomic complexity and sluggish blood flow during atrial arrhythmias, the LAA is presumed to be the source of thromboembolism in most cases of AF. In nonvalvular AF, thrombi are localized within the LAA on 80% to 90% of occasions.[3] By comparison, localization outside the LAA occurs in 56% of cases with valvular AF.[3] In nonvalvular AF, the best validated methods of identifying patients at risk of stroke are based largely on clinical risk factors such as the CHADS2 score, which attributes risk based on the presence of Congestive heart failure, history of Hypertension, Age greater than 75 years, Diabetes mellitus, and prior Stroke or transient ischemic attack.[12,13] Each factor adds 1 point to the risk score, except for stroke or transient ischemic attack (TIA), which

adds 2 points. The CHA2DS2-VASc score[14] also incorporates vascular disease (defined as prior myocardial infarction, peripheral artery disease, or aortic plaque), age 65 to 74 years, and female gender as additional risk factors to the CHADS2 score, and may have improved performance in identifying further subsets at increased risk for thromboembolism.[15] Increasing CHADS2 score has been shown to be associated with increasing likelihood of having LAA thrombus or sludge (ie, dense spontaneous echo contrast present throughout the cardiac cycle) on transesophageal echocardiography (TEE),[16] which is thought to reflect a prethrombotic state from sluggish LAA flow and is a known risk factor for stroke.[17–19] Structural changes in the LAA, with endothelial damage, inflammation and fibrosis, left atrial dilatation, blood stasis, and abnormal prothrombotic changes in platelet function and the coagulation system, have all been described in AF and have been suggested to provide the link between AF burden,[19,20] clinical risk factors for stroke, and the presence of atrial thrombus in this population.[21,22]

Of importance, the risk factors for stroke in AF are also risk factors for atherosclerosis. Patients with AF may have LAA-dependent (LAA thromboembolism)[2,23] and LAA-independent (aortic arch, carotid, and intracerebral artery disease) stroke mechanisms (Fig. 1).[24] Given that warfarin does not significantly affect atheroembolic or arterial

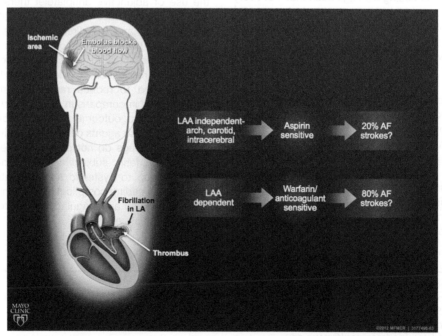

Fig. 1. Left atrial appendage (LAA)-dependent and LAA-independent stroke in atrial fibrillation (AF). (*Reprinted from* the Mayo Foundation; with permission.)

occlusive disease yet dramatically reduces stroke in AF, it is reasonable to expect that an LAA-occlusion strategy will prevent most warfarin-sensitive strokes in AF.[25,26] Based on this premise, a recently completed prospective, randomized trial (see later discussion) found noninferiority of LAA exclusion compared with warfarin therapy,[5] providing proof of concept that in patients with nonvalvular AF in whom warfarin reduces stroke risk, the LAA is the most likely source of thrombus. Finally, further evidence of the role of intra-atrial thrombus in the etiology of stroke comes from a randomized trial reporting similar event rates after electrical cardioversion when TEE was used to exclude thrombus in a comparison with conventional anticoagulation.[27]

LAA STRUCTURE AND FUNCTION

The LAA has traditionally not been attributed any significant role in cardiac function, although it is now recognized as the major source of production of atrial natriuretic peptide and may also contribute to atrial reservoir and booster functions.[28] The LAA is structurally complex, and varies anatomically in size and shape among individuals (**Fig. 2**).[29–32] It arises from the free wall of the left atrium and extends superiorly, lying freely in the pericardial sac.[33] It bears a close anatomic relationship to important adjacent structures. The left phrenic nerve runs along the overlying pericardium.[33] The LAA ostium is situated anterolateral to the left aortic sinus and main coronary artery, and

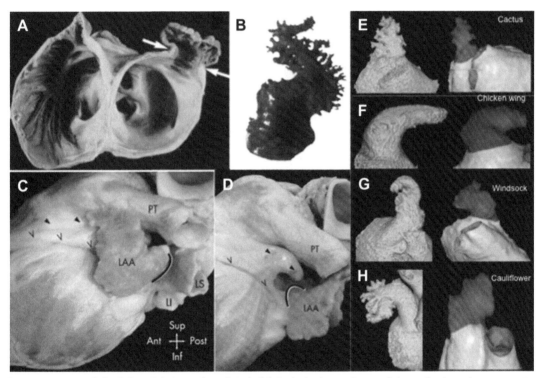

Fig. 2. Anatomy of the left atrial appendage (LAA). (*A*) Pathologic specimen of the atria viewed anteroposteriorly. This appendage has 2 lobes. Arrows identify the ostium. Note the pectinate muscles in the appendage body. (*B*) Synthetic resin cast of the LAA demonstrating the complex microanatomy with multiple recesses. (*C*, *D*) Anatomic relations of the LAA, viewed from the left. The arc identifies the site of the ostium. Arrows track the course of the left anterior descending artery, and the letters V track the great cardiac vein. LI, left inferior pulmonary vein; LS, left superior pulmonary vein; PT, pulmonary trunk. In *D*, the appendage is deflected up to reveal its undersurface. (*E–H*) Variation in LAA shape and size, with 3-dimensional computed tomography (*left*) and magnetic resonance imaging (*right*) reconstructions. The seemingly less complex configuration, chicken wing (*F*), is associated with less atrial fibrillation than the other morphologies (see text for discussion). (*From* [*A*] Agmon Y, Khandheria BK, Gentile F, et al. Echocardiographic assessment of the left atrial appendage. J Am Coll Cardiol 1999;34(7):1867–77, with permission; [*B*] Ernst G, Stollberger C, Abzieher F, et al. Morphology of the left atrial appendage. Anat Rec 1995;242(4):553–61, with permission; [*C*, *D*] Su P, McCarthy KP, Ho SY. Occluding the left atrial appendage: anatomical considerations. Heart 2008;94(9):1166–70, with permission; [*E–H*] Di Biase L, Santangeli P, Anselmino M, et al. Does the left atrial appendage morphology correlate with the risk of stroke in patients with atrial fibrillation? Results from a multicenter study. J Am Coll Cardiol 2012;60(6):531–38, with permission.)

is separated from the left superior pulmonary vein by a narrow tissue invagination (wherein lies the ligament of Marshal, which is important in AF arrhythmogenesis[34,35]), while inferior to the ostium lie the great cardiac vein and circumflex artery.[32] The circumflex artery is usually less than 2 mm from the LAA ostium.[36] In a minority of patients, the sinus node artery arising from the circumflex artery runs nearby.[32]

In general, LAA size increases until the end of the second decade of life, and thereafter no significant differences with age and gender is seen, although the ostium is wider in taller individuals.[30] Morphologically the invagination created by the superior pulmonary vein results in a clearly defined superoposterior border endocardially; the other borders are less well defined.[32] The ostium is usually oval, although there is marked individual variation in shape.[37] The rim of the ostium itself is smooth, and the appendage body contains a variable number and size of pectinate muscles.[30] Atrial tissue immediately surrounding the outside of the ostium may be pitted and focally thin.[32]

The appendage body has marked variability in size and shape, including the degree of curvilinearity and, when resin casts are made, the amount of "branches and twigs" formed by outpouchings and lobes.[29,32] The number of lobes also varies, with 20% to 70% of individuals having a single lobe, 16% to 54% having 2, and the remainder having up to 4 lobes.[37,38] Some investigators have described classifications based on computed tomography (CT) imaging characteristics of orientation of the LAA ostium to either the left superior pulmonary vein[36] or structure of the main body (see **Fig. 2**).[37]

An understanding of these concepts is integral to either designing or deploying mechanical therapies directed at the LAA. Eccentrically shaped ostia may be challenging to close with a circular mechanical plug, or multilobed, complex body geometries may be difficult to encompass with an external loop. Moreover, LAA morphology, microstructure, and function may be related to risk of thrombosis and stroke. LAA emptying velocity assessed on Doppler TEE is associated with dense echo contrast and cardioembolic events.[39,40] Recently, LAA morphology was characterized by CT or magnetic resonance imaging (MRI) in 932 patients and was found to be associated with risk of cerebrovascular events, independent of CHADS2 score, age, and AF subtype.[41] The morphologies described, with their associated rate of cerebrovascular events, were cactus (30%, event rate 12.6% [35/278]), chicken wing (48%, event rate 4.4% [20/451]), windsock (19%, event rate 10.6% [19/179]), and cauliflower (3%, event rate 16.7% [4/24]) (see **Fig. 2**). The chicken wing was found to confer significantly less event risk than the others (odds ratio 0.21, $P = .036$), and compared with the chicken wing, the odds ratio for an event was 4.1 for cactus, 4.5 for windsock, and 8.0 for cauliflower morphologies.[41] The role of LAA morphology in clinical risk stratification remains undefined at present.

LAA CLOSURE TO REDUCE CARDIOEMBOLIC RISK

Several clinical and preclinical studies have reported on closure of the LAA for stroke prevention in AF. In general, this can be performed surgically or percutaneously. Percutaneous approaches can be divided into 3 broad categories: transseptally placed endocardial plug devices, percutaneous epicardial procedures, and hybrid approaches that use transseptal and epicardial access.[42] The availability of multiple approaches allows tailoring of the approach for a given patient based on clinical, physiologic, and anatomic considerations. For LAA closure to become an attractive option for patients with nonvalvular AF, it must be safe and effective in elderly patients who have AF, and permit elimination of the risks of bleeding and challenges of compliance with long-term anticoagulant therapy.

SURGICAL APPROACH

Surgical exclusion or excision of the LAA is performed by many centers at the time of cardiac surgery, and has been recommended as routine practice in patients undergoing mitral valve surgery.[43] The various surgical techniques, including endocardial or epicardial exclusion with sutures, staple excision, or surgical amputation and oversewing, are reviewed in detail elsewhere (**Fig. 3**).[44,45] A retrospective study of 205 patients undergoing mitral valve replacement has reported a reduction in embolic events with appendage ligation from 17% to 3%.[46] A larger retrospective study of 2067 patients undergoing either coronary bypass or valve surgery compared the rate of postoperative stroke in a subset of 260 patients with AF, of whom 145 had LAA ligation.[34] Rates of stroke were 0% with ligation compared with 6.1% without ligation ($P = .003$).

There have been 2 randomized clinical trials of surgical LAA ligation, LAAOS (the Left Atrial Appendage Occlusion Study)[47] and LAAOS II.[48] LAAOS randomized 77 patients with AF and risk factors for stroke undergoing coronary bypass grafting (without concomitant valvular surgery) to

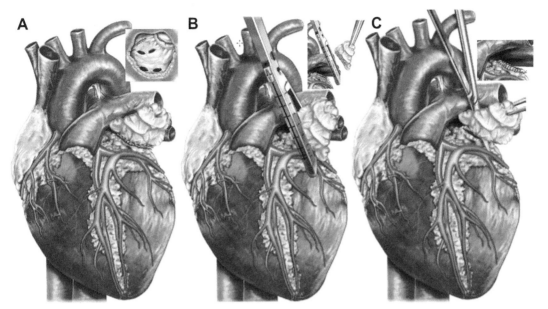

Fig. 3. Techniques for surgical ligation of the left atrial appendage (LAA). (*A*) Suture exclusion, either epicardial (*main panel*) or endocardial (*inset*). (*B*) Stapled excision, with inset demonstrating the removed LAA and intact stump. (*C*) Excision by removal and oversew by scissors (pictured) or electrocautery, with inset demonstrating residual sutured LAA stump. (*From* Chatterjee S, Alexander JC, Pearson PJ, et al. Left atrial appendage occlusion: lessons learned from surgical and transcatheter experiences. Ann Thorac Surg 2011;92(6):2283–92; with permission.)

ligation versus no ligation in a 2:1 fashion.[47] Of note, the surgeon determined feasibility of ligation based on surgical appendage anatomy before randomization. Although the study was underpowered to detect a difference in thromboembolic events (overall 2.6% had an event at 13 ± 7 months), LAA occlusion was reported to be safe. A major finding of the study was the significant rate of incomplete closure and the importance of surgical technique, with an increased rate of successful ligation with staples in comparison with exclusion with sutures (87% vs 43% on TEE; *P* = .14). Similar results were found in a subsequent retrospective study of 137 patients who had TEE following LAA surgical excision or ligation with either sutures or staples.[49] In this study only 40% of closures were successful. It is not clear whether confirmation of closure with TEE was performed at the time of surgery. Failure with sutures usually results from persistent Doppler flow into the appendage, whereas with stapling failure is due to residual appendage tissue beyond the staple line.[20,45,49] In part this may be due to difficulties in identifying the internal ostium of the LAA surgically, or lack of confirmation of closure at the time of surgery.

A study performed at Mayo Clinic, Minnesota, identified 94 patients over a 10-year period who had surgical LAA closure at the time of cardiac

surgery (20% aortic, 68% mitral, and 36% coronary bypass grafting) who also underwent TEE-guided electrical cardioversion for acute postoperative AF.[50] Although none of the patients included in this analysis had an atrial thrombus identified on intraoperative TEE, thrombus was present in 26 of 94 patients (27.7%) at the time of cardioversion, with significantly higher prevalence when the LAA was incompletely closed on TEE (16 of 34 [47%] vs 7 of 60 [12%] with closed LAA, *P* = .002). Patency rates were much higher in suture exclusions than in amputation (51% vs 17%, *P*<.0001), as were total thrombus rates (33% vs 14%, *P* not significant). As a further insight into mechanistic factors, the only 3 patients with thrombus outside the LAA (ie, in the body of the LA) had undergone Maze procedures, and 2 had also undergone mitral valve surgery (Michael Cullen, MD, personal communication, 2013, Mayo Clinic).

The recently published LAAOS II trial randomized 51 patients undergoing coronary bypass surgery or valve surgery without prosthetic valve implantation to LAA occlusion and aspirin (no anticoagulation unless for a non-AF indication) versus no LAA occlusion and oral anticoagulation therapy. This trial was underpowered to detect any significant difference in clinical events between the groups, but was presented as a feasibility study before conducting a larger, adequately powered trial. Of note, the investigators undertook several measures following the results of the first LAAOS study to minimize thrombus formation resulting from incomplete closure or residual stump: (1) simple oversewing or suture ligation was not permitted, and the LAA had to be either amputated and closed or stapled; (2) intraoperative TEE was used to monitor for successful closure with absent Doppler flow across the closure line; and (3) any residual stump had to be smaller than 1 cm. Combined 1-year event rates of death, myocardial infarction, occlusion versus nonocclusion, vascular embolism, or major bleeding was, as expected given the small numbers, not significantly different (occlusion vs nonocclusion: 4 [15.4%] vs 5 [20.0%], P = .61).

Whether novel devices placed at the time of cardiac surgery in lieu of the techniques described here will increase the success of LAA exclusion remains to be conclusively determined. The Atri-Clip device (Atricure, West Chester, OH, USA) is placed epicardially at the base of the appendage under direct vision, leading to successful LAA exclusion in all 36 patients on 3-year follow-up in an initial European study (although of the initial 40 patients, 4 [10%] died in the immediate postoperative setting from causes thought to be unrelated to the use of the AtriClip device)[51] and 67 of 70 patients (96%) in a subsequent United States study,[52] with no procedural complications. Fumoto and colleagues[53] have also reported on preclinical experience with an atrial clip. The Tiger-Paw system (LAAx Inc, Livermore, CA, USA) is a cliplike system with interrupted barbs that puncture and seal the LAA base grasped between the jaws of the delivery forceps. Sixty patients undergoing cardiac surgery were treated, with successful closure in all 54 who had subsequent TEE.[54] The Endoloop suture (Johnson & Johnson, Cincinnati, OH, USA), a circular epicardial ligature, was tested in 12 patients and was associated with failure in 9 patients (75%) on contrast CT evaluation at 3 months.[55] Long-term follow-up data are not currently available for these devices.

The thromboembolic risk associated with incomplete surgical closure of appendage is attested to by studies demonstrating recurrent thrombus formation in up to 50% and thromboembolic clinical events in 8% of patients with incomplete closure.[56] This finding may explain why cumulative experience from 5 clinical trials and 1 randomized controlled trial, with a total of 1400 patients, has failed to show a clinical benefit of surgical appendage occlusion.[57] Moreover, a major limitation in these studies was the only 55% to 66% occlusion rate achieved. In addition, it is

difficult to justify the risks of an open surgical procedure specifically to target the LAA in patients who are not undergoing cardiac surgery for other reasons.

Clinical experience with video-assisted thoracoscopy has been reported.[23] Fifteen patients with AF, risk factors for stroke, and either persistent LAA clot on warfarin or an absolute contraindication to warfarin underwent thoracoscopic LAA closure with either an Endoloop or staple exclusion, with TEE confirmation of successful closure. The procedure was successful in 14 of 15 patients, and the rate of stroke was 4.0% per patient-year.[23] This initial experience has been followed by 2 subsequent reports wherein the LAA was excised[58] or closed with an Endoloop circular suture,[59] and with adjunctive pulmonary vein isolation. A preclinical study with expandable silicone bands in dogs has also been reported.[60]

In summary, surgical LAA closure is currently recommended at the time of mitral valve surgery. Previous studies have reported disappointing success rates for closure, possibly related to inadequate confirmation of closure at the time of surgery, difficulty with assessing closure during bypass when the heart is empty, or limitations of the techniques used in the published reports. Ongoing studies in which the surgeon's attention is focused on closure may resolve the question of surgical closure at the time of concomitant cardiac surgery. The often frail and elderly nature of patients with AF may limit isolated surgical LAA exclusion as a widespread strategy for stroke prevention.

PERCUTANEOUS LAA CLOSURE

Percutaneous LAA closure is less invasive than surgical closure, typically uses concomitant confirmation of closure at the time of procedure, and may be better tolerated in an often frail and elderly population. However, as with surgical strategies, the evidence demonstrating stroke prevention remains limited, and significant complications may occur. Three percutaneous approaches have been developed (**Table 1**): transseptal, epicardial, and hybrid (transseptal with epicardial).

Transseptal Approach

To date, clinical experience with several endovascular transseptal devices has been reported, all of which involve endocardial deployment of a plug into the LAA to exclude it from the central circulation. However, thus far no study has compared one percutaneous device with another in a randomized trial, although there is one small nonrandomized prospective study that compared 2

Table 1
Overview of percutaneous approaches for left atrial appendage (LAA) closure

Device/ Method	Advantages	Limitations
Transseptal device placement	Transseptal technique widely available Available in the setting of previous cardiac surgery Validated as noninferior to warfarin for stroke prevention (WATCHMAN)	Need for procedural and short-term anticoagulation and/or antithrombotic regimen until endothelialization occurs Foreign body left in central circulation (small risk of embolization, erosion, dislodgment) Device must be sized to match LAA Previous atrial-septal defect closure may preclude transseptal delivery
Epicardial	No foreign body left behind No need for procedural anticoagulation because no contact with central circulation and no transseptal puncture (which exposes blood to tissue factor) Adjustable size loop to accommodate variable LAA shape/morphology without need for sizing Pericardial control facilitates management of effusion should one develop	Human experience very limited Previous cardiac surgery limits pericardial access and maneuverability Epicardial access techniques less widely available than transseptal puncture
Hybrid	No foreign body left behind Pericardial control facilitates management of effusion should one develop	Need for transseptal and epicardial access with risks of both, and delivery failure if cannot achieve both Superiorly directed LAA, multiple lobes, and pectus excavatum may preclude use

From Friedman PA, Holmes DR. Non-surgical left atrial appendage closure for stroke prevention in atrial fibrillation. J Cardiovasc Electrophysiol 2011;22(10):1184–91; with permission.

of the devices (see later discussion). Because of the presence of a foreign body in contact with blood, some form of anticoagulation or antiplatelet therapy is administered until endothelialization occurs. Devices developed include the PLAATO (ev3 Endovascular, Inc, Plymouth, MN, USA; subsequently withdrawn from the market),[61–65] WATCHMAN (**Fig. 4**, Atritech, Plymouth, MN, USA),[66–69] AGA or AMPLATZER Cardiac Plug (**Fig. 4**, St Jude Medical, Plymouth, MN, USA; currently not available for use in the United States),[70,71] and Transcatheter Patch (Custom Medical Devices, Athens, Greece).[72] A novel device, the Lifetech (Lifetech Scientific Corp, Shenzhen, China) LAmbre Device, is at the stage of preclinical feasibility study,[73] and incorporates an articulation at the waist between the component that is introduced into LAA and rests over the ostium, which is intended to allow for a degree of self-orientation. The device is designed to be fully retrievable and repositionable. Human trials are reportedly under way (clinical trials.gov/NCT01920412 with a planned completion date of September 2013).

PLAATO

The PLAATO device (ev3 Endovascular) was the first device designed specifically for LAA occlusion. It is no longer available because the manufacturer has discontinued production, despite initially promising clinical results. It consisted of a self-expanding nitinol cage (range of diameter 15–32 mm) covered with a blood-impermeable material, which sealed the LAA. It was delivered into the LAA following femoral vein catheterization and puncture of the interatrial septum with a 12F sheath. Following its deployment, additional pharmacologic thromboembolic prophylaxis was not administered.

In the initial European PLAATO feasibility trial, the device was successfully deployed in 101 of 103 patients.[74] Adverse outcomes included 8 pericardial effusions that required treatment, 3 nonprocedural deaths, 2 strokes, and 2 TIAs, at a mean follow-up of 10 months. In the combined American and European feasibility study, the device was successful in 108 of 111 patients with nonvalvular AF, high risk of stroke, and contraindications to warfarin.[62] Adverse events included 4 deaths, 2 strokes, 1 emergency cardiac surgery,

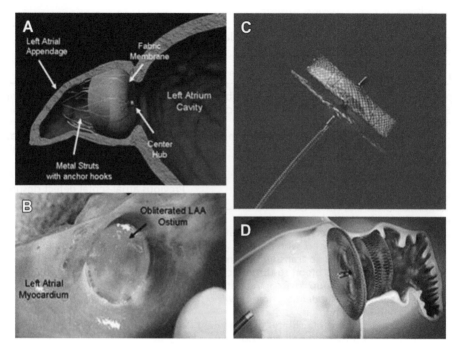

Fig. 4. Transseptal left atrial appendage (LAA) closure devices. (*A*) The WATCHMAN device deployed in the LAA. (*B*) Canine model following chronic WATCHMAN placement with endothelialization. Following endothelialization, the polyester membrane no longer makes contact with the central circulation, and anticoagulation is not needed. (*C*) The AGA or AMPLATZER cardiac plug on its delivery shaft. The distal lobe is designed to provide retention and stability, and the proximal disk LAA occlusion. (*D*) The cardiac plug deployed in the LAA. ([*A, B*] Copyright © Boston Scientific Corporation or its affiliates. All rights reserved. Used with permission of Boston Scientific Corporation; [*C, D*] *Courtesy of* St Jude Medical, Plymouth, MN; with permission.)

3 pericardiocenteses for hemopericardium,1 hemothorax, 1 brachial plexus palsy, and 1 deep venous thrombosis The annual stroke rate was 2.2%, comparing favorably with the CHADS2 predicted stroke rate of 6.3%. In a 5-year follow-up report of 64 patients in the North American subgroup, the annual rate of stroke or TIA was 3.8%, compared with a predicted rate of 6.6% based on CHADS2 score.[61] In the European PLAATO Study of 180 patients the stroke rate was 2.3% per year compared with 6.6% predicted by the CHADS2 score, and 12 patients had major adverse events of which 8 were procedure related.[75]

WATCHMAN

The WATCHMAN device (Atritech) is made of a self-expanding nitinol frame with fixation barbs and a permeable polyester fabric cover, and is available in sizes between 21 and 33 mm in diameter (see **Fig. 4**). It is delivered through a 12F sheath (outer diameter 14F) following transseptal puncture under TEE guidance after a pigtail catheter is maneuvered into the LAA to perform an LAA angiogram. Proper positioning and stability

of the device are verified by TEE and angiography before device release.[5,68]

The WATCHMAN device has been tested in the only randomized prospective, controlled trial of percutaneous LAA closure, the PROTECT-AF study.[5] This noninferiority study compared device appendage closure with warfarin in patients with nonvalvular AF, increased risk of stroke, and no contraindication to anticoagulation. The composite end point of stroke, cardiovascular death, and systemic embolism was not significantly different in the 463 patients randomized to WATCHMAN, with subsequent discontinuation of warfarin, in comparison with the 244 patients randomized to continued warfarinization alone (3.0 vs 4.9 per 100 patient-years, relative risk 0.62, 95% confidence interval [CI] 0.35–1.25, probability of noninferiority in excess of 99.9%). With the WATCHMAN device, 86% of patients were able to stop warfarin therapy at 45 days and 93% were off warfarin at 12 months while aspirin was continued for life. The principal criterion used for determining feasibility of withdrawal of warfarin was less than 5 mm of peridevice flow on TEE.[5,68]

Placement of a device in the LAA shifted the stroke mechanisms. Thrombus was identified on the device in 3.7% of patients, including one in whom it was detected 6 days after an ischemic stroke. During the trial, ischemic stroke was more common in the device group (3.0% vs 2.0% for control), and tended to occur early. Approximately 5% of patients developed a periprocedural pericardial effusion, and although this did not affect the clinical end points it did increase hospital stay.[76] However, the hemorrhagic risk was significantly lower in the device group (relative risk 0.009, 95% CI 0.00–0.45), and during follow-up the benefit of device therapy accumulated over time owing to the progressive cumulative risk of hemorrhagic stroke and bleeding on warfarin therapy. Patients randomized to device therapy more often reported an improvement in quality of life from baseline to 12 months compared with those randomized to warfarin (34.9% vs 24.7%, P = .01).[77] Data from the 2.3-year follow-up of the PROTECT-AF trial report sustained benefit from LAA closure and, in those who were able to discontinue warfarin, fewer primary end points and less functional impact of

events compared with those randomized to warfarin.[78] Preliminary data after a mean 3.8-year follow-up are reported to demonstrate a reduction in the trial's primary end point of stroke, cardiovascular death, and systemic embolism with the WATCHMAN group in comparison with the warfarin group (2.3 vs 3.8 events per 100 patient-years; hazard ratio 0.61, 95% CI 0.38–0.97, P = .03).[76] A microsimulation modeling study has predicted that compared with warfarin and dabigatran, WATCHMAN has increased cost-effectiveness.[79]

Major procedural complications were reported in 12% of patients and included pericardial effusion requiring drainage, embolic stroke, device migration (**Fig. 5**), and device sepsis. Incomplete endothelialization at 10 months in a patient requiring device explantation attributable to thromboembolism is also described.[80] With increased procedural experience and device redesign, the complication rate has significantly fallen by more than 50%, with periprocedural stroke falling from 0.9% to 0% in a subsequent

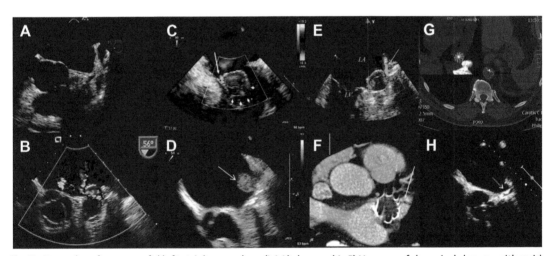

Fig. 5. Examples of unsuccessful left atrial appendage (LAA) closure. (*A, B*) Unsuccessful surgical closure, with residual stump (*A*) and persistent flow into the appendage (*B*). (*C*) Peridevice leak (*arrow*) in a patient with a WATCHMAN device. (*D*) Thrombus on a deployed WATCHMAN device (*arrow*). (*E, F*) Peridevice leak with a deployed PLAATO device. Yellow arrows point to leak identified by color flow Doppler imaging (*E*) and computed tomography (CT) contrast (*F*). (*G*) Embolization of WATCHMAN device (*arrows*) to descending aorta demonstrated on CT. (*H*) Unsuccessful surgical closure with residual LAA stump containing thrombus (*arrow*). (*From* [*A, B*] Kanderian AS, Gillinov AM, Pettersson GB, et al. Success of surgical left atrial appendage closure: assessment by transesophageal echocardiography. J Am Coll Cardiol 2008;52(11):924–9, with permission; [*C*] Viles-Gonzalez JF, Kar S, Douglas P, et al. The clinical impact of incomplete left atrial appendage closure with the Watchman Device in patients with atrial fibrillation: a PROTECT AF (Percutaneous Closure of the Left Atrial Appendage Versus Warfarin Therapy for Prevention of Stroke in Patients with Atrial Fibrillation) substudy. J Am Coll Cardiol 2012;59(10):923–9, with permission; [*E, F*] Viles-Gonzalez JF, Reddy VY, Petru J, et al. Incomplete occlusion of the left atrial appendage with the percutaneous left atrial appendage transcatheter occlusion device is not associated with increased risk of stroke. J Interv Card Electrophysiol 2012;33(1):69–75, with permission; and *Courtesy of* [*D*] Dr David Luria, MD, Leviev Heart Center, Tel Hashomer, Israel; [*G*] Drs Béla Merkely, MD, PhD, and László Gellér, MD, PhD, Heart Centre, Semmelweis University, Budapest, Hungary; [*H*] Dr William Novak, MD, Heart Care Midwest, Bloomington, IL.)

report of 542 patients in the PROTECT-AF and 460 patients in the Continued Access Protocol (CAP) registry ($P = .04$).[68]

One limitation of the WATCHMAN study is its recruitment of a large proportion of patients with CHADS2 score of 1 and paroxysmal AF. Whether a similar success can be achieved in a higher-risk population (CHADS2 score ≥ 2) is being tested by the PREVAIL study, the results of which are awaited (ClinicalTrials.gov identifier NCT00129545). The ASA-Plavix (ASAP) feasibility study prospectively evaluated WATCHMAN in 150 AF patients with CHADS-2 score of 1 or greater and a contraindication for oral anticoagulation in a nonrandomized single-group allocation design.[81] Following device implantation, patients were administered clopidogrel or ticlopidine for 6 months, and lifelong aspirin. At 14.4 ± 8.6 months follow-up there was a rate of ischemic stroke of 1.7% per year, which is approximately 70% to 80% lower than expected in patients with similar CHADS2 score.[81] A similar study in Europe evaluated 59 consecutive patients with AF and anticoagulation contraindication, using a strategy to oversize the device by 15% to 30% in comparison with the LAA diameter[82]; this was aimed at minimizing device repositioning, leakage, and embolization. A 3% rate of pericardial effusion and 5% rate of thrombi at the device occurred during the first 45 days of dual-antiplatelet therapy. There were no cases of late reopening or residual leaks greater than 5 mm around the device. In the patients with device thrombi, there was 1 minor thromboembolic event during 6-month follow-up, and all patients were able to stop dual-antiplatelet therapy after 6 months.

Peridevice leak in WATCHMAN and PLAATO

Because of the eccentric, oval shape of the LAA ostium and circular shape of closure plugs, peridevice leaks are common. The clinical significance of discontinuing warfarin in patients with persistent peridevice leaks was analyzed using PROTECT-AF data.[83] In patients with adequate Doppler TEE images available, peridevice leak was noted in 41%, 34%, and 32% at 45 days, 6 months, and 12 months, respectively ($P = .001$ for decrease over time). The majority had moderate flow (1–3 mm flow width, 60%) and major flow (>3 mm, 32%). There was no difference in primary end point of the trial or embolic rates between those with or without periprosthetic flow, with no interaction with increased flow severity or discontinuation of warfarin.

A smaller study of 58 patients undergoing WATCHMAN implantation from a single center reported peridevice leak on Doppler TEE in 28% at the time of implantation, 29% at 45 days, and 35% at 12 months.[66] The study was underpowered to detect a difference in stroke rate (with only 2 patients developing stroke), although it did report that leaks enlarged with time, in contrast to the experience from PROTECT-AF.

Peridevice leakage from PLAATO has also been reported. In the combined European and American study, successful occlusion on TEE Doppler was seen in 98% at implantation, 100% at 1 month, and 98% at 6 months.[62] In the European PLAATO Study, successful occlusion on TEE Doppler was seen in 90% of patients 2 months.[75] In 22 patients from a single center, peridevice leak was detected in 59% using contrast CT, although again this study was underpowered to detect a difference in stroke (experienced by 4 patients).[83] This study, though small, reported increased sensitivity at detecting leaks with contrast CT when compared with TEE in the 13 patients who underwent both studies; in 2 patients with no evidence of leak on CT the finding was confirmed on TEE, while in 11 patients with leak on CT 3 patients had no leak on TEE.

In aggregate, the available data indicate that peridevice leaks are common, affecting up to 30% to 60% of patients, and that when small (<5 mm) they do not adversely affect device effectiveness in stroke prevention. However, the poor quality of the data (which consist of retrospective analysis, and include only subsets of populations) and low event rates limit the strength of this conclusion. Nonetheless, at first sight the results with percutaneous endocardial device LAA closure appear discordant to those with surgical approaches, in which incomplete closure is associated with increased stroke risk, as noted earlier. Of importance, the velocity of the leak, the degree of residual exposed LAA anatomic complexity, and the ability of the leak to accommodate a thrombus may be quite different between patients with a surgical leak and those with a peridevice leak (see **Fig. 5**). The smaller leaks with higher-velocity flow seen around devices may be less thrombogenic than the larger leaks that have been reported following surgical closure. Indeed, a large LAA ostium (before closure) has been associated with risk of stroke.[22] A direct comparison between outcomes in patients with LAA leaks following surgical versus percutaneous device closure has never been performed. Nonetheless, patients with surgical leaks are typically anticoagulated, whereas a small but growing experience supports the use of antiplatelet agents for small peridevice leaks (<5 mm by TEE).

AMPLATZER

The AGA or AMPLATZER Cardiac Plug (St Jude Medical) has been approved for use in Europe for several years, with mounting experience from several centers. In the United States it is now approved for investigative use only, and patients are currently being recruited into the ACP trial, a randomized, open-label, noninferiority study (clinical trials.gov/NCT01118299). The AMPLATZER Cardiac Plug is a nitinol device composed of a lobe designed to prevent migration and a proximal disk that occludes the LAA orifice, with an interconnecting articulating waist to facilitate adequate positioning in variable ostial configurations (see **Fig. 4**D, E). There are 12 stabilizing wires equally spaced circumferentially around the main disk to improve device placement and retention. It is available in 8 sizes from 16 to 30 mm diameter. The size of the chosen device should be at least 2 mm larger than the diameter of the LAA "landing zone." The device is designed to close cardiac structures with a minimum depth of 10 mm and is delivered via transseptal puncture and TEE/fluoroscopic guidance, with deployment into the LAA by stepwise retraction of the covering sheath. It can be recaptured and redeployed. Following device implantation, dual-antiplatelet therapy with aspirin and clopidogrel for 1 month and aspirin monotherapy thereafter is recommended.[84]

There has been increasing clinical experience published to date of the use of this device in patients with contraindications to oral anticoagulant therapies. In a European registry, successful deployment was reported in 132 of 137 patients.[71] Complications were seen in 7% and included 3 ischemic stroke, 3 device embolization, and 5 clinically significant pericardial effusions. One center in Germany, which also contributed to the aforementioned initial report, recently published its 10-year experience with endovascular LAA occlusion.[85] A total of 152 patients had attempted LAA closure; the investigators used nondedicated devices in 32 (patent foramen ovale, atrial septal defect, and ventricular septal defect occluders) and the AMPLATZER cardiac plug in the remaining 120 patients. Procedure-related complications (pericardial effusion, device embolization, and procedure-related stroke) and major bleeds were seen in 8 patients (6.7%) with cardiac plug and in 7 (22%) with nondedicated devices ($P = .0061$), the major difference being due to the difference in device embolization rates (2 [1.6%] vs 5 [12%], $P = .0048$). Thus, in successfully treated patients, the annual incidence of stroke and major bleeding was 0.8% after a mean follow-up of 2.6 years.

Cumulative experience with the AMPLATZER cardiac plug was also reported from 7 centers in Canada on 52 patients with 98.1% acute procedural success, with serious adverse effects of device embolization (1.9%) and pericardial effusion (1.9%).[86] At a mean follow-up of 20 months, the rates of death, stroke, systemic embolism, pericardial effusion, and major bleeding were 5.8%, 1.9%, 0%, 1.9%, and 1.9%, respectively. The presence of mild peridevice leak was observed in 16.2% of patients at the 6-month follow-up as evaluated by TEE. There were no cases of device thrombosis. In an Italian study, successful closure was reported in 34 of 37 cases (92%) and the 1-year stroke rate was 2.9% (1 patient).[87] In a Brazilian series, 85 of 86 patients had successful deployment.[88] There was 1 complication with tamponade and 1 unrelated death. On follow-up, 6 patients had thrombus formation on the device. There were no strokes or device embolization. In a single-center series of 35 consecutive patients from Spain, there were no immediate complications.[89] On follow-up, 5 patients developed device thrombi, there was 1 transient cerebrovascular event, and 3 patients died of noncardiac causes. In a Chinese series, the LAA was successfully occluded in 19 of 20 patients, with 1 catheter-related thrombus formation, 1 coronary artery air embolism, and 1 TEE-attributed esophageal injury.[90] In a single-operator series from Israel, successful deployment was reported in all 100 patients, with 2 serious complications (1 periprocedural tamponade, 1 postprocedural acute pulmonary edema) and no deaths.[91] An unusual complication of pulmonary artery tear causing tamponade during device implantation has also been reported.[92] Several clinical trials with the AMPLATZER device are under way (see later discussion).

A small study consisting of 80 patients prospectively compared the AMPLATZER Cardiac Plug with the WATCHMAN in a 1:1 fashion. There were no significant differences between the group with respect to procedural times, success, or serious adverse events (1 air embolism and 1 delayed tamponade in each group). All patients received antithrombotic therapy for 6 weeks. After repeat TEE, patients were switched to aspirin. No thromboembolic events were observed in either group after a median follow-up of 1 year.

Transcatheter patch

The Transcatheter Patch (Custom Medical Devices)[72] is a frameless bioabsorbable device used for the occlusion of heart defects. Device apposition is accomplished by balloon inflation, and the patch adheres to cardiac tissues over 48 hours via fibrin formation. Efforts are under way to accelerate the adhesion process (with surgical glue) and to permit immediate patch deployment (via catheter-driven detachment). Experience in 17 patients is reported.[72] In 3 patients, the patch did not attach and in 1 it was placed beyond the LAA ostium. Sheath thrombosis was seen in 1 patient. There were no strokes at 1-year follow-up.

Epicardial Approach

Major limitations of the transseptal approach are the mechanical risks of transseptal puncture, the exposure of blood to tissue factor following puncture (with attendant thrombotic risk), and the need for adjunctive anticoagulation both during and following the procedure owing to the presence of a potentially thrombogenic foreign body in the central circulation. In addition, there is potential for any foreign body to dislodge, erode through tissues, or become infected.[42] An epicardial approach to the LAA offers the promise of overcoming these limitations. This approach was first reported with video-assisted thoracoscopy and subsequent left lung collapse with surgical pericardiotomy to access the LAA.[23]

Results of preclinical studies of LAA ligation devices introduced through a subxiphoid percutaneous pericardial approach are available (Aegis Medical, Vancouver, Canada; Epitek, Minneapolis, MN, USA).[93,94] Following pericardial access, an appendage grabber is introduced (**Fig. 6**). Embedded electrodes within the jaws permit electrical navigation onto the appendage via bipolar electrograms that identify the electrical activity of the tissue captured by the jaws. A hollow suture preloaded with a support wire to permit remote suture-loop manipulation and fluoroscopic visualization is advanced to the appendage base and looped around the appendage. The loop can be variably sized to accommodate multiple LAA lobes and shapes. Following loop closure, the wire is removed leaving only suture behind, which is remotely locked with a clip to maintain closure. A firm closure is confirmed by the elimination of LAA electrical activity, which occurs within seconds.[94] A loop may be opened and repositioned

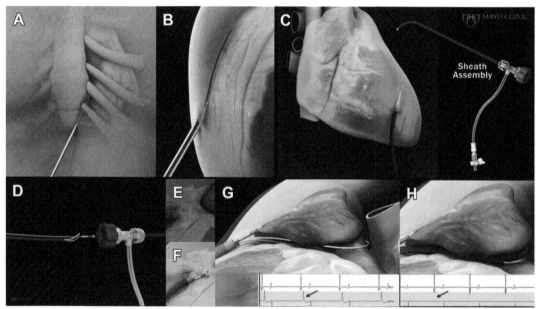

Fig. 6. Epicardial system for percutaneous left atrial appendage (LAA) closure. (*A, B*) Percutaneous puncture to gain access to the pericardial space. (*C*) Placement of sheath in pericardial space using Seldinger technique. (*D*) Introduction of multielectrode LAA grabber with a preloaded looped suture into sheath. (*E, F*) Positioning of grabber toward LAA using electrograms from the electrodes embedded in and immediately proximal to the grabber jaws. (*G*) The grabber is used to identify the appendage and record its electrograms, while the hollow suture loop delivery tool is used to place the loop around the base of the LAA. (*H*) On tightening of the suture, the LAA ostium is closed. The arrows show the LAA electrogram obtained from electrodes embedded in the grabber jaws. Within seconds of closure, the LAA electrical activity is eliminated (note absence of electrogram at *arrow*) and the surface P wave becomes shorter because the LAA no longer contributes to the P wave (not shown). Simultaneous transesophageal echocardiography is used to confirm placement at the LAA ostium and its complete closure. (*Reprinted from* the Mayo Foundation; with permission).

if the initial closure is unsatisfactory, or additional loops may be placed for multilobed LAAs that are not fully closed with the first loop, using the suture tails from the first loop as a rail.

In addition to avoiding vascular entry, the need for systemic anticoagulation, and placement of a foreign body in the central circulation, potential advantages of this technique include having access to the pericardial space in the event of complication, identification of adequate closure via LAA electrogram elimination, and use of a variably sized loop to accommodate LAA anatomic variability. Within seconds of complete LAA closure, electrical activity is eliminated (see **Fig. 6**) and the surface electrocardiogram P wave is shortened. Chronically the LAA involutes and becomes atretic.[93] Whether LAA elimination by this means will affect rhythm control (by eliminating a mass of fibrillating atrial tissue) is not known. A small series has demonstrated feasibility in humans.[95] This approach will likely be limited to patients with prior cardiac surgery or recurrent pericarditis caused by the formation of pericardial adhesions, which would limit intrapericardial navigation.

Hybrid Approach

Human experience with a hybrid strategy whereby percutaneous epicardial LAA ligation is guided by an endocardial magnet-tipped wire placed in the LAA has been reported, using the LAARIAT system (SentreHEART, Inc, Palo Alto, CA, USA).[26,96] The technique involves defining the anatomy of the appendage with a contrast injection, and placing a magnet-tipped wire within the appendage via the transseptal approach (**Fig. 7**). A second magnet-tipped wire is placed epicardially following percutaneous epicardial access, and positioned in continuity with the transseptal endocardial wire, thereby forming a rail over which an epicardial suture loop is advanced and then closed. TEE confirms appendage closure. A prescreening CT scan is performed to assess appendage size and morphology. patients with superiorly oriented appendages (approximately 10% of screened patients) are excluded because such morphology may complicate withdrawal of the delivery tool, and patients with appendages greater than 40 mm in diameter are excluded because they may not fit within the first-

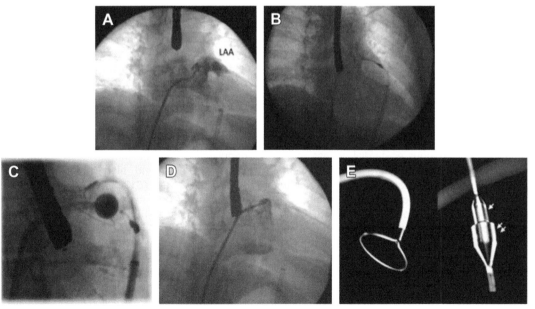

Fig. 7. Hybrid approach to left atrial appendage (LAA) closure using the LAARIAT system (SentreHEART, Inc, Palo Alto, CA). (*A*) Contrast injection identifies the LAA. (*B*) End-to-end connection of the magnet-tipped epicardial (percutaneous pericardial access) and endocardial (transseptal access) wires is used for alignment and stability. (*C*) Inflation of a balloon in LAA orifice is used to guide snare positioning at LAA base. (*D*) Contrast injection following closure. (*E*) *Left*: The LARIAT suture delivery system comprising an adjustable, pretied size-0 Teflon-coated, braided polyester suture and radiopaque closure snare. *Right*: A 0.025-inch endocardial (*single arrow*) and 0.035-inch epicardial (*double arrow*) guide wire, each with a magnet tip of opposite polarity. (*From [A–D]* Friedman PA, Holmes DR. Non-surgical left atrial appendage closure for stroke prevention in atrial fibrillation. J Cardiovasc Electrophysiol 2011;22(10):1184–91, with permission; [*E*] Singh SM, Dukkipati SR, d'Avila A, et al. Percutaneous left atrial appendage closure with an epicardial suture ligation approach: a prospective randomized pre-clinical feasibility study. Heart Rhythm 2010;7(3):370–6, with permission.)

generation loop size. Prescreening TEE is performed to confirm the absence of mobile left atrial thrombus.

In the earliest experience, the device was pretested in 2 patients undergoing mitral valve replacement before testing in 11 patients undergoing AF ablation percutaneously, of whom the initial 2 had a minimally invasive surgical pericardial window of less than 20 mm.[96] Intraprocedural left atrial angiography and TEE were used to assess for effective closure, lack of perforation or diverticulum, and lack of involvement of the left upper pulmonary vein. Ten of the 11 patients (9 with percutaneous epicardial access) had successfully acute appendage ligation confirmed on left atrial angiography and TEE, while 1 patient had a residual 1-mm jet on color Doppler but with normal atriography.[96] Mean procedure time was 85.7 minutes and mean fluoroscopy time 16.2 minutes. Two patients could not complete the procedure, one because of inadequate echocardiographic visualization of the marker balloon within the left atrial ostium and the other because of preexisting pericardial adhesions. Complications were reported in 1 patient with a small hemopericardium after requiring 2 attempts to access the pericardial space, with no clinical consequence. Durability to 60 days was assessed with TEE in 6 patients, of whom 4 had persistent closure and 2 had reopening of up to 2 mm.

Subsequently, a larger series found that 85 of 89 (96%) patients who passed a screening CT underwent successful closure.[97] Three patients had a residual leak of 2 mm or less, and 1 had a leak of less than 3 mm. There were 2 complications related to percutaneous epicardial access and 1 related to transseptal puncture. Adverse events include severe pericarditis postoperatively (n = 2), late pericardial effusion (n = 1), and late strokes thought to be nonembolic (n = 2). There were also 2 unexplained sudden deaths: one in a patient with documented bradycardias who refused pacemaker implant 12 months after LAA closure, and another 3 months after closure, after the patient presented with weakness, no heart failure, and negative initial workup.

More recently, in a report of 27 patients with AF and a high risk of stroke, and unable to take anticoagulation medications, acute procedural success was seen in 25 patients, in 22 of whom TEE confirmed persistent closure at 4 months. Complications included 1 LAA perforation, 3 cases of pericarditis, 1 periprocedural cerebrovascular accident (CVA) from thrombus formation on the transseptal sheath, and 1 late CVA thought to be noncardioembolic.[98] Other isolated cases with

complications reported in the literature include early reopening of the appendage,[99] and de novo thrombus forming on the endocardial surface of the device in a patient with ongoing AF.[100]

Specific advantages of the hybrid approach include the ability to reposition the snare once closed, and a likely lower learning curve provided by the endocardial and epicardial magnet-tipped wires, which form a stable rail over which the loop can be deployed. Limitations include the need for a simultaneous endoluminal approach with transseptal puncture (with the risk of systemic thromboembolism and the need for procedural anticoagulation) and epicardial approach, introducing the risk of both strategies; limited utility in appendages superiorly directed or with multiple lobes; and difficulty of use in patients with pectus excavatum.[26,42] It is estimated that 90% of LAAs have morphologies amenable to closure via this system.

ONGOING CLINICAL TRIALS OF LAA EXCLUSION

Several studies of percutaneous LAA exclusion are at various stages of progress (ClinicalTrials.gov). The AMPLATZER Cardiac Plug Clinical Trial (NCT01118299) is an open-label, noninferiority randomized study comparing 45-day adverse events attributable to the device with optimal medical therapy, and is set to complete by December 2015. The ELIGIBLE study (NCT01628068) is a prospective, multicenter, randomized study of percutaneous LAA closure with the AMPLATZER device and subsequent aspirin and clopidogrel therapy versus standard treatment with oral anticoagulants in patients with a history of gastrointestinal bleeding and high embolic risk. The ISAR-AF study (NCT01363895) is a randomized comparison of percutaneous closure of the LAA with AF catheter ablation. The AMPLATZER Cardiac Plug Clinical Trial (NCT01118299) is a randomized, open-label safety study to evaluate the device in nonvalvular AF compared with warfarin. The EVOLVE study (NCT01196897) is a nonrandomized single-group evaluation of the next-generation WATCHMAN device in nonvalvular AF patients. The fourth-generation WATCHMAN device is available in 22-, 26-, and 31-mm sizes, with an increased number of device spines for improved radial strength, and design changes aimed at improving device stability, permitting multiple recaptures and redeployments.[101] The PLACE III study (NCT01680757) will be a prospective, multicenter registry of patients undergoing LAA ligation with the LARIAT system, which aims to enroll 100 patients.

Several studies have been designed to address questions relating to a surgical approach to LAA exclusion. The Left Atrial Appendage Occlusion Study III (LAAOS III, NCT01561651) aims to randomize 3500 patients with AF undergoing heart surgery to LAA excision versus no excision. The Exclusion of the Left Atrial Appendage (LAA) With the LAAx, Inc. TigerPaw System study (NCT00962702) is a nonrandomized single-group evaluation of safety and efficacy of this LAA closure cliplike device in patients undergoing cardiac surgery. The Evaluation of the Cardioblate Closure Device in Facilitating Occlusion of the Left Atrial Appendage study (NCT00841529) was to test appendage closure via placement of an occlusion band at the time of cardiac surgery, but has been terminated after recruitment of 40 patients. The RESTORE SR II study (NCT00566176) is a nonrandomized, single-group assignment study assessing thoracoscopic epicardial pulmonary vein isolation using the AtriCure Bipolar System (Medtronic, Minneapolis, MN, USA) combined with LAA exclusion.

Two registered studies will examine the effects of LAA occlusion using WATCHMAN on cardiac function including neurohormonal changes, the Effects of Left Atrial Appendage Occlusion study (NCT00510900) and the Atrial and Brain Natriuretic Peptide Secretion After Percutaneous Closure of the Left Atrial Appendage study (NCT01522911).

TOWARD THE FUTURE

Although ongoing studies are poised to answer several important questions related to LAA closure in reduction of stroke risk, several unknown factors remain, the first of which is determining when the appendage is adequately closed; whether the definition should be anatomic, electrical, or functional[26,42]; and whether transesophageal or intracardiac echocardiography, CT, or MRI is the optimal imaging study.[102–108] All closure devices and techniques will leave a small "beak" where tissues are approximated or adjacent to a device; whether such a situation affects stroke prevention is not known. In addition, accessory lobes, pectinate muscles, or other structures may exist proximal to a device or closure; their impact is uncertain. How closure will affect atrial function, subsequent intervention to the atrium, such as catheter ablation, and vice versa are unknown. The optimal antithrombotic strategy is not yet defined, and it is not known whether AF burden and type (valvular vs nonvalvular) affect the closure decision. What has become clear is that LAA closure is emerging as an option for stroke prevention in nonvalvular AF in patients at high

risk of bleeding on anticoagulants. Current European guidelines recommend device closure in patients with high risk of stroke and contraindications for long-term anticoagulation (Class IIb, level of evidence B).[15]

In the future, as new devices are tested and procedural competence, clinical experience, and trial data grow, LAA closure may become an increasingly attractive option for stroke prevention in the often older and frail population at highest risk for stroke from AF, as it eliminates the long-term cumulative bleeding risks and adherence challenges of anticoagulant therapy. For patients with previous cardiac surgery, recurrent pericarditis, or thoracic irradiation, endovascular strategies will be attractive, as pericardial access and manipulation may be somewhat limited. For patients with a strict contraindication to anticoagulation or with a high risk of infection, epicardial/nondevice strategies are appealing, as entry to the central circulation is avoided. Ultimately, the availability of multiple approaches will allow the physician to select the optimal approach for a given patient based on physiologic, anatomic, and clinical considerations.

REFERENCES

1. Fuster V, Ryden LE, Cannom DS, et al. ACC/AHA/ESC 2006 Guidelines for the management of patients with atrial fibrillation: a report of the American College of Cardiology/American Heart Association Task Force on Practice Guidelines and the European Society of Cardiology Committee for Practice Guidelines (Writing Committee to Revise the 2001 Guidelines for the Management of Patients With Atrial Fibrillation): developed in collaboration with the European Heart Rhythm Association and the Heart Rhythm Society. Circulation 2006;114(7):e257–354.
2. Blackshear JL, Odell JA. Appendage obliteration to reduce stroke in cardiac surgical patients with atrial fibrillation. Ann Thorac Surg 1996;61(2):755–9.
3. Mahajan R, Brooks AG, Sullivan T, et al. Importance of the underlying substrate in determining thrombus location in atrial fibrillation: implications for left atrial appendage closure. Heart 2012;98(15):1120–6.
4. Bungard TJ, Ackman ML, Ho G, et al. Adequacy of anticoagulation in patients with atrial fibrillation coming to a hospital. Pharmacotherapy 2000;20(9):1060–5.
5. Holmes DR, Reddy VY, Turi ZG, et al. Percutaneous closure of the left atrial appendage versus warfarin therapy for prevention of stroke in patients with atrial fibrillation: a randomised non-inferiority trial. Lancet 2009;374(9689):534–42.

6. Albers GW, Diener HC, Frison L, et al. Ximelagatran vs warfarin for stroke prevention in patients with nonvalvular atrial fibrillation: a randomized trial. JAMA 2005;293(6):690–8.

7. Connolly SJ, Ezekowitz MD, Yusuf S, et al. Dabigatran versus warfarin in patients with atrial fibrillation. N Engl J Med 2009;361(12):1139–51.

8. Patel MR, Mahaffey KW, Garg J, et al. Rivaroxaban versus warfarin in nonvalvular atrial fibrillation. N Engl J Med 2011;365(10):883–91.

9. Granger CB, Alexander JH, McMurray JJ, et al. Apixaban versus warfarin in patients with atrial fibrillation. N Engl J Med 2011;365(11):981–92.

10. Brass LM, Krumholz HM, Scinto JM, et al. Warfarin use among patients with atrial fibrillation. Stroke 1997;28(12):2382–9.

11. Onalan O, Lashevsky I, Hamad A, et al. Nonpharmacologic stroke prevention in atrial fibrillation. Expert Rev Cardiovasc Ther 2005;3(4):619–33.

12. Gage BF, Waterman AD, Shannon W, et al. Validation of clinical classification schemes for predicting stroke: results from the National Registry of Atrial Fibrillation. JAMA 2001;285(22):2864–70.

13. Rietbrock S, Heeley E, Plumb J, et al. Chronic atrial fibrillation: incidence, prevalence, and prediction of stroke using the Congestive heart failure, Hypertension, Age >75, Diabetes mellitus, and prior Stroke or transient ischemic attack (CHADS2) risk stratification scheme. Am Heart J 2008;156(1):57–64.

14. Lip GY, Nieuwlaat R, Pisters R, et al. Refining clinical risk stratification for predicting stroke and thromboembolism in atrial fibrillation using a novel risk factor-based approach: the euro heart survey on atrial fibrillation. Chest 2010; 137(2):263–72.

15. Camm AJ, Lip GY, De Caterina R, et al. 2012 focused update of the ESC Guidelines for the management of atrial fibrillation: an update of the 2010 ESC Guidelines for the management of atrial fibrillation. Developed with the special contribution of the European Heart Rhythm Association. Eur Heart J 2012;33(21):2719–47.

16. Puwanant S, Varr BC, Shrestha K, et al. Role of the CHADS2 score in the evaluation of thromboembolic risk in patients with atrial fibrillation undergoing transesophageal echocardiography before pulmonary vein isolation. J Am Coll Cardiol 2009; 54(22):2032–9.

17. Jones EF, Calafiore P, McNeil JJ, et al. Atrial fibrillation with left atrial spontaneous contrast detected by transesophageal echocardiography is a potent risk factor for stroke. Am J Cardiol 1996;78(4): 425–9.

18. Bernhardt P, Schmidt H, Hammerstingl C, et al. Patients with atrial fibrillation and dense spontaneous echo contrast at high risk a prospective and serial follow-up over 12 months with transesophageal echocardiography and cerebral magnetic resonance imaging. J Am Coll Cardiol 2005;45(11): 1807–12.

19. Wysokinski WE, Ammash N, Sobande F, et al. Predicting left atrial thrombi in atrial fibrillation. Am Heart J 2010;159(4):665–71.

20. Healey JS, Connolly SJ, Gold MR, et al. Subclinical atrial fibrillation and the risk of stroke. N Engl J Med 2012;366(2):120–9.

21. Watson T, Shantsila E, Lip GY. Mechanisms of thrombogenesis in atrial fibrillation: Virchow's triad revisited. Lancet 2009;373(9658):155–66.

22. Beinart R, Heist EK, Newell JB, et al. Left atrial appendage dimensions predict the risk of stroke/ TIA in patients with atrial fibrillation. J Cardiovasc Electrophysiol 2011;22(1):10–5.

23. Blackshear JL, Johnson WD, Odell JA, et al. Thoracoscopic extracardiac obliteration of the left atrial appendage for stroke risk reduction in atrial fibrillation. J Am Coll Cardiol 2003;42(7): 1249–52.

24. Hart RG, Pearce LA, Miller VT, et al. Cardioembolic vs. noncardioembolic strokes in atrial fibrillation: frequency and effect of antithrombotic agents in the stroke prevention in atrial fibrillation studies. Cerebrovasc Dis 2000;10(1):39–43.

25. Chimowitz MI, Lynn MJ, Howlett-Smith H, et al. Comparison of warfarin and aspirin for symptomatic intracranial arterial stenosis. N Engl J Med 2005;352(13):1305–16.

26. Syed FF, Asirvatham SJ. Left atrial appendage as a target for reducing strokes: justifiable rationale? Safe and effective approaches? Heart Rhythm 2011;8(2):194–8.

27. Klein AL, Grimm RA, Murray RD, et al. Use of transesophageal echocardiography to guide cardioversion in patients with atrial fibrillation. N Engl J Med 2001;344(19):1411–20.

28. Gibson DN, Price MJ, Ahern TS, et al. Left atrial appendage occlusion for the reduction of stroke and embolism in patients with atrial fibrillation. J Cardiovasc Med (Hagerstown) 2012;13(2): 131–7.

29. Ernst G, Stollberger C, Abzieher F, et al. Morphology of the left atrial appendage. Anat Rec 1995;242(4):553–61.

30. Veinot JP, Harrity PJ, Gentile F, et al. Anatomy of the normal left atrial appendage: a quantitative study of age-related changes in 500 autopsy hearts: implications for echocardiographic examination. Circulation 1997;96(9):3112–5.

31. Ramaswamy P, Lytrivi ID, Srivastava S, et al. Left atrial appendage: variations in morphology and position causing pitfalls in pediatric echocardiographic diagnosis. J Am Soc Echocardiogr 2007; 20(8):1011–6.

32. Su P, McCarthy KP, Ho SY. Occluding the left atrial appendage: anatomical considerations. Heart 2008;94(9):1166–70.

33. Lachman N, Syed FF, Habib A, et al. Correlative anatomy for the electrophysiologist, part II: cardiac ganglia, phrenic nerve, coronary venous system. J Cardiovasc Electrophysiol 2011;22(1):104–10.

34. De Simone CV, Noheria A, Lachman N, et al. Myocardium of the superior vena cava, coronary sinus, vein of Marshall, and the pulmonary vein ostia: gross anatomic studies in 620 hearts. J Cardiovasc Electrophysiol 2012;23(12):1304–9.

35. Macedo PG, Kapa S, Mears JA, et al. Correlative anatomy for the electrophysiologist: ablation for atrial fibrillation. Part I: pulmonary vein ostia, superior vena cava, vein of Marshall. J Cardiovasc Electrophysiol 2010;21(6):721–30.

36. Wongcharoen W, Tsao HM, Wu MH, et al. Morphologic characteristics of the left atrial appendage, roof, and septum: implications for the ablation of atrial fibrillation. J Cardiovasc Electrophysiol 2006;17(9):951–6.

37. Wang Y, Di Biase L, Horton RP, et al. Left atrial appendage studied by computed tomography to help planning for appendage closure device placement. J Cardiovasc Electrophysiol 2010; 21(9):973–82.

38. Heist EK, Refaat M, Danik SB, et al. Analysis of the left atrial appendage by magnetic resonance angiography in patients with atrial fibrillation. Heart Rhythm 2006;3(11):1313–8.

39. Goldman ME, Pearce LA, Hart RG, et al. Pathophysiologic correlates of thromboembolism in nonvalvular atrial fibrillation: I. Reduced flow velocity in the left atrial appendage (The Stroke Prevention in Atrial Fibrillation [SPAF-III] study). J Am Soc Echocardiogr 1999;12(12):1080–7.

40. Agmon Y, Khandheria BK, Gentile F, et al. Echocardiographic assessment of the left atrial appendage. J Am Coll Cardiol 1999;34(7): 1867–77.

41. Di Biase L, Santangeli P, Anselmino M, et al. Does the left atrial appendage morphology correlate with the risk of stroke in patients with atrial fibrillation? Results from a multicenter study. J Am Coll Cardiol 2012;60(6):531–8.

42. Friedman PA, Holmes DR. Non-surgical left atrial appendage closure for stroke prevention in atrial fibrillation. J Cardiovasc Electrophysiol 2011; 22(10):1184–91.

43. Bonow RO, Carabello BA, Chatterjee K, et al. ACC/AHA 2006 guidelines for the management of patients with valvular heart disease: a report of the American College of Cardiology/American Heart Association Task Force on Practice Guidelines (writing Committee to Revise the 1998 guidelines for the management of patients with valvular heart disease) developed in collaboration with the Society of Cardiovascular Anesthesiologists endorsed by the Society for Cardiovascular Angiography and Interventions and the Society of Thoracic Surgeons. J Am Coll Cardiol 2006;48(3):e1–148.

44. Gillinov AM, Pettersson G, Cosgrove DM. Stapled excision of the left atrial appendage. J Thorac Cardiovasc Surg 2005;129(3):679–80.

45. Chatterjee S, Alexander JC, Pearson PJ, et al. Left atrial appendage occlusion: lessons learned from surgical and transcatheter experiences. Ann Thorac Surg 2011;92(6):2283–92.

46. Garcia-Fernandez MA, Perez-David E, Quiles J, et al. Role of left atrial appendage obliteration in stroke reduction in patients with mitral valve prosthesis: a transesophageal echocardiographic study. J Am Coll Cardiol 2003;42(7):1253–8.

47. Healey JS, Crystal E, Lamy A, et al. Left Atrial Appendage Occlusion Study (LAAOS): results of a randomized controlled pilot study of left atrial appendage occlusion during coronary bypass surgery in patients at risk for stroke. Am Heart J 2005; 150(2):288–93.

48. Whitlock RP, Vincent J, Blackall MH, et al. Left Atrial Appendage Occlusion Study II (LAAOS II). Can J Cardiol 2013;29(11):1443–7.

49. Kanderian AS, Gillinov AM, Pettersson GB, et al. Success of surgical left atrial appendage closure: assessment by transesophageal echocardiography. J Am Coll Cardiol 2008;52(11):924–9.

50. Cullen MW, Stulak J, Li Z, et al. Value of transesophageal echocardiography to guide cardioversion in patients with atrial fibrillation after cardiac surgery. J Am Coll Cardiol 2013;61(10):E967.

51. Emmert MY, Puippe G, Baumuller S, et al. Safe, effective and durable epicardial left atrial appendage clip occlusion in patients with atrial fibrillation undergoing cardiac surgery: first long-term results from a prospective device trial. Eur J Cardiothorac Surg 2013;45(1):126–31.

52. Ailawadi G, Gerdisch MW, Harvey RL, et al. Exclusion of the left atrial appendage with a novel device: early results of a multicenter trial. J Thorac Cardiovasc Surg 2011;142(5):1002–9, 1009 e1.

53. Fumoto H, Gillinov AM, Ootaki Y, et al. A novel device for left atrial appendage exclusion: the third-generation atrial exclusion device. J Thorac Cardiovasc Surg 2008;136(4):1019–27.

54. Slater AD, Tatooles AJ, Coffey A, et al. Prospective clinical study of a novel left atrial appendage occlusion device. Ann Thorac Surg 2012;93(6):2035–8 [discussion: 2038–40].

55. Adams C, Bainbridge D, Goela A, et al. Assessing the immediate and sustained effectiveness of circular epicardial surgical ligation of the left atrial appendage. J Card Surg 2012;27(2):270–3.

56. Katz ES, Tsiamtsiouris T, Applebaum RM, et al. Surgical left atrial appendage ligation is frequently incomplete: a transesophageal echocardiographic study. J Am Coll Cardiol 2000;36(2):468–71.

57. Dawson AG, Asopa S, Dunning J. Should patients undergoing cardiac surgery with atrial fibrillation have left atrial appendage exclusion? Interact Cardiovasc Thorac Surg 2010;10(2):306–11.

58. Wolf RK, Schneeberger EW, Osterday R, et al. Video-assisted bilateral pulmonary vein isolation and left atrial appendage exclusion for atrial fibrillation. J Thorac Cardiovasc Surg 2005;130(3): 797–802.

59. Yilmaz A, Van Putte BP, Van Boven WJ. Completely thoracoscopic bilateral pulmonary vein isolation and left atrial appendage exclusion for atrial fibrillation. J Thorac Cardiovasc Surg 2008;136(2):521–2.

60. McCarthy PM, Lee R, Foley JL, et al. Occlusion of canine atrial appendage using an expandable silicone band. J Thorac Cardiovasc Surg 2010; 140(4):885–9.

61. Block PC, Burstein S, Casale PN, et al. Percutaneous left atrial appendage occlusion for patients in atrial fibrillation suboptimal for warfarin therapy: 5-year results of the PLAATO (Percutaneous Left Atrial Appendage Transcatheter Occlusion) Study. JACC Cardiovasc Interv 2009;2(7):594–600.

62. Ostermayer SH, Reisman M, Kramer PH, et al. Percutaneous left atrial appendage transcatheter occlusion (PLAATO system) to prevent stroke in high-risk patients with non-rheumatic atrial fibrillation: results from the international multi-center feasibility trials. J Am Coll Cardiol 2005;46(1): 9–14.

63. Park JW, Leithauser B, Gerk U, et al. Percutaneous left atrial appendage transcatheter occlusion (PLAATO) for stroke prevention in atrial fibrillation: 2-year outcomes. J Invasive Cardiol 2009;21(9): 446–50.

64. Ussia GP, Mangiafico S, Privitera A, et al. Percutaneous left atrial appendage transcatheter occlusion in patients with chronic nonvalvular atrial fibrillation: early institutional experience. J Cardiovascular Medicine (Hagerstown) 2006;7(8):569–72.

65. Ussia GP, Mule M, Cammalleri V, et al. Percutaneous closure of left atrial appendage to prevent embolic events in high-risk patients with chronic atrial fibrillation. Catheter Cardiovasc Interv 2009; 74(2):217–22.

66. Bai R, Horton RP, di Biase L, et al. Intraprocedural and long-term incomplete occlusion of the left atrial appendage following placement of the WATCHMAN device: a single center experience. J Cardiovasc Electrophysiol 2012;23(5):455–61.

67. Holmes DR Jr, Fountain R. Stroke prevention in atrial fibrillation: WATCHMAN versus warfarin. Expert Rev Cardiovasc Ther 2009;7(7):727–9.

68. Reddy VY, Holmes D, Doshi SK, et al. Safety of percutaneous left atrial appendage closure: results from the Watchman Left Atrial Appendage System for Embolic Protection in Patients with AF (PROTECT AF) clinical trial and the Continued Access Registry. Circulation 2011; 123(4):417–24.

69. Viles-Gonzalez JF, Kar S, Douglas P, et al. The clinical impact of incomplete left atrial appendage closure with the Watchman Device in patients with atrial fibrillation: a PROTECT AF (Percutaneous Closure of the Left Atrial Appendage Versus Warfarin Therapy for Prevention of Stroke in Patients With Atrial Fibrillation) substudy. J Am Coll Cardiol 2012;59(10):923–9.

70. Meier B, Palacios I, Windecker S, et al. Transcatheter left atrial appendage occlusion with Amplatzer devices to obviate anticoagulation in patients with atrial fibrillation. Catheter Cardiovasc Interv 2003; 60(3):417–22.

71. Park JW, Bethencourt A, Sievert H, et al. Left atrial appendage closure with Amplatzer cardiac plug in atrial fibrillation: initial European experience. Catheter Cardiovasc Interv 2011;77(5):700–6.

72. Toumanides S, Sideris EB, Agricola T, et al. Transcatheter patch occlusion of the left atrial appendage using surgical adhesives in high-risk patients with atrial fibrillation. J Am Coll Cardiol 2011;58(21):2236–40.

73. Lam YY, Yan BP, Doshi SK, et al. Preclinical evaluation of a new left atrial appendage occluder (Lifetech LAmbre Device) in a canine model. Int J Cardiol 2013;168(4):3996–4001.

74. Sousa JE, Costa MA, Tuzcu EM, et al. New frontiers in interventional cardiology. Circulation 2005; 111(5):671–81.

75. Bayard YL, Omran H, Neuzil P, et al. PLAATO (Percutaneous Left Atrial Appendage Transcatheter Occlusion) for prevention of cardioembolic stroke in non-anticoagulation eligible atrial fibrillation patients: results from the European PLAATO study. EuroIntervention 2010;6(2):220–6.

76. Holmes DR Jr, Lakkireddy DR, Whitlock RP, et al. Left atrial appendage occlusion: opportunities and challenges. J Am Coll Cardiol 2013. http://dx.doi.org/10.1016/j.jacc.2013.08.1631. [Epub ahead of print].

77. Alli O, Doshi S, Kar S, et al. Quality of life assessment in the randomized PROTECT AF (Percutaneous Closure of the Left Atrial Appendage Versus Warfarin Therapy for Prevention of Stroke in Patients With Atrial Fibrillation) trial of patients at risk for stroke with nonvalvular atrial fibrillation. J Am Coll Cardiol 2013;61(17):1790–8.

78. Reddy VY, Doshi SK, Siever H, et al. Percutaneous left atrial appendage closure for stroke prophylaxis in patients with atrial fibrillation: 2.3 year follow-up

of the PROTECT AF trial. Circulation 2013;127(6): 720–9.

79. Singh SM, Micieli A, Wijeysundera HC. Economic evaluation of percutaneous left atrial appendage occlusion, dabigatran, and warfarin for stroke prevention in patients with nonvalvular atrial fibrillation. Circulation 2013;127(24):2414–23.

80. Massarenti L, Yilmaz A. Incomplete endothelialization of left atrial appendage occlusion device 10 months after implantation. J Cardiovasc Electrophysiol 2012;23(12):1384–5.

81. Reddy VY, Mobius-Winkler S, Miller MA, et al. Left atrial appendage closure with the Watchman device in patients with a contraindication for oral anticoagulation: the ASAP study (ASA Plavix Feasibility Study With Watchman Left Atrial Appendage Closure Technology). J Am Coll Cardiol 2013; 61(25):2551–6.

82. Meincke F, Schmidt-Salzmann M, Kreidel F, et al. New technical and anticoagulation aspects for left atrial appendage closure using the WATCHMAN(R) device in patients not taking warfarin. EuroIntervention 2013;9(4):463–8.

83. Viles-Gonzalez JF, Reddy VY, Petru J, et al. Incomplete occlusion of the left atrial appendage with the percutaneous left atrial appendage transcatheter occlusion device is not associated with increased risk of stroke. J Interv Card Electrophysiol 2012; 33(1):69–75.

84. Jain AK, Gallagher S. Percutaneous occlusion of the left atrial appendage in non-valvular atrial fibrillation for the prevention of thromboembolism: NICE guidance. Heart 2011;97(9):762–5.

85. Nietlispach F, Gloekler S, Krause R, et al. Amplatzer left atrial appendage occlusion: single center 10-year experience. Catheter Cardiovasc Interv 2013;82(2):283–9.

86. Urena M, Rodes-Cabau J, Freixa X, et al. Percutaneous left atrial appendage closure with the AMPLATZER cardiac plug device in patients with nonvalvular atrial fibrillation and contraindications to anticoagulation therapy. J Am Coll Cardiol 2013;62(2):96–102.

87. Danna P, Proietti R, Sagone A, et al. Does left atrial appendage closure with a cardiac plug system reduce the stroke risk in nonvalvular atrial fibrillation patients? A single-center case series. Pacing Clin Electrophysiol 2013;36(3):347–53.

88. Guerios EE, Schmid M, Gloekler S, et al. Left atrial appendage closure with the Amplatzer Cardiac Plug in patients with atrial fibrillation. Arq Bras Cardiol 2012;98(6):528–36.

89. Lopez-Minguez JR, Eldoayen-Gragera J, Gonzalez-Fernandez R, et al. Immediate and one-year results in 35 consecutive patients after closure of left atrial appendage with the Amplatzer cardiac plug. Rev Esp Cardiol 2013;66(2):90–7.

90. Lam YY, Yip GW, Yu CM, et al. Left atrial appendage closure with AMPLATZER cardiac plug for stroke prevention in atrial fibrillation: initial Asia-Pacific experience. Catheter Cardiovasc Interv 2012;79(5):794–800.

91. Meerkin D, Butnaru A, Dratva D, et al. Early safety of the Amplatzer Cardiac Plug for left atrial appendage occlusion. Int J Cardiol 2013;168(4):3920–5.

92. Bianchi G, Solinas M, Gasbarri T, et al. Pulmonary artery perforation by plug anchoring system after percutaneous closure of left appendage. Ann Thorac Surg 2013;96(1):e3–5.

93. Bruce CJ, Stanton CM, Asirvatham SJ, et al. Percutaneous epicardial left atrial appendage closure: intermediate-term results. J Cardiovasc Electrophysiol 2011;22(1):64–70.

94. Friedman PA, Asirvatham SJ, Dalegrave C, et al. Percutaneous epicardial left atrial appendage closure: preliminary results of an electrogram guided approach. J Cardiovasc Electrophysiol 2009;20(8):908–15.

95. Bruce CJ, Friedman PA, Asirvatham SJ, et al. Novel percutaneous left atrial appendage closure. Cardiovascular Revascularization Medicine 2013;14: 164–6.

96. Bartus K, Bednarek J, Myc J, et al. Feasibility of closed-chest ligation of the left atrial appendage in humans. Heart Rhythm 2011;8(2):188–93.

97. Bartus K, Han FT, Bednarek J, et al. Percutaneous left atrial appendage suture ligation using the LARIAT device in patients with atrial fibrillation: initial clinical experience. J Am Coll Cardiol 2013; 62(2):108–18.

98. Stone D, Byrne T, Pershad A. Early results with the LARIAT device for left atrial appendage exclusion in patients with atrial fibrillation at high risk for stroke and anticoagulation. Catheter Cardiovasc Interv 2013. http://dx.doi.org/10.1002/ccd.25065. [Epub ahead of print].

99. Di Biase L, Burkhardt JD, Gibson DN, et al. 2D and 3D TEE evaluation of an early reopening of the LARIAT epicardial left atrial appendage closure device. Heart Rhythm 2013. http://dx.doi.org/10. 1016/j.hrthm.2013.08.023. [Epub ahead of print].

100. Giedrimas E, Lin AC, Knight BP. Left atrial thrombus after appendage closure using LARIAT. Circulation 2013;6(4):e52–3.

101. Singh IM, Holmes DR Jr. Left atrial appendage closure. Curr Cardiol Rep 2010;12(5):413–21.

102. Krishnaswamy A, Patel NS, Ozkan A, et al. Planning left atrial appendage occlusion using cardiac multidetector computed tomography. Int J Cardiol 2012;158(2):313–7.

103. Lockwood SM, Alison JF, Obeyesekere MN, et al. Imaging the left atrial appendage prior to, during, and after occlusion. JACC Cardiovasc Imaging 2011;4(3):303–6.

104. Mohrs OK, Wunderlich N, Petersen SE, et al. Contrast-enhanced CMR in patients after percutaneous closure of the left atrial appendage: a pilot study. J Cardiovasc Magn Reson 2011;13:33.

105. Nucifora G, Faletra FF, Regoli F, et al. Evaluation of the left atrial appendage with real-time 3-dimensional transesophageal echocardiography: implications for catheter-based left atrial appendage closure. Circ Cardiovasc Imaging 2011;4(5):514–23.

106. Chue CD, de Giovanni J, Steeds RP. The role of echocardiography in percutaneous left atrial appendage occlusion. Eur J Echocardiogr 2011;12(10):i3–10.

107. MacDonald ST, Newton JD, Ormerod OJ. Intracardiac echocardiography off piste? Closure of the left atrial appendage using ICE and local anesthesia. Catheter Cardiovasc Interv 2011; 77(1):124–7.

108. Budge LP, Shaffer KM, Moorman JR, et al. Analysis of in vivo left atrial appendage morphology in patients with atrial fibrillation: a direct comparison of transesophageal echocardiography, planar cardiac CT, and segmented three-dimensional cardiac CT. J Interv Card Electrophysiol 2008;23(2): 87–93.

Cryptogenic Stroke
When and How Should You Look for Arrhythmias?

Zachary Laksman, MD*, George Klein, MD

KEYWORDS

- Cryptogenic stroke • Atrial fibrillation • Arrhythmia • Mobile cardiac outpatient telemetry

KEY POINTS

- Subclinical atrial fibrillation (AF) is a common cause of cryptogenic stroke.
- Longer monitoring improves detection rates of subclinical AF.
- Incorporation of risk factors predicting patients at higher risk of stroke can be used to target populations suitable for longer-term monitoring.
- Although longer duration of AF would be expected to increase the risk of stroke, the exact cutoff for duration of clinical significance is not yet established.
- It seems probable that a combination of clinical risk factors and duration of AF will provide the best prediction of future clinical stroke.

CRYPTOGENIC STROKE

Cryptogenic stroke specifically encompasses patients who have had brain infarction of unknown etiology after an extensive cardiac, vascular, and serologic evaluation has failed to identify a recognized cause.[1] This category continues to account for 30% to 40% of ischemic strokes[2,3] despite a growing armamentarium and refinement of diagnostic modalities. Early angiographic studies demonstrated that most of these events were not attributable to large-artery thrombosis.[4] Serial angiographic studies reinforced the hypothesis that many of these strokes were related to embolic material that would disappear within a few days of the initial insult.[5,6] Embolic occlusions undergoing spontaneous thrombolysis could be seen in most of these patients, with more than 80% having demonstrable potential embolic sources in one study.[7]

THE IMPORTANCE OF ATRIAL FIBRILLATION

Atrial fibrillation (AF) is the most common cardioembolic source of ischemic stroke, and can be found in 1 in 4 patients presenting with their first episode of stroke.[8,9] Unfortunately, only 5% of patients present with AF on their electrocardiogram (ECG) or on telemetry during their index hospitalization, leaving a large proportion of AF undetected.[10] Patients who experience an AF-related stroke will benefit from anticoagulation as a measure for secondary prevention. Anticoagulation therapy after detection of AF provides an additional 40% reduction in risk compared with antiplatelet therapy alone,[11] and overall a 65% relative risk reduction for stroke.[12] Patients with cardioembolic strokes suffer the greatest long-term mortality in comparison with other stroke subtypes, even after adjusting for comorbidities and stroke severity,[13] thus making the identification of AF in patients

---

The authors have nothing to disclose.
Cardiac Electrophysiology, University Hospital, London Health Sciences Centre, 339 Windermere Road, London, Ontario N6G 2V4, Canada
* Corresponding author. University Hospital, London Health Sciences Centre, 6th floor, Arrhythmia Service, 339 Windermere Road, London, Ontario N6G 2V4, Canada.
E-mail address: zlaksman@uwo.ca

Card Electrophysiol Clin 6 (2014) 161–167
http://dx.doi.org/10.1016/j.ccep.2013.10.001
1877-9182/14/$ – see front matter © 2014 Elsevier Inc. All rights reserved.

who have suffered a stroke of paramount importance.

AF is often paroxysmal and can be asymptomatic or associated with vague symptomatology, making it difficult to document in a patient presenting with stroke. Patients with paroxysmal AF (PAF) have a similar risk of stroke when compared with patients with chronic AF, and experience similar reduction in the risk of recurrent strokes.[13] Subclinical AF is thought to be associated with a 2.5-fold increased risk of ischemic stroke or systemic embolus, and many speculate that it accounts for a significant proportion of patients with cryptogenic strokes.[14] This article outlines the current evidence and indications for ECG monitoring in documenting subclinical AF in patients with cryptogenic stroke. In addition, evidence to date regarding risk factors of AF that may inform further testing is briefly reviewed.

Because only a proportion of patients with suspected AF are identified on their index hospitalization for stroke, the search for AF often extends to the outpatient setting. Of note, despite ubiquitous inpatient telemetry for patients admitted with an acute ischemic stroke, a health care worker is generally required to appropriately recognize and act on an episode of AF, a task not without obstacles in a busy hospital setting. In one study, 6% of patients admitted to a stroke unit at an academic medical center had AF that was missed on

telemetry but was detected by concurrent Holter monitoring once reviewed by an overreading physician.[15] AF detection usually relies on outpatient ECG monitoring, which may extend the yield of AF to an additional 6% to 8% of patients, with longer recordings producing greater yield.[16] This approach provides the rationale for longer periods of surveillance, the duration of which is to be determined. Outpatient monitoring is currently highly variable and is dictated by physician preference, local availability, and infrastructure.

OPTIONS FOR OUTPATIENT ELECTROCARDIOGRAPHIC SCREENING OF ATRIAL FIBRILLATION

Since the development of the Holter monitor in the 1940s, there has been progressive improvement and refinement in ambulatory ECG monitoring. In 1999, the American College of Cardiology and the American Heart Association released practice guidelines categorizing ambulatory monitors as either continuous short-term recorders (24–48 h) or intermittent longer-term recorders, the latter being loop recorders with or without the requirement for patient activation.[17] Current systems typically consist of 3 to 5 ECG electrodes yielding 2 ECG vectors and a third derived ECG (**Fig. 1**). The ECG signals are acquired at up to 1000 samples per second in an effort to obtain high-fidelity

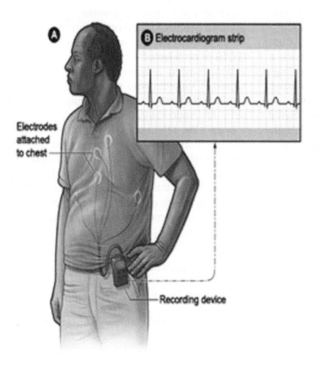

Fig. 1. (*A*) How a Holter or event monitor attaches to a patient. In this example, the monitor is clipped to the patient's belt and electrodes are attached to his chest. (*B*) An electrocardiogram strip, which maps the data from the Holter or event monitor. (*From* What to expect while using a Holter or event monitor. National Heart, Lung, and Blood Institute Web site. Available at: http://www.nhlbi.nih.gov/health/health-topics/topics/holt/while.html. Accessed October 1, 2013.)

tracings. Assuming that the recordings are adequate, AF can be diagnosed and quantified in terms of total burden and episode duration.[18] The yield of 3 to 7 days of ambulatory Holter monitoring is estimated to be 6% after an episode labeled as cryptogenic stroke.[16,19]

Intermittent longer-term recorders can be used for weeks at a time with similar electrode requirements, or "leadless" systems whereby leads are incorporated into the recording unit carried by the patient. The disadvantage of a leadless system is that it requires patient activation, and is therefore not suitable for the diagnosis of subclinical arrhythmias. The iPhone 4S has shown the potential to act as a monitoring device to detect symptomatic PAF, and with the current ubiquitous nature of hand-held devices, this type of strategy has global implications.[20] Loop recorders can be activated by patient events or can be programmed to auto-trigger recordings, for example to capture episodes of tachycardia that may be AF. Once triggered, the patient is notified with preemptive instructions to transmit for review. Alternatively, auto-triggered loop recorders can be designed for wireless transmission to a local device, which can then be relayed to a central monitoring station over a preexisting network.

To overcome some of the limitations of the aforementioned monitoring systems, and with the concept that longer monitoring is of greater benefit, ambulatory telemetry and patch-monitoring systems have been developed. These systems have the capability of frequent wireless transmissions and storage of up to 30 days of data, and have been shown to significantly increase the likelihood of detecting AF.[21] Recently, water-resistant patches have been developed (Zio Patch; iRhyth Technologies, San Francisco, CA) that can store up to 14 days of continuous single-lead ECG data. This class of long-term outpatient monitoring devices, often referred to as mobile cardiac outpatient telemetry (MCOT), is associated with reasonable compliance rates (approximately 70%), often a shortcoming of traditional long-term Holter monitoring.[22] The yield of MCOTs can be as high as 23% for the detection of PAF in patients with cryptogenic stroke.[23] The duration of episodes can often be short, and hence of uncertain clinical significance. In one of the landmark MCOT studies, 85% of episodes recorded were shorter than 30 seconds.[24,25]

IMPLANTED DEVICES

Pacemakers and implantable cardioverter-defibrillators provide the most definitive and permanent continuous monitoring. These devices are capable of identifying and recording AF unambiguously, especially if atrial ECGs are available. Patients who receive these devices are often older, have preexisting conduction-system disease, and have comorbidities that increase their risk of AF. In an unselected population of patients without known AF undergoing device implantation, 30% were diagnosed with PAF within 1 year.[26] Another study demonstrated that patients with implantable devices who had subclinical AF of at least 6 minutes' duration had a 2.5-fold increased risk of stroke or systemic embolism (**Fig. 2**).[27] Although it appears that longer durations of AF are associated with the greatest risk, the aforementioned study was underpowered to evaluate this outcome. Episodes lasting less than 5 minutes per day were associated with lower risk of thromboembolic events when compared with episodes of greater than >24 hours' duration in a pacemaker population.[28] However, episodes as short as 5 minutes are also associated with increased risk of stroke.[29]

An alternative in patients without an indication for a permanent implantable device is the implantable loop recorder (ILR). These devices diagnose AF principally by variability of the RR intervals in current models, which are not usually well suited to record atrial activity. ILRs are implanted subcutaneously in the anterior chest wall, and can be connected to leadless monitoring devices for the detection of bradyarrhythmias and tachyarrhythmias. The implantation procedure is generally well tolerated, with minimal complications or side effects. In addition, they are compatible with magnetic resonance imaging.[30] Current ILRs automatically detect AF with sensitivity of 96% and specificity of 85%, and can remain in place for up to 3 years.[31] The specificity can be improved in practice with manual review of stored electrograms. Approximately 1 in 4 patients with cryptogenic stroke, after a thorough search for a cause has failed to bear fruit, will have AF documented within 1 year of ILR implantation.[32,33] The time from the first documented episode of AF is on average 5 months after the index stroke event, underlining the importance of long-term cardiac monitoring in patients with suspected AF. Not surprisingly, ILR insertion leads to substantially improved detection of AF when compared with 7-day outpatient Holter monitoring.[31]

OTHER RISK FACTORS FOR STROKE

When considering ILR implantation for the diagnosis of subclinical AF in patients with cryptogenic stroke, it might be reasonable to consider factors

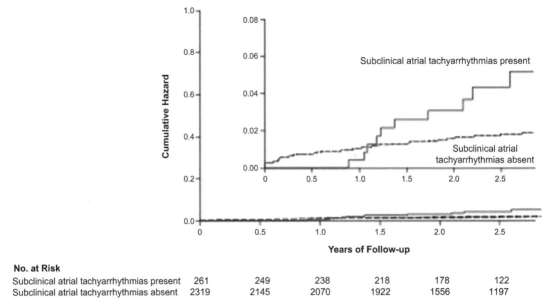

The figure shows cumulative hazard curves with "No. at Risk" data below:

No. at Risk

Subclinical atrial tachyarrhythmias present	261	249	238	218	178	122
Subclinical atrial tachyarrhythmias absent	2319	2145	2070	1922	1556	1197

Fig. 2. Risk of ischemic stroke or systemic embolism after the 3-month visit, according to whether subclinical atrial tachyarrhythmias were or were not detected between enrollment and the 3-month visit. The inset shows the same data on an enlarged y-axis. (*From* Healey JS, Connolly SJ, Gold MR, et al. Subclinical atrial fibrillation and the risk of stroke. N Engl J Med 2012;366(2):126; with permission.)

that would identify patients at the higher risk of AF to increase yield. Multiple predictors of PAF in patients with cryptogenic stroke have been identified, and include diabetes, female gender, more than 100 premature atrial complexes (PACs) on 24-hour Holter, left atrial dilation, left ventricular dysfunction, nonlacunar anterior circulation infarcts, and multiple infarcts seen on neuroimaging.[24,34–36] The predictors make pathophysiologic sense and do not require testing beyond standard practice. Scoring systems for the prediction of PAF using these risk factors have been developed, although they have not become part of standard practice.[37,38] Of these risk factors, dilated left atrium and frequent PACs have stood out as the strongest predictors.[39]

Although multiple genetic polymorphisms have been implicated in the pathogenesis of AF, they do not increase the yield of AF detection when added to conventional risk factors.[40,41] Alternatively, investigators have examined molecular markers to differentiate stroke subtypes for targeted secondary prevention. Genetic profiling has been used successfully to differentiate cardioembolic stroke from large-vessel stroke, with greater than 90% sensitivity and specificity. In addition, genetic profiling can differentiate cardioembolic strokes caused by AF from non-AF causes with similar sensitivity and specificity (**Fig. 3**).[42] These tools, in addition to the potential for new biomarkers, may facilitate targeted screening in the future.

SUMMARY

The trend in outpatient electrocardiographic monitoring for AF in patients with cryptogenic stroke has moved toward longer monitoring periods, resulting in an increased detection rate of

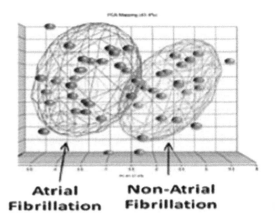

Atrial Fibrillation   Non-Atrial Fibrillation

Fig. 3. Principal components analysis of the 37 genes that differentiated cardioembolic stroke attributable to atrial fibrillation (AF) from non-AF causes. Each sphere represents a single subject. The ellipsoid surrounding the spheres represents 2 standard deviations from the group mean. (*Adapted from* Jickling GC, Xu H, Stamova B, et al. Signatures of cardioembolic and large-vessel ischemic stroke. Ann Neurol 2010;68: 681–692; with permission.)

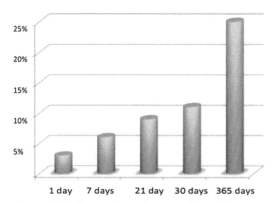

Fig. 4. Yield of outpatient electrocardiographic monitoring for AF in cryptogenic stroke. The x-axis shows the duration of monitoring and the y-axis shows the percentage of patients diagnosed with AF. Note that this analysis includes multiple studies, and multiple study definitions of AF.

subclinical PAF (**Fig. 4**). This abundance of patient data raises new questions, leaving clinical decision making uninformed. One of the heaviest burdens placed on clinicians is a decision regarding anticoagulation when faced with shorter episodes of AF in asymptomatic individuals. There is no compelling evidence that treating such patients with subclinical AF and very brief episodes captured by long-term monitoring will improve outcomes. It is abundantly clear that anticoagulation has a known risk of bleeding complications, patient dissatisfaction, and cost. Essentially one is left with the fact that studies to date have assigned arbitrary designations to the duration of PAF required for diagnosis, and the clinically significant burden, namely the frequency and duration of PAF that warrants anticoagulation, remains unknown.

Likely the best predictors of embolic stroke for both primary and secondary prevention will be a combination of AF screening, quantification, and the identification of other risk factors for embolic stroke. Stepwise population-based risk-factor screening programs for AF are feasible and efficacious in identifying candidates for oral anticoagulation.[43] New models incorporating biomarkers have been, and undoubtedly will continue to be developed in the attempt to refine our prognostic ability in identifying patients with subclinical AF at the highest risk of stroke who may benefit from anticoagulation.[44] For the time being, clinicians may reasonably use traditional risk factors for stroke to aid in the decision of initiating anticoagulation when faced with newly identified AF considered to be of borderline frequency or duration.[45,46]

REFERENCES

1. Adams HP Jr, Bendixen BH, Kappelle LJ, et al. Classification of subtype of acute ischemic stroke. Definitions for use in a multicenter clinical trial. TOAST. Trial of Org 10172 in Acute Stroke Treatment. Stroke 1993;24(1):35–41 PubMed PMID: 7678184.

2. Kolominsky-Rabas PL, Weber M, Gefeller O, et al. Epidemiology of ischemic stroke subtypes according to TOAST criteria: incidence, recurrence, and long-term survival in ischemic stroke subtypes: a population-based study. Stroke 2001;32(12):2735–40 PubMed PMID: 11739965.

3. Lee BI, Nam HS, Heo JH, et al, Yonsei Stroke Team. Yonsei Stroke Registry. Analysis of 1,000 patients with acute cerebral infarctions. Cerebrovasc Dis 2001;12(3):145–51 PubMed PMID: 11641577.

4. Sacco RL, Ellenberg JH, Mohr JP, et al. Infarcts of undetermined cause: the NINCDS stroke data bank. Ann Neurol 1989;25(4):382–90 PubMed PMID: 2712533.

5. Dalal PM, Shah PM, Aiyar RR. Arteriographic study of cerebral embolism. Lancet 1965;2(7408):358–61 PubMed PMID: 14328794.

6. Liebeskind A, Chinichian A, Schechter MM. The moving embolus seed during serial cerebral angiography. Stroke 1971;2(5):440–3 PubMed PMID: 5111580.

7. Fieschi C, Argentino C, Lenzi GL, et al. Clinical and instrumental evaluation of patients with ischemic stroke within the first six hours. J Neurol Sci 1989;91(3):311–21 PubMed PMID: 2671268.

8. White H, Boden-Albala B, Wang C, et al. Ischemic stroke subtype incidence among whites, blacks, and Hispanics: the Northern Manhattan Study. Circulation 2005;111(10):1327–31 PubMed PMID: 15769776.

9. Marini C, De Santis F, Sacco S, et al. Contribution of atrial fibrillation to incidence and outcome of ischemic stroke: results from a population-based study. Stroke 2005;36(6):1115–9 PubMed PMID: 15879330.

10. Liao J, Khalid Z, Scallan C, et al. Noninvasive cardiac monitoring for detecting paroxysmal atrial fibrillation or flutter after acute ischemic stroke: a systematic review. Stroke 2007;38(11):2935–40 PubMed PMID: 17901394.

11. Hart RG, Pearce LA, Aguilar MI. Meta-analysis: antithrombotic therapy to prevent stroke in patients who have nonvalvular atrial fibrillation. Ann Intern Med 2007;146(12):857–67 PubMed PMID: 17577005.

12. Wann LS, Curtis AB, Ellenbogen KA, et al. 2011 ACCF/AHA/HRS focused update on the management of patients with atrial fibrillation (update on dabigatran): a report of the American College of Cardiology Foundation/American Heart Association

Task Force on practice guidelines. J Am Coll Cardiol 2011;57(11):1330–7 PubMed PMID: 21324629.

13. Stead LG, Gilmore RM, Bellolio MF, et al. Cardioembolic but not other stroke subtypes predict mortality independent of stroke severity at presentation. Stroke Res Treat 2011;2011:281496 PubMed PMID: 22007347. PubMed Central PMCID: 3191739.

14. King A. Atrial fibrillation: could subclinical AF be a missing link in the etiology of cryptogenic stroke? Nat Rev Cardiol 2012;9(3):126 PubMed PMID: 22290237.

15. Lazzaro MA, Krishnan K, Prabhakaran S. Detection of atrial fibrillation with concurrent Holter monitoring and continuous cardiac telemetry following ischemic stroke and transient ischemic attack. J Stroke Cerebrovasc Dis 2012;21(2):89–93 PubMed PMID: 20656504.

16. Jabaudon D, Sztajzel J, Sievert K, et al. Usefulness of ambulatory 7-day ECG monitoring for the detection of atrial fibrillation and flutter after acute stroke and transient ischemic attack. Stroke 2004;35(7):1647–51 PubMed PMID: 15155965.

17. Crawford MH, Bernstein SJ, Deedwania PC, et al. ACC/AHA guidelines for ambulatory electrocardiography. A report of the American College of Cardiology/American Heart Association Task Force on Practice Guidelines (Committee to Revise the Guidelines for Ambulatory Electrocardiography). Developed in collaboration with the North American Society for pacing and Electrophysiology. J Am Coll Cardiol 1999;34(3):912–48 PubMed PMID: 10483977.

18. Mittal S, Movsowitz C, Steinberg JS. Ambulatory external electrocardiographic monitoring: focus on atrial fibrillation. J Am Coll Cardiol 2011;58(17):1741–9 PubMed PMID: 21996384.

19. Schuchert A, Behrens G, Meinertz T. Impact of long-term ECG recording on the detection of paroxysmal atrial fibrillation in patients after an acute ischemic stroke. Pacing Clin Electrophysiol 1999;22(7):1082–4 PubMed PMID: 10456638.

20. McManus DD, Lee J, Maitas O, et al. A novel application for the detection of an irregular pulse using an iPhone 4S in patients with atrial fibrillation. Heart Rhythm 2013;10(3):315–9 PubMed PMID: 23220686. PubMed Central PMCID: 3698570.

21. Rothman SA, Laughlin JC, Seltzer J, et al. The diagnosis of cardiac arrhythmias: a prospective multicenter randomized study comparing mobile cardiac outpatient telemetry versus standard loop event monitoring. J Cardiovasc Electrophysiol 2007;18(3):241–7 PubMed PMID: 17318994.

22. Bernstein RA. Detection of atrial fibrillation after cryptogenic stroke. Curr Treat Options Cardiovasc Med 2012;14(3):298–304 PubMed PMID: 22562457.

23. Sinha AM, Diener HC, Morillo CA, et al. Cryptogenic Stroke and underlying Atrial Fibrillation (CRYSTAL AF): design and rationale. Am Heart J 2010;160(1):36–41.e1 PubMed PMID: 20598970.

24. Tayal AH, Tian M, Kelly KM, et al. Atrial fibrillation detected by mobile cardiac outpatient telemetry in cryptogenic TIA or stroke. Neurology 2008;71(21):1696–701 PubMed PMID: 18815386.

25. Bernstein RA, Passman R. Prevention of stroke in patients with high-risk atrial fibrillation. Curr Neurol Neurosci Rep 2010;10(1):34–9 PubMed PMID: 20425224.

26. Ziegler PD, Glotzer TV, Daoud EG, et al. Incidence of newly detected atrial arrhythmias via implantable devices in patients with a history of thromboembolic events. Stroke 2010;41(2):256–60 PubMed PMID: 20044517.

27. Healey JS, Connolly SJ, Gold MR, et al. Subclinical atrial fibrillation and the risk of stroke. N Engl J Med 2012;366(2):120–9 PubMed PMID: 22236222.

28. Boriani G, Botto GL, Padeletti L, et al. Improving stroke risk stratification using the CHADS2 and CHA2DS2-VASc risk scores in patients with paroxysmal atrial fibrillation by continuous arrhythmia burden monitoring. Stroke 2011;42(6):1768–70 PubMed PMID: 21493904.

29. Botto GL, Padeletti L, Santini M, et al. Presence and duration of atrial fibrillation detected by continuous monitoring: crucial implications for the risk of thromboembolic events. J Cardiovasc Electrophysiol 2009;20(3):241–8 PubMed PMID: 19175849.

30. Haeusler KG, Koch L, Ueberreiter J, et al. Safety and reliability of the insertable Reveal XT recorder in patients undergoing 3 Tesla brain magnetic resonance imaging. Heart Rhythm 2011;8(3):373–6 PubMed PMID: 21070885.

31. Ritter MA, Kochhauser S, Duning T, et al. Occult atrial fibrillation in cryptogenic stroke: detection by 7-day electrocardiogram versus implantable cardiac monitors. Stroke 2013;44(5):1449–52 PubMed PMID: 23449264.

32. Etgen T, Hochreiter M, Mundel M, et al. Insertable cardiac event recorder in detection of atrial fibrillation after cryptogenic stroke: an audit report. Stroke 2013;44(7):2007–9 PubMed PMID: 23674523.

33. Cotter PE, Martin PJ, Ring L, et al. Incidence of atrial fibrillation detected by implantable loop recorders in unexplained stroke. Neurology 2013;80(17):1546–50 PubMed PMID: 23535493. PubMed Central PMCID: 3662328.

34. Miller DJ, Khan MA, Schultz LR, et al. Outpatient cardiac telemetry detects a high rate of atrial fibrillation in cryptogenic stroke. J Neurol Sci 2013;324(1–2):57–61 PubMed PMID: 23102659.

35. Bhatt A, Majid A, Razak A, et al. Predictors of occult paroxysmal atrial fibrillation in cryptogenic strokes detected by long-term noninvasive cardiac monitoring. Stroke Res Treat 2011;2011:172074 PubMed PMID: 21423555. PubMed Central PMCID: 3056431.

36. Gaillard N, Deltour S, Vilotijevic B, et al. Detection of paroxysmal atrial fibrillation with transtelephonic

EKG in TIA or stroke patients. Neurology 2010; 74(21):1666–70 PubMed PMID: 20498434.

37. Malik S, Hicks WJ, Schultz L, et al. Development of a scoring system for atrial fibrillation in acute stroke and transient ischemic attack patients: the LADS scoring system. J Neurol Sci 2011;301(1–2):27–30 PubMed PMID: 21130468.

38. Suissa L, Bertora D, Lachaud S, et al. Score for the targeting of atrial fibrillation (STAF): a new approach to the detection of atrial fibrillation in the secondary prevention of ischemic stroke. Stroke 2009;40(8): 2866–8 PubMed PMID: 19461041.

39. Khan M, Miller DJ. Detection of paroxysmal atrial fibrillation in stroke/TIA patients. Stroke Res Treat 2013;2013:840265 PubMed PMID: 23662246. PubMed Central PMCID: 3622405.

40. Ellinor PT, Lunetta KL, Albert CM, et al. Meta-analysis identifies six new susceptibility loci for atrial fibrillation. Nat Genet 2012;44(6):670–5 PubMed PMID: 22544366. PubMed Central PMCID: 3366038.

41. Smith JG, Newton-Cheh C, Almgren P, et al. Genetic polymorphisms for estimating risk of atrial fibrillation in the general population: a prospective study. Arch Intern Med 2012;172(9):742–4 PubMed PMID: 22782207.

42. Sharp FR, Jickling GC, Stamova B, et al. Molecular markers and mechanisms of stroke: RNA studies of blood in animals and humans. J Cereb Blood Flow Metab 2011;31(7):1513–31 PubMed PMID: 21505474. PubMed Central PMCID: 3137473.

43. Engdahl J, Andersson L, Mirskaya M, et al. Stepwise screening of atrial fibrillation in a 75-year-old population: implications for stroke prevention. Circulation 2013;127(8):930–7 PubMed PMID: 23343564.

44. Singer DE, Chang Y, Borowsky LH, et al. A new risk scheme to predict ischemic stroke and other thromboembolism in atrial fibrillation: the ATRIA study stroke risk score. J Am Heart Assoc 2013;2(3): e000250 PubMed PMID: 23782923.

45. Gage BF, Waterman AD, Shannon W, et al. Validation of clinical classification schemes for predicting stroke: results from the National Registry of Atrial Fibrillation. JAMA 2001;285(22):2864–70 PubMed PMID: 11401607.

46. Lip GY, Nieuwlaat R, Pisters R, et al. Refining clinical risk stratification for predicting stroke and thromboembolism in atrial fibrillation using a novel risk factor-based approach: the Euro Heart Survey on Atrial Fibrillation. Chest 2010;137(2):263–72 PubMed PMID: 19762550.

Neurointerventional Therapies for Stroke in Atrial Fibrillation
Illustrated Cases

Amit B. Sharma, MD[a], Enoch B. Lule, MD[a],
Anmar Razak, MD[b], Syed I. Hussain, MD[b],
Shalini Sharma, MD[c], Peerawut Deeprasertkul, MD[a],
Ranjan K. Thakur, MD, MPH, MBA, FHRS[a],*

KEYWORDS

- Stroke • Atrial fibrillation • Ischemic stroke • Intracranial hemorrhage • Thromboembolism

KEY POINTS

- Stroke is the leading cause of disability in adults and the most serious complication of atrial fibrillation (AF). Strokes may be ischemic (80%) or hemorrhagic (20%). AF is the leading cause of cardioembolic strokes; these strokes are caused by large thromboemboli and are more disabling.
- Distinction between ischemic and hemorrhagic strokes at the time of presentation is critical because approaches to treatment are different. This distinction can be made rapidly with a noncontrast computed tomography scan.
- The goal of treatment of acute ischemic stroke is reperfusion of ischemic brain tissue, whereas the treatment of hemorrhagic stroke is supportive therapy and correction of the underlying condition that may have lead to bleeding.
- The treatment of acute ischemic strokes is similar to treatment of acute myocardial infarction, which requires timely reperfusion for optimal results. The main reperfusion strategies include intravenous and/or intra-arterial thrombolysis, mechanical thrombectomy, and (rarely) angioplasty and/or stent.

INTRODUCTION

Approximately 800,000 strokes occur in the United States every year, resulting in 200,000 deaths, making stroke the leading cause of disability in adults.[1,2] In general, ischemia accounts for 80% of acute strokes and the remainder are hemorrhagic events.[1,2] Early distinction between these types of strokes is critical because the approaches to treatment are different. The goal for acute ischemic stroke is reperfusion of ischemic brain tissue, whereas the treatment of hemorrhagic stroke is supportive therapy and correction of the underlying conditions that may have led to bleeding, such as uncontrolled hypertension, reversal of anticoagulation, ruptured aneurysms, and bleeding into an ischemic stroke. Treatment may be complicated by concomitant occurrence of ischemia and hemorrhage; an initial ischemic event may lead to secondary hemorrhage and vice versa. In these cases, treatment is prioritized

Disclosures: None.
[a] Sparrow Thoracic and Cardiovascular Institute, Michigan State University, 1200 East Michigan Avenue, Lansing, MI 48912, USA; [b] Department of Neurology and Ophthalmology, Michigan State University, Lansing, MI, USA; [c] Department of Radiology, Michigan State University, Lansing, MI, USA
* Corresponding author. Sparrow Thoracic and Cardiovascular Institute, 1200 East Michigan Avenue, Suite 580, Lansing, MI 48912.
E-mail address: thakur@msu.edu

to the management of hemorrhage and supportive therapy for the ischemic component.

Acute ischemic strokes may be thrombotic or embolic. Acute embolic strokes are usually caused by thromboembolism from the heart or atheroembolism from the aorta, carotid or vertebral arteries. Emboli from the heart (cardioembolism), account for 10% to 30% of all strokes.[3] Strokes caused by atrial fibrillation (AF) are generally ischemic events (ischemia may be complicated by secondary hemorrhage) caused by cardiogenic thromboembolism and are the most serious complication of AF, in part because these strokes are larger and more disabling.[4,5] The treatment of acute ischemic strokes is similar to treatment of acute myocardial infarction (AMI), which requires timely reperfusion for optimal results. Like AMI, reperfusion strategies include intravenous (IV) and/or intra-arterial thrombolysis and catheter-based therapies. However, unlike AMI, not many patients with stroke receive reperfusion therapy because of late presentation (>4.5 hours from symptom onset), few qualified hospitals and specialists, and unavailability of rapidly accessible advanced neuroimaging facilities in most hospitals. Even if an intervention is possible, reasons for not intervening include small vessel occlusion (lacunar stroke), transient ischemic attacks (TIA), end-of-life strokes, and mild strokes outweighing the risks of intervention. As a result of these factors, few neurointerventional procedures are performed for acute strokes.

Interventional therapies for acute stroke include IV and/or intra-arterial thrombolysis, mechanical thrombectomy, angioplasty, and stent. The following cases are examples of the use of these therapies in patients with strokes caused by AF.

CASE 1

A 76-year-old woman with a history of hypertension and hyperlipidemia (CHADS$_2$, 2; CHA$_2$DS$_2$-Vasc, 4) was brought to the hospital with slurred speech, left facial droop, and right-sided weakness 5 hours after onset of symptoms. Initial head computed tomography (CT) was normal (**Fig. 1**). Electrocardiogram (ECG) showed AF with rapid ventricular rate at 160/min. Duration of AF was unknown and she was asymptomatic with respect to AF. She was not on any anticoagulation therapy. Rate control was achieved with IV diltiazem.

A diagnosis of acute right middle cerebral artery (MCA) ischemic stroke was made. On the National Institutes of Health Stroke Scale (NIHSS), the stroke severity was graded to be 15. CT

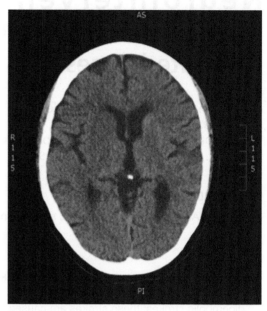

Fig. 1. CT of the head on presentation of the patient in case 1 shows no abnormalities.

angiography (CTA) of head and neck showed acute occlusion in the right MCA. CT perfusion showed mismatch between mean transit time and cerebral blood volume, indicating penumbra in the right MCA area.

She was out of the window of the IV thrombolysis and it was decided to take her to the catheterization laboratory for mechanical thrombectomy. Right MCA occlusion was shown with Thrombolysis in Cerebral Infarction (TICI) flow graded as 0 (see **Fig. 2**); this was treated with Trevo stent retriever along with aspiration using a Penumbra System, Neuron 5MAX aspiration catheter (**Fig. 3**). After 1 pass, the clot was retrieved. End result with angiography showed TICI 2a perfusion with persistent small M3 superior division branch occlusion (**Fig. 4**). Follow-up CT showed hemorrhagic transformation of infarct in the right basal ganglia including the head of the right caudate nucleus with moderate mass effect on the right lateral ventricle (**Fig. 5**).

She continued to have left-sided neglect, right gaze preference, and weakness in upper and lower extremities, although primarily in the left upper extremity. Oral intake was also poor, so a percutaneous endoscopic gastrostomy tube was placed and she continued to receive oral diltiazem. On the fourth day, she spontaneously converted to sinus rhythm.

With physical therapy, she was able to stand with assistance but not ambulate. She had a high blood lactate dehydrogenase level and a renal

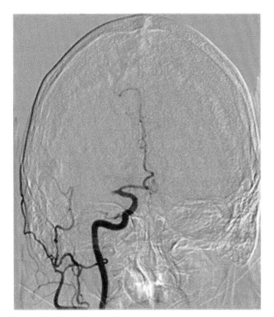

Fig. 2. Right MCA occlusion on catheter angiogram.

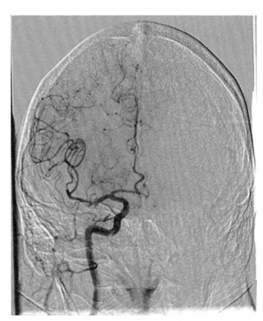

Fig. 4. Recanalization of the main right MCA trunk.

infarct was identified on CT of abdomen/pelvis, but renal function remained normal. Anticoagulation was not started in view of hemorrhagic transformation of the infarct in the basal ganglia. She was discharged with partial improvement; NIHSS on discharge was 12.

Discussion

Acute stroke management requires assessment of location, severity, and cause of the stroke. The NIHSS score provides a uniform, consistent (interobserver and test-retest) quantitative assessment of the severity of stroke.[6,7] The score is divided into 11 items, each of which is graded between 0 and 4, with cumulative score varying between 0 and 42 (**Table 1**).[8] A score of 0 for an item indicates normal function and increasing scores correspond with increasing level of dysfunction. Total scores of less than 4 are considered minor strokes, 5 to 15 are considered

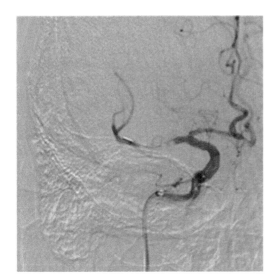

Fig. 3. Trevo retriever in the right MCA thrombus.

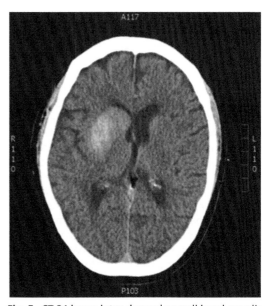

Fig. 5. CT 24 hours later showed a small basal ganglia hemorrhage with preservation of cortex.

Table 1	
The NIHSS score	
1. Level of Consciousness	
Responsiveness	0–3
Questions	0–2
Commands	0–2
2. Horizontal eye movement	0–2
3. Visual field test	0–3
4. Facial palsy	0–3
5. Motor: arm	0–4
6. Motor: leg	0–4
7. Limb ataxia	0–2
8. Sensory	0–2
9. Language	0–3
10. Speech	0–2
11. Extinction and inattention	0–2

moderate strokes, and greater than 15 are considered severe strokes. Patients with NIHSS scores between 8 and 20 are more likely to benefit from reperfusion and are less likely to experience hemorrhagic transformation, making them ideal candidates for an appropriate reperfusion therapy (thrombolysis or percutaneous intervention).[9]

A patient presenting with stroke symptoms should undergo an expeditious noncontrast CT to rule out intracranial hemorrhage. In addition, CT perfusion imaging may help define the anatomic extent of the stroke and whether there is surrounding region where blood flow is reduced but the tissue may be salvageable (penumbra).[10] CT perfusion imaging or CTA are not necessary to treat patients presenting early, within the first 3 to 4.5 hours, who may be suitable candidates for IV thrombolysis. However, they are beneficial for risk-benefit stratification in patients presenting beyond 4.5 hours after the onset of stroke symptoms. Magnetic resonance imaging (MRI) with diffusion-weighted and perfusion-weighted imaging can also identify mismatch, which indicates penumbra with ischemic but salvageable tissue. An infarct without penumbra does not improve with intervention and intervention may cause hemorrhagic transformation. Imaging information can therefore be useful to guide therapy (thrombolysis or percutaneous intervention) and prevent harm.

Although advanced imaging information can be useful, most stroke trials to date have used only non–contrast-enhanced CT to rule out hemorrhage, for enrollment. Thus, the simple brain CT remains the only imaging study required before

administration of IV thrombolysis and has the best level of evidence to recommend it.[11]

Recombinant tissue plasminogen activator (rtPA) is the only US Food and Drug Administration (FDA)–approved agent for IV thrombolysis in patients with stroke presenting within 3 hours of symptoms.[12] The European Cooperative Acute Stroke Study III showed that IV alteplase (rtPA) administered up to 4.5 hours after symptom onset in ischemic stroke was also safe and effective.[13] However, IV thrombolytics may take more than 2 hours to recanalize the occlusion.[14] Thus, percutaneous endovascular interventions are appropriate first-line stroke therapies outside the 4.5-hour window during which IV thrombolytic therapy may be ineffective.[15]

Intravenous thrombolysis is less likely to be effective for large cerebral arteries or proximal occlusions, including intracranial internal carotid artery and the proximal MCA. Intra-arterial thrombolysis has been shown to be effective in only 1 trial, using prourokinase, and thus all available thrombolytics can be used intra-arterially on an off-label basis.[16] However, intra-arterial thrombolytics are more likely to be effective for these lesions.

A meta-analysis of 53 studies showed that spontaneous or therapeutic recanalization and reperfusion in acute ischemic stroke was associated with improved functional status and lower mortality.[17] In patients presenting outside the 4.5-hour window, mechanical thrombectomy devices may be considered. Mechanical devices may have additional advantages: rapid recanalization, suitability for large vessels, and lower risk of hemorrhage.

Although several foreign-body retrieval devices have been studied in the acute stroke setting, 4 devices are currently FDA approved (Penumbra Aspiration System by Penumbra Inc; Solitaire FR Revascularization Device by EV3; Stryker Trevo Pro Retrieval System by Concentric Medical; and Merci Retriever by Concentric Medical). Procedural success is usually measured using the TICI flow grade at the site of occlusion (**Box 1**).[18]

This patient's occlusion was treated with a Trevo stent retriever and an aspiration catheter. A deployed stent entraps the thrombus between the struts of the stent and the vessel wall, restoring blood flow past the occlusion. Stent retrievers allow thrombectomy to be performed by pulling the deployed stent back into the guide catheter and the retracted material is removed via the aspiration catheter. The stent can be used repeatedly in this fashion and this technique is applicable even in small vessels. Another advantage of this technique is that anticoagulation or antiplatelet

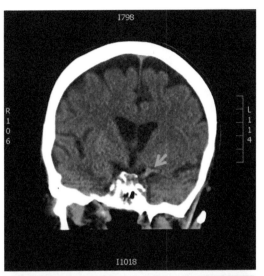

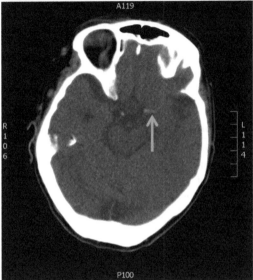

Fig. 6. In the patient in case 2, CT on arrival showed left carotid terminus/MCA thrombus (*arrows*).

CASE 2

A 79-year-old woman with a history of AF presented with acute-onset aphasia and right hemiplegia. She had been on warfarin, but it had been discontinued 6 months previously because of noncompliance. Her $CHADS_2$ score was 1 and CHA_2DS_2VASc score was 3. Home medications included sotalol 80 mg twice a day, sertraline 50 mg, loperamide 2 mg, and gabapentin 300 mg. CT scan in the emergency department showed a hyperdense left MCA lesion consistent with a thrombus (**Fig. 6**). NIHSS score was 13. ECG showed AF with ventricular rate of 142/min. Echocardiography showed preserved left ventricular ejection fraction (LVEF) with grade II diastolic dysfunction and left atrial (LA) size of 4.5 cm. Sotalol was stopped and IV diltiazem was started for rate control.

She presented within the window for rtPA and received 0.9 mg/kg IV infusion (10% bolus and 90% infusion over 1 hour). Repeat CT at 24 hours showed no hemorrhage and a few hypodensities in the left basal ganglia, consistent with infarction (**Fig. 7**).

On the day of discharge, the patient was able to speak in full sentences, follow commands, and showed only mild right-sided weakness; NIHSS score was 4. She was started on Pradaxa 150 mg twice a day in addition to sustained-release diltiazem and the plan was to do a transesophageal

agents are not needed because the stent is not left in situ.

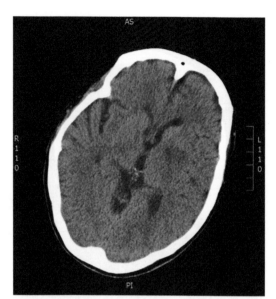

Fig. 7. CT 24 hours later shows hypodensities in the basal ganglia, consistent with infarction. The cortex is preserved.

echocardiogram after 6 weeks, cardiovert, and start oral amiodarone.

Discussion

For eligible patients, IV rtPA is recommended for acute stroke if it can be initiated within 4.5 hours of onset of symptoms (**Box 2**).[13,19–21] Concerns arise about the use of IV thrombolytics if the differential diagnosis of the patient's acute symptoms might include stroke mimics, such as seizure disorder, migraine, or conversion reaction. If the patient is otherwise eligible without any contraindications, it is recommended that therapy be administered because none of the patients with stroke mimics who received thrombolytic therapy developed hemorrhagic complications.[22,23]

CASE 3

An 86-year-old woman with history of hypertension, hyperlipidemia, and paroxysmal AF (CHADS$_2$, 2; CHA$_2$DS$_2$VASc, = 4) was brought to the hospital with slurred speech and right-sided weakness. Warfarin had been stopped several months earlier because of her history of frequent falls. A diagnosis of left MCA thromboembolic stroke with NIHSS score of 14 was made. ECG at the time of admission showed sinus rhythm at a rate of 80 beats per minute (bpm) with evidence of old inferior wall myocardial infarction. A two-dimensional (2D) echocardiogram showed LVEF of 40% with basal and midinferoseptal hypokinesia, and LA diameter was 3.8 cm.

> **Box 2**
> **Eligibility criteria for treatment of acute ischemic stroke with rtPA**
>
> *Inclusion criteria:*
>
> Age greater than or equal to 18 years
>
> Clinical diagnosis of acute stroke with measurable neurologic deficit
>
> Duration less than 4.5 hours, from onset of symptoms to initiation of IV rtPA
>
> *Exclusion criteria:*
>
> Significant stroke or head trauma in the last 3 months
>
> History of intracranial hemorrhage, neoplasm, arteriovenous malformation, or aneurysm
>
> Recent intracranial or intraspinal surgery
>
> Arterial puncture at a noncompressible site in less than 7 days
>
> Symptoms suggesting subarachnoid hemorrhage
>
> Persistent hypertension (systolic ≥185 mm Hg; diastolic ≥110 mm Hg)
>
> Serum glucose less than 50 mg/dL
>
> Active internal bleeding
>
> Acute bleeding diatheses including platelet count less than 100,000/mm^3, INR greater than 1.7, heparin use in the last 48 hours, and current use of a direct thrombin inhibitor or a factor Xa inhibitor
>
> Evidence of intracranial hemorrhage on CT
>
> Evidence of infarction involving more than 33% of cerebral hemisphere
>
> *Relative exclusion criteria:*
>
> Minor and isolated neurologic signs
>
> Spontaneously clearing stroke symptoms
>
> Major surgery or serious trauma in the last 14 days
>
> Gastrointestinal or urinary tract bleeding in the last 21 days
>
> Myocardial infarction in the last 3 months
>
> Seizure at the onset of stroke with postictal neurologic impairment
>
> Pregnancy

Initial brain CT was normal (**Fig. 8**), but the MRI showed left hemispheric stroke (**Fig. 9**). CTA showed left internal carotid artery (ICA) terminus occlusion and distal occlusion (**Fig. 10**), likely caused by a fragment from the proximal embolus.

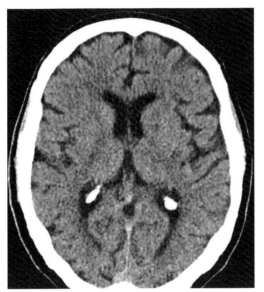

Fig. 8. In the patient in case 3, initial CT of the head was negative.

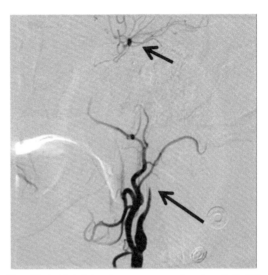

Fig. 10. Initial lateral angiogram showing left ICA pseudo-occlusion (*lower arrow*) caused by distal embolus occlusion (*upper arrow*); TICI flow 0.

She was outside the 4.5-hour window for IV rtPA. She was taken to the catheterization laboratory and received 30 mg of intra-arterial rtPA with mechanical thrombectomy using Penumbra aspiration and Solitaire retriever. At first, TICI flow was 0, which was recanalized to flow grade 2b (**Fig. 11**). At discharge, brain CT was normal

(**Fig. 12**) and the NIHSS score improved to 5. She was started on rivaroxaban 15 mg daily at discharge.

Discussion

Intra-arterial thrombolysis may be considered in patients who are poor candidates for IV thrombolysis or have thrombotic occlusion of large vessels.[15,19,24–26] Because administration is performed under angiographic visualization, at the site of the occlusion, the dose of the drug is much smaller. In general, the dose of intra-arterial therapy is one-third of the IV dose. However, intra-arterial administration does not seem

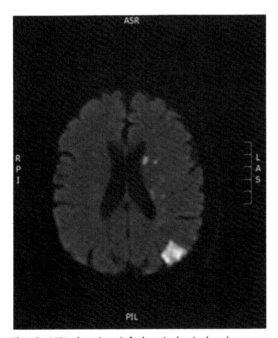

Fig. 9. MRI showing left hemispheric border zone stroke.

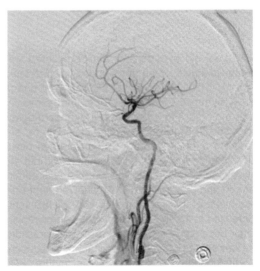

Fig. 11. Post mechanical thrombectomy, TICI flow 2b.

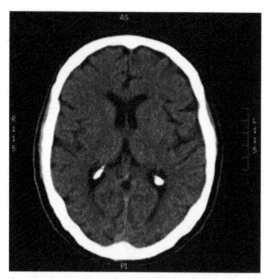

Fig. 12. Repeat CT 24 hours after embolectomy with no significant infarct.

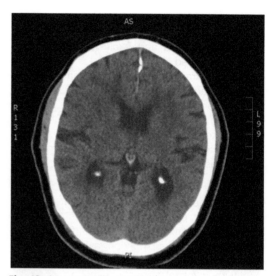

Fig. 13. In case 4, CT on arrival was normal.

to be superior to IV administration.[27] Some studies have reported higher intracranial hemorrhage rates with intra-arterial thrombolytic therapy, but this may in part be because of the greater stroke severity in patients undergoing intra-arterial therapy.[28] Some have suggested using a combination of IV and intra-arterial thrombolytic therapy to achieve higher recanalization rates and better stroke outcomes. However, clinical trials have not supported this approach.[29] The approach for now is to use IV thrombolysis within the 4.5-hour window and consider percutaneous catheter-based therapies (possibly with adjuvant intra-arterial thrombolysis, if indicated) outside this window or if there are contra-indications to IV thrombolysis.

CASE 4

A 68-year-old hypertensive man presented with acute weakness of left arm and leg with left facial droop; NIHSS score was 10. ECG showed normal sinus rhythm. CT of the brain at time of admission was normal (**Fig. 13**). A 2D echocardiogram showed LVEF of 65%, LA diameter 3.5 cm, and negative bubble study for patent foramen ovale. CTA of head and neck was negative, without any significant stenosis. Intravenous rtPA was administered and post-rtPA CT brain showed right parietal bleed of 3.7 × 2.5 cm (**Fig. 14**). NIHSS score increased to 16 and he underwent a hemicraniectomy because of increased intracranial pressure. He was sent to inpatient rehabilitation for recovery.

Although he presented in sinus rhythm, ECG 24 hours later showed AF at 110 bpm. CHADS$_2$

was 1, and CHA$_2$DS$_2$Vasc was 2. On the fourth day, he spontaneously converted to sinus rhythm and was started on oral amiodarone loading. Anticoagulation could not be started because of the massive bleed, and the patient was discharged to the rehabilitation facility on amiodarone 200 mg daily.

Discussion

Before administration of IV rtPA, the following should be confirmed:

1. Treatment is being started within the 4.5-hour window from onset of symptoms to administration of rtPA

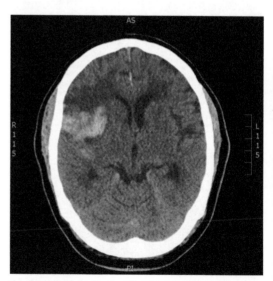

Fig. 14. CT of the brain after IV tPA shows a right parietal bleed, 3.7 × 2.5 cm.

2. A persistent and measurable neurologic deficit is present; hypoglycemia has been ruled out
3. Eligibility criteria and exclusion criteria have been reviewed
4. A noncontrast CT brain or MRI has ruled out hemorrhage
5. Blood pressure is less than 185/110 mm Hg (see **Box 2**)
6. Two large-bore IV lines are in place
7. Accurate body weight has been determined for rtPA dosing

The dose of rtPA is 0.9 mg/kg of body weight, with a maximum dose of 90 mg, administered intravenously. Ten percent of the dose is given as a bolus over 1 minute and the remainder is infused over 1 hour. A follow-up noncontrast head CT is recommended after 24 hours, before initiating treatment with antiplatelet agents or anticoagulants.[19]

Intracranial hemorrhage (ICH) is the most serious complication of thrombolytic therapy. Most clinical trials and community-based studies have shown a symptomatic ICH rate of 5% to 6%.[12,30–34] A meta-analysis of clinical trials with rtPA administered in the 4.5-hour to 6-hour window suggested a significantly higher risk of ICH (odds ratio, 2.96; 95% confidence interval, 1.55–5.66]).[35]

ICH should be suspected if there is sudden neurologic deterioration, such as a decline in the level of consciousness, a new headache, nausea and vomiting, or a sudden increase in blood pressure (Cushing reflex). A noncontrast head CT or MRI should be obtained immediately along with laboratory studies to assess coagulation status. If ICH is confirmed, reversal of thrombolytic and antiplatelet effects should be considered.[35] Ten units of cryoprecipitate to increase fibrinogen and factor VIII levels and 6 to 8 units of platelets have been recommended, although not proven to be effective.[36,37]

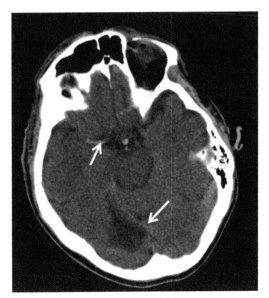

Fig. 15. Initial CT scan shows right carotid terminus/MCA thrombus as well as an old right occipital stroke. Initial CT scan shows right carotid terminus/MCA thrombus (*top arrow*) as well as an old right occipital stroke (*bottom arrow*).

This patient underwent a craniotomy to decompress the brain, in order to avert herniation. Neurosurgical evacuation for intracerebral bleeding caused by thrombolysis is controversial, although, in the GUSTO-I trial of thrombolysis for myocardial infarction, the 30-day survival was significantly higher with evacuation than without (65% vs 35%) and there was a trend toward better functional outcomes (20% vs 12% respectively).[38]

CASE 5

A 77-year-old man with history of ischemic cardiomyopathy, hypertension, status post implantable cardioverter defibrillator (ICD) placement,

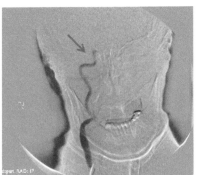
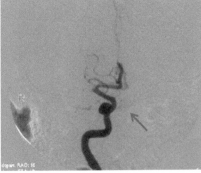

Fig. 16. Mechanical thrombectomy with minimal recanalization of ICA terminus but continued occlusion of the middle and anterior cerebral arteries. Initial CT scan shows right carotid terminus/MCA thrombus (*top arrow*) as well as an old right occipital stroke (*bottom arrow*).

congestive heart failure, and paroxysmal AF ($CHADS_2$, 3; CHA_2DS_2VASc, 4) presented to the emergency department with a syncopal episode at home. He stated that he was walking around the house when he developed a "funny feeling" and then lost consciousness and found himself on the floor. He reported that he felt his ICD discharge. ECG shows atrial sensed, ventricular paced rhythm. ICD interrogation showed an appropriate shock for ventricular tachycardia. He was on warfarin with an International Normalized Ratio (INR) of 1.6. He was admitted for observation.

The next day, he developed weakness in the left upper and lower extremities. A noncontrast head CT scan showed right carotid terminus/MCA thrombus as well as an old right occipital stroke (**Fig. 15**). Mechanical thrombectomy was attempted with minimal recanalization of ICA terminus and persistent occlusion of the middle and anterior cerebral arteries (**Fig. 16**). A CT scan 24 hours later showed massive right hemispheric infarct with large subfalcine herniation to the left (**Fig. 17**). He went into respiratory arrest and died the next day.

Discussion

Stroke in patients with AF, treated with warfarin, but with a subtherapeutic INR, as shown by this case, is a common clinical problem. It has been estimated that only half of the patients with nonvalvular AF, who are suitable candidates for warfarin, are treated with warfarin, and the warfarin-treated patients are in the therapeutic INR range only about half the time.[39–44] Although clinical trials have shown new anticoagulants to

be as effective as warfarin for stroke prevention in patients with nonvalvular AF, the clinical outcomes in the community setting may be better than those for warfarin because of persistent anticoagulant effect, without subtherapeutic periods.[45–47]

SUMMARY

Strokes may be ischemic (80%) or hemorrhagic (20%) events. Strokes caused by AF are generally ischemic events, caused by cardiogenic thromboemboli. These emboli may be large and occlude large vessels, such as the intracranial ICA. In general, strokes caused by AF are larger and result in more neurologic deficits. Time is of the essence to get optimal results, because the treatment of acute ischemic strokes is similar to treatment of AMI, which requires timely reperfusion for optimal results. Like AMI, reperfusion strategies include IV and/or intra-arterial thrombolysis and catheter-based therapies. Unlike AMI, not many patients with stroke receive reperfusion therapy because of late presentation (>4.5 hours), few qualified hospitals and specialists, and unavailability of expeditious advanced neuroimaging facilities in most hospitals.

REFERENCES

1. Heart and stroke statistics. Available at: http://www.heart.org/HEARTORG/General/Heart-and-Stroke-Association-Statistics_UCM_319064_SubHomePage.jsp. Accessed October 1, 2013.
2. Lloyd-Jones D, Adams RJ, Brown TM, et al. Heart disease and stroke statistics – 2010 update: a report from the American Heart Association. Circulation 2010;121:e46–215.
3. Duvuyst G, Bogousslavsky J. Which cardiac diagnosis tests apply in the acute phase of stroke and when are they useful?. In: Bogousslavsky J, editor. Acute stroke treatment. London: Martin Dunitz; 1997. p. 65–78.
4. Lin HJ, Wolf PA, Kelly-Hayes M, et al. Stroke severity in atrial fibrillation. The Framingham Study. Stroke 1996;27(10):1760–4.
5. Miller PS, Andersson FL, Kalra L. Are cost benefits of anticoagulation in atrial fibrillation underestimated? Stroke 2005;36(2):360–6.
6. Brott T, Adams HP, Olinger CP, et al. Measurements of acute cerebral infarction—a clinical examination scale. Stroke 1989;20:864–70.
7. Goldstein LB, Bartels C, Davis JN. Interrater reliability of the NIH Stroke Scale. Arch Neurol 1989;46:660–2.
8. National Institutes of Health Stroke Scale (NIHSS). Available at: http://www.ninds.nih.gov/doctors/NIH_Stroke_Scale.pdf. Accessed October 1, 2013.

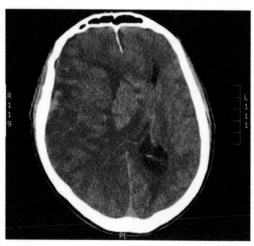

Fig. 17. A CT scan 24 hours later shows massive right hemispheric infarct with large subfalcine herniation to the left.

9. White CJ, Abou-Chebl A, Cates CU, et al. Stroke intervention: catheter-based therapy for acute ischemic stroke. J Am Coll Cardiol 2011;58:101–16.

10. Lin K, Do KG, Ong P, et al. Perfusion CT improves diagnostic accuracy for hyperacute ischemic stroke in the 3-hour window: study of 100 patients with diffusion MRI confirmation. Cerebrovasc Dis 2009; 28:72–9.

11. Adams HP Jr, del Zoppo G, Alberts MJ, et al, American Heart Association/American Stroke Association Stroke Council, American Heart Association/American Stroke Association Clinical Cardiology Council, American Heart Association/American Stroke Association Cardiovascular Radiology and Intervention Council, Atherosclerotic Peripheral Vascular Disease Working Group, Quality of Care Outcomes in Research Interdisciplinary Working Group. Guidelines for the early management of adults with ischemic stroke: a guideline from the American Heart Association/American Stroke Association Stroke Council, Clinical Cardiology Council, Cardiovascular Radiology and Intervention Council, and the Atherosclerotic Peripheral Vascular Disease and Quality of Care Outcomes in Research Interdisciplinary Working Groups: the American Academy of Neurology affirms the value of this guideline as an educational tool for neurologists. Stroke 2007;38:1655–711.

12. Tissue plasminogen activator for acute ischemic stroke. The National Institutes of Neurological Disorders and Stroke rtPA Stroke Study Group. N Engl J Med 1995;333:1581–7.

13. Hacke W, Kaste M, Bluhmki E, et al, for the ECASS Investigators. Thrombolysis with 3 to 4.5 hours after acute ischemic stroke. N Engl J Med 2008;359: 1317–29.

14. Alvarez-Sabin J, Molina CA, Ribo M, et al. Impact of admission hyperglycemia on stroke outcome after thrombolysis: risk stratification in relation to time to reperfusion. Stroke 2004;35:2493–8.

15. Meyers PM, Schumacher HC, Hagashida RT, et al. Indications for the performance of intracranial endovascular neurointerventional procedures: a scientific statement from the American Heart Association Council on Cardiovascular Radiology and Intervention, Stroke Council, Council on Cardiovascular Surgery and Anesthesia, Interdisciplinary Council on Peripheral Vascular Disease, and Interdisciplinary Council on Quality of Care and Outcomes Research. Circulation 2009;119:2235–49.

16. Furlan A, Hagashida R, Wechsler L, et al. Intra-arterial prourokinase for acute ischemic stroke: the PROACT II study: a non-randomized controlled trial: prolyse in acute cerebral thromboembolism. JAMA 1999;282:2003–11.

17. Rha JH, Saver JL. The impact of recanalization on ischemic stroke outcome: a meta-analysis. Stroke 2007;38:967–73.

18. Hagashida RT, Furlan AJ, Roberts H, for the Technology Assessment Committees of the American Society of Interventional and Therapeutic Neuroradiology and the Society of Interventional Radiology. Trial design and reporting standards for intraarterial cerebral thrombolysis for acute ischemic stroke. Stroke 2003;34:e109–37.

19. Jauch EC, Saver JL, Adams HP Jr. Guidelines for the early management of patients with acute ischemic stroke: a guideline for healthcare professionals from the American Heart Association/American Stroke Association. Stroke 2013;44:870.

20. Lansberg MG, O'Donnell MJ, Khatri P. Antithrombotic and thrombolytic therapy for ischemic stroke: antithrombotic therapy and prevention of thrombosis, 9th edition: American College of Chest Physicians evidence-based clinical practice guidelines. Chest 2012;141:e601S.

21. del Zoppo GJ, Saver JL, Jauch EC. Expansion of the time window for treatment of acute ischemic stroke with intravenous tissue plasminogen activator. A science advisory from the American Heart Association/American Stroke Association. Stroke 2009;40:2945.

22. Chernyshev OY, Martin-Schild S, Albright KC. Safety of tPA in stroke mimics and neuroimaging-negative cerebral ischemia. Neurology 2010;74:1340.

23. Tsivgoylis G, Alexandrov AV, Chang J. Safety and outcomes of intravenous thrombolysis in stroke mimics: a 6-year, single-care center study and pooled analysis of reported series. Stroke 2011;42:1771.

24. Khalessi AA, Natarajan SK, Orion D, et al. Acute stroke intervention. JACC Cardiovasc Interv 2011; 4:261.

25. Meyers PM, Schumacher HC, Connolly ES, et al. Current status of endovascular stroke treatment. Circulation 2011;123:2591.

26. Chimowitz MI. Endovascular treatment for acute ischemic stroke – still unproven. N Engl J Med 2013;368:952.

27. Ciccone A, Valvassori L, Nichleatti M, et al. Endovascular treatment for acute ischemic stroke. N Engl J Med 2013;368:904.

28. del Zoppo GJ, Higashida RT, Furlan AJ, et al, for the PROACR investigators. PROACT: a phase II randomized trial of recombinant prourokinase by direct arterial delivery in acute middle cerebral artery stroke: prolyse in acute cerebral thromboembolism. Stroke 1998;29:4.

29. Broderick JP, Palesch YY, Demchuk AM, et al. Endovascular therapy after intravenous t-PA versus t-PA alone for stroke. N Engl J Med 2013;368:893.

30. Lees KR, Bluhmki E, von Kummer R, et al. Time to treatment with intravenous alteplase and outcome in stroke: an updated pooled analysis of ECASS, ATLANTIS, NINDS, and EPITHET trials. Lancet 2010;375:1695.

31. Albers GW, Bates VE, Clark WM, et al. Intravenous tissue-type plasminogen activator for treatment of acute stroke: the Standard Treatment with Alteplase to Reverse Stroke (STARS) study. JAMA 2000;283: 1145.

32. LaMonte MP, Bahouth MN, Magder LS, et al. A regional system of stroke care provides thrombolytic outcomes comparable with the NINDS stroke trial. Ann Emerg Med 2009;54:319.

33. Hill MD, Buchan AM, Canadian Alteplase for Stroke Effectiveness Study (CASES) Investigators. Thrombolysis for acute ischemic stroke: results of the Canadian Alteplase for Stroke Effectiveness Study. CMAJ 2005;172:1307.

34. Wahlgren N, Ahmed N, Davalos A, et al. Thrombolysis with alteplase for acute ischemic stroke in the Safe Implementation of Thrombolysis in Stroke-Monitoring Study (SITS-MOST): an observational study. Lancet 2007;369:275.

35. Millan M, Dorado L, Davalos A. Fibrinolytic therapy in acute stroke. Curr Cardiol Rev 2010;6:218–26.

36. Broderick J, Connolly S, Feldman E, et al. Guidelines for the management of spontaneous intracerebral hemorrhage in adults: 2007 update: a guideline from the American Heart Association/American Stroke Association Stroke Council, High Blood Pressure Research Council, and the Quality of Care and Outcomes in Research Interdisciplinary Working Group. Stroke 2007;38:2001.

37. Goldstein JN, Marrero M, Masrur S, et al. Management of thrombolysis-associated symptomatic intracerebral hemorrhage. Arch Neurol 2010;67: 965.

38. Mahaffey KW, Granger CB, Sloan MA, et al. Neurosurgical evacuation of intracerebral hemorrhage after thrombolysis therapy for acute myocardial infarction: experience from the GUSTO-I trial. Global Utilization of Streptokinase and Tissue-Plasminogen Activator (tPA) for Occluded Coronary Arteries. Am Heart J 1999;138:493.

39. Go AS, Hylek EM, Borowsky LH, et al. Warfarin use among ambulatory patients with nonvalvular atrial fibrillation. Ann Intern Med 1999;131:927–34.

40. Rose AJ, Hylek EM, Ozonoff A, et al. Risk-adjusted percent time in therapeutic range as a quality indicator for outpatient oral anticoagulation. Results of the Veterans Affairs Study to Improve Anticoagulation (VARIA). Circ Cardiovasc Qual Outcomes 2011; 4(1):22–9.

41. Baker WL, Cios DA, Sander SD, et al. Meta-analysis to assess the quality of warfarin control in atrial fibrillation patients in the United States. J Manag Care Pharm 2009;15(3):244–52.

42. Rose AJ, Ozonoff A, Henalult LE, et al. Warfarin for atrial fibrillation in community-based practice. J Thromb Haemost 2008;6(10):1647–54.

43. Sarawate C, Sikirica MV, Willey VJ, et al. Monitoring anticoagulation in atrial fibrillation. J Thromb Thrombolysis 2006;21(2):191–8.

44. McCormick D, Gurwitz JH, Goldberg RJ, et al. Prevalence and quality of warfarin use for patients with atrial fibrillation in the long-term care setting. Arch Intern Med 2001;161(20):2458–63.

45. Connolly SJ, Ezekowitz MD, Yusuf S, et al, for the RE-LY Steering Committee and Investigators. Dabigatran versus warfarin in patients with atrial fibrillation. N Engl J Med 2009;361:1139–51.

46. Patel M, Mahaffey KW, Garg J, et al, for the ROCKET AF Steering Committee for the ROCKET AF investigators. Rivaroxaban versus warfarin in nonvalvular atrial fibrillation. N Engl J Med 2011; 365:883–91.

47. Connolly SJ, Eikelboom J, Joyner C, et al, for the AVERROES Steering Committee and Investigators. Apixaban in patients with atrial fibrillation. N Engl J Med 2011;364:806–17.

Index

Note: Page numbers of article titles are in **boldface** type.

A

Ablation. *See* Atrial fibrillation (AF) ablation
ACS. *See* Acute coronary syndrome (ACS)
Acute coronary syndrome (ACS)
    previous
        anticoagulants in AF management related to,
            80–81
Adherence problems
    anticoagulants in AF management and
        how to deal with, 82
AF. *See* Atrial fibrillation (AF)
Age
    as factor in AF, 2, 31
Air embolism
    SCLs during AF ablation related to, 90
AMPLATZER
    in percutaneous LAA closure, 151–152
Anticoagulant(s)
    in AF management
        questions related to, **79–86**
            frail populations–related, 82–83
            how to assess anti-coagulation effect,
               81–82
            how to deal with adherence problems, 82
            how to deal with surgery, 81
            how to deal with systemic thrombolysis for
               ischemic stroke or ST elevation MI, 82
            how to manage bleeding, 83–84
            introduction, 79–80
            who should not switch, 80–81
            who should switch, 80
    oral
        in stroke prevention in AF
            underuse of, 64–67
    postablation
        in cerebrovascular complications prevention in
            AF ablation, 119
    in stroke prevention in AF, 10–11, 64–67, 71–75
        aspirin with, 75
        clinical trials with, 75
Anticoagulation. *See also* Anticoagulant(s)
    AF ablation and
        issues related to, **95–100**. *See also* Atrial
            fibrillation (AF) ablation, anticoagulation
            issues in
Aortic atheroma
    cardiogenic embolism due to, 46–49
Aortic heart disease
    evaluation of

        in stroke prevention, 23
            strands, 23–24
Apixaban
    reversing, 98
    in stroke prevention in AF, 71–72, 74–75
Aspirin
    during AF ablation, 97
    in stroke prevention in AF, 68–71
        with anticoagulants, 75
Atheroma(s)
    aortic
        cardiogenic embolism due to, 46–49
Atrial fibrillation (AF), **1–4**
    abnormal blood constituents in, 7
    abnormal blood stasis in, 6
    age as factor in, 31
    age at diagnosis, 2
    asymptomatic
        device detection of
            in patients with prior stroke, 137
    cardiovascular disease and, 2–3
    cerebrovascular events and, 32–33
    characteristics of, 43–44
    costs related to, 1, 5–6
    cryptogenic stroke and, 33, 161–162
    dementia and, 35–37
    device-detected
        in patients with stroke risk factors, 37–38
        stroke events related to, 135–137
    diagnosis of, 2–3
    early detection of
        impact on stroke outcomes, **125–132**
            future directions in, 129–130
            introduction, 125–126
            in patients with implanted cardiac rhythm
               management devices, 127–128
            in primary prevention of stroke, 128–129
    ECG screening of
        outpatient, 162–163
    economic impact of, 3
    epidemiology of, 31–32
    gender as factor in, 1
    inflammation in, 7
    introduction, 5–6, 101
    LA function assessment and, 18–21
        CT in, 20–21
        MRI in, 20–21
        TEE in, 18–20
        TTE in, 18

Printed and bound by CPI Group (UK) Ltd, Croydon, CR0 4YY

03/10/2024

01040377-0018